Nutrition for Elite Athletes

Nutrition for Elite Athletes

Edited by
Eric S. Rawson, PhD, FACSM, CSCS
Bloomsburg University
Bloomsburg, Pennsylvania, USA

Stella Lucia Volpe, PhD, RD, LDN, FACSM
Drexel University
Philadelphia, Pennsylvania, USA

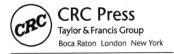

CRC Press
Taylor & Francis Group
Boca Raton London New York

CRC Press is an imprint of the
Taylor & Francis Group, an **informa** business

CRC Press
Taylor & Francis Group
6000 Broken Sound Parkway NW, Suite 300
Boca Raton, FL 33487-2742

Version Date: 20150720

International Standard Book Number-13: 978-1-4665-5798-7 (Hardback)

This book contains information obtained from authentic and highly regarded sources. Reasonable efforts have been made to publish reliable data and information, but the author and publisher cannot assume responsibility for the validity of all materials or the consequences of their use. The authors and publishers have attempted to trace the copyright holders of all material reproduced in this publication and apologize to copyright holders if permission to publish in this form has not been obtained. If any copyright material has not been acknowledged please write and let us know so we may rectify in any future reprint.

Visit the Taylor & Francis Web site at
http://www.taylorandfrancis.com

and the CRC Press Web site at
http://www.crcpress.com

To my family, friends, colleagues, and mentors for their inspiration, guidance, and humor. In memory of Priscilla Clarkson, PhD, who continues to teach me.

Eric S. Rawson

To my husband, Gary R. Snyder, and our German shepherd dogs, Sasha and Bear, as well as my entire family, for their constant support.

In memory of my parents, Antonio and Felicetta Volpe, who, through their love and example, taught me, and continue to teach me, the value of hard work.

Stella Lucia Volpe

Contents

Preface

We have been friends and colleagues for many years. When CRC Press asked us to edit a book, we thought it would be a great opportunity for us to bring together wonderful colleagues and friends from around the world, who are also experts in the field.

This book is meant to be a text for sports nutritionists, exercise physiologists, professors/scientists, and practitioners in related fields. We hope that it will help bring science to practice and/or bring about new research ideas that will continue to move this field forward.

In this book, global experts discuss a number of topics within sports nutrition. These chapters provide in-depth evaluations of each area. The book begins with "Foundations of Energy Metabolism," which provides an excellent basis for this topic. The next two chapters focus on endurance athletes, while Chapters 4 and 5 discuss nutrition and dietary supplements for strength power athletes. Chapter 6 focuses on "Nutrition and Dietary Supplements for Team Sport Athletes," a chapter not often found in sports nutrition books. In addition, Chapter 7 is both a unique and comprehensive chapter on "Nutrition and Dietary Supplements for Aesthetic and Weight-Class Sport Athletes." Dietary supplements, as well as food safety for athletes, followed by the interactions of drugs, nutrients, and exercise, provide complete information in these important areas in sports. Chapter 10 focuses on "Nutrition, Exercise, and Immunology," providing the reader with an excellent overview in this area. A thorough background in hydration is provided in Chapter 11, "Hydration for High-Level Athletes." Finally, "Minerals and Athletic Performance" is described in Chapter 12.

This book is unique and will provide the reader with a strong background in all of the aforementioned areas. We hope you enjoy it and that it informs your research, teaching, and/or practice.

Eric S. Rawson, PhD, FACSM
Stella Lucia Volpe, PhD, RD, LDN, FACSM

Acknowledgments

We would like to thank all of the authors of this book who provided us with excellent and timely topics on sports nutrition. The authors of this book are amazing researchers and practitioners who have had a major impact on sports nutrition.

We would also like to acknowledge our colleagues, mentors, and students over the years. All have influenced us, and we thank them!

Acknowledgments

Editors

Eric S. Rawson, PhD, FACSM, is professor and chair of the Department of Exercise Science at Bloomsburg University, Pennsylvania. He earned his PhD in exercise science from the University of Massachusetts, Amherst where he studied under the direction of Dr. Priscilla Clarkson. He is a certified strength and conditioning specialist from the National Strength and Conditioning Association. Dr. Rawson's research focuses on the interactions between nutrition and skeletal muscle. In particular, Dr. Rawson has studied the effects of dietary supplements on muscle function.

Stella Lucia Volpe, PhD, RD, LDN, FACSM, is professor and chair of the Department of Nutrition Sciences at Drexel University, Philadelphia, Pennsylvania. Her BS in exercise science is from the University of Pittsburgh. Dr. Volpe earned her MS in exercise physiology and her PhD in nutrition, both from Virginia Tech. She is also a certified exercise specialist from the American College of Sports Medicine and a registered dietitian. Dr. Volpe's area of research is in obesity and diabetes prevention, as well as in sports nutrition.

Contributors

Lawrence E. Armstrong, PhD, FACSM
Korey Stringer Institute
Department of Kinesiology
University of Connecticut
Storrs, Connecticut

Charles E. Brightbill, MS
Department of Exercise Science
Bloomsburg University
Bloomsburg, Pennsylvania

**Louise Burke, OAM, PhD, APD,
    FACSM**
Australian Institute of Sport
Belconnen, Canberra, Australia

and

MacKillop Institute for Health Research
Australian Catholic University
Melbourne, Victoria, Australia

**Jennifer Burris, MS, RD, CSG,
    CNSC, CSSD, CDE**
Steinhardt School of Culture, Education
    and Human Development
Department of Nutrition, Food Studies
    and Public Health
New York University
New York, New York

Patrícia Lopes Campos-Ferraz, PhD
School of Physical Education and
    Sports
Laboratory of Nutrition Applied to
    Physical Activity and Metabolism
University of São Paulo
São Paulo, Brazil

**Douglas J. Casa, PhD, ATC, FACSM,
    FNATA**
Korey Stringer Institute
Department of Kinesiology
University of Connecticut
Storrs, Connecticut

Anne E. Eudy, PharmD
U.S. Department of Veterans Affairs
Eastern Colorado Health Care System
Denver, Colorado

Rodrigo Branco Ferraz, MSc
School of Physical Education and Sports
Laboratory of Nutrition Applied to
    Physical Activity and Metabolism
University of São Paulo
São Paulo, Brazil

Mathew S. Ganio, PhD
Department of Health, Human
    Performance and Recreation
University of Arkansas
Fayetteville, Arkansas

Jayme Hostetter, PharmD Candidate
Eshelman School of Pharmacy
University of North Carolina at
    Chapel Hill
Chapel Hill, North Carolina

Stavros A. Kavouras, PhD, FACSM
Department of Health, Human
    Performance and Recreation
University of Arkansas
Fayetteville, Arkansas

Rachel C. Kelley, MS
Department of Nutrition Sciences
Drexel University
Philadelphia, Pennsylvania

Antonio Herbert Lancha, PhD
School of Physical Education and
   Sports
Laboratory of Nutrition Applied to
   Physical Activity and Metabolism
University of São Paulo
São Paulo, Brazil

**Luciana Oquendo Pereira Lancha,
   PhD, RD**
School of Physical Education and Sports
Laboratory of Nutrition Applied to
   Physical Activity and Metabolism
University of São Paulo
São Paulo, Brazil

Mariana Lucena, PharmD Candidate
Eshelman School of Pharmacy
University of North Carolina at
   Chapel Hill
Chapel Hill, North Carolina

Ronald J. Maughan, PhD, FACSM
School of Sport, Exercise and
   Health Sciences
Loughborough University
Leicestershire, United Kingdom

Mary P. Miles, PhD, FACSM
Department of Health and Human
   Development
Montana State University
Bozeman, Montana

Caoileann H. Murphy, MSc, RD
Department of Kinesiology
McMaster University
Hamilton, Ontario, Canada

Adam M. Persky, PhD, FACSM
Eshelman School of Pharmacy
University of North Carolina at
   Chapel Hill
Chapel Hill, North Carolina

**Stuart M. Phillips, PhD, FACSM,
   FACN**
Department of Kinesiology
McMaster University
Hamilton, Ontario, Canada

Eric S. Rawson, PhD, FACSM
Department of Exercise Science
Bloomsburg University
Bloomsburg, Pennsylvania

Rebecca L. Stearns, PhD, ATC
Korey Stringer Institute
Department of Kinesiology
University of Connecticut
Storrs, Connecticut

Cortney N. Steele, MS
Department of Exercise Science
Bloomsburg University
Bloomsburg, Pennsylvania

**Stella Lucia Volpe, PhD, RD, LDN,
   FACSM**
Department of Nutrition Sciences
Drexel University
Philadelphia, Pennsylvania

Melvin H. Williams, PhD, FACSM
Department of Human Movement
   Sciences
Old Dominion University
Norfolk, Virginia

Jonathan E. Wingo, PhD
Department of Kinesiology
University of Alabama
Tuscaloosa, Alabama

Kathleen Woolf, PhD, RD, FACSM
Steinhardt School of Culture, Education
and Human Development
Department of Nutrition, Food Studies
and Public Health
New York University
New York, New York

1 Foundations of Energy Metabolism

Adam M. Persky, PhD, FACSM
Eshelman School of Pharmacy, University of North
Carolina at Chapel Hill, Chapel Hill, North Carolina

Anne E. Eudy, PharmD
U.S. Department of Veterans Affairs, Eastern
Colorado Health Care System, Denver, Colorado

CONTENTS

INTRODUCTION

Proper nutrition underpins our ability to function within the confines of activities of daily living (e.g., showering, walking, preparing meals), but also is foundational to peak exercise performance. The compounds contained within food provide the fuel for physiologic work and the elements needed for the synthesis of new tissue or the repair of existing tissues. For example, the fat found within eggs can provide energy for respiratory muscles to maintain our ventilation while the protein within the egg can be incorporated into building new muscle tissue or repairing the microscopic injuries that occur when we lift weights.

This chapter reviews: (1) energetics on a molecular level through the common pathways in which energy is derived from macronutrients such as carbohydrates, fats, and proteins; (2) energetics on a systems level via the components of total daily energy expenditure, and (3) the relationship between exercise intensity and substrate utilization. These foundational concepts will support the more advanced discussions of the roles of macro- and micronutrients in exercise performance found later in this book.

ENERGY

In general, energy is considered the ability to perform work. Work is the process of using some form of energy to invoke change on a system. For instance, in order to perform one concentric contraction during a bicep curl (i.e., to move the weight from a resting position with the elbow extended toward the body by bending the elbow using the muscles in your upper arm), energy will be utilized from stored fuel sources such as glycogen to elicit muscle contraction in your bicep muscles. The work done is a function of the amount of weight in the hand and how far that weight travels, which will depend on the length of the arm.

Energy exists in a variety of forms: mechanical, chemical, heat, and electrical. The human body utilizes all four types of energy and all are linked. Mechanical energy is the easiest form to recognize because we can see it happen. This type of energy is used to move the body, such as when jumping or swinging a bat to hit a ball. While we can see the results of mechanical energy, we can feel and sometimes see heat energy. The body produces heat to maintain the appropriate internal body temperature, or releases heat through sweat for the same reason. Mechanical energy and heat energy can be linked by using the example of shivering. When we shiver, we are attempting to generate heat through the mechanics of muscle contraction. Chemical and electrical energy are more relevant to internal body processes such as producing usable energy from the catabolism of glucose or coordinating contractions of the atrium and ventricles during a cardiac cycle, respectively.

Energy comes from the food we eat and is required by our bodies. This is based on Newton's first law of thermodynamics, also referred to as the conservation of energy. The law states that energy cannot be created or destroyed but is simply transformed from one form into another (e.g., carbohydrate from pasta is turned into energy to kick a ball). Metabolism is the process that allows the human body to functionally convert food to usable forms of energy; that is, transfer energy from one form into another. This process is a conglomeration of different pathways that are constantly in process within the body using various enzymes and substrates yielding high-energy products. Later in this chapter, we will focus on the detailed relationship of energy and metabolism. First, it is important to understand how our body uses the energy provided by metabolism.

Doing work requires energy input and results in the expenditure of energy. As noted earlier, energy can never be created or destroyed; it simply changes forms. Therefore, energy can be considered on a continuum (Knuttgen 1995). Before the energy confined in foodstuffs can do work for us, it must be stored in a functional form within the body, which then has the potential to do that work. Energy stores are derived from the food we eat. We store some of the energy from food in the form of a molecule called phosphocreatine (or creatine phosphate), but this accounts for a very small percentage; details of this molecule will be discussed later in the chapter. We store much more energy in glycogen (storage form of carbohydrate), fat (storage of lipids), and muscle (storage of proteins). When needed, we can break these stores down and retrieve energy to do work.

The energy from these storage forms is actually released when doing work either as the work itself (e.g., moving weight in the bicep curl) or as a heat by-product (Figure 1.1). When the body does mechanical work, usually contraction of a muscle, any energy that is not directly consumed as movement of the muscle is expelled as heat. Because the body is not 100% efficient, it cannot convert completely all energy stores to mechanical energy (Knuttgen 1995). This also is true for the energy used in anabolic processes such as synthesizing glycogen or muscle tissue or transport processes such as moving metabolic intermediates into and out of the mitochondrial spaces.

UNITS OF ENERGY

Energy can be described in many units because it exists in so many forms. In general, energy is defined in terms of work and work is the product of force and distance. In the International System of Units, the gold standard unit for energy is the joule (J). Joules are very small units and it is often useful to relate them as kilojoules (1 kilojoule [kJ] = 1000 joules [J]). As an example of work, if a basketball player runs the length of the court (approximately 94 ft), he will have done approximately 5 times more work than if he ran to the free-throw line (19 ft) at the same speed. Conversely, if he wore a 50-lb weighted vest and ran the length of the court, he would have done more work than without the vest because he needed to generate more force.

Work should not be confused with power. Power is the ratio of work and time and usually has units of watts. For example, if an athlete runs the length of the court in 10 sec, he would have generated more power than if he did it in 20 sec; however, he would have done the same amount of work.

Another unit used to describe energy is the calorie, or cal. Instead of measuring force and distance, the calorie only relates two variables—heat and mass. A calorie portrays the amount of heat required to increase the temperature of 1 g of pure

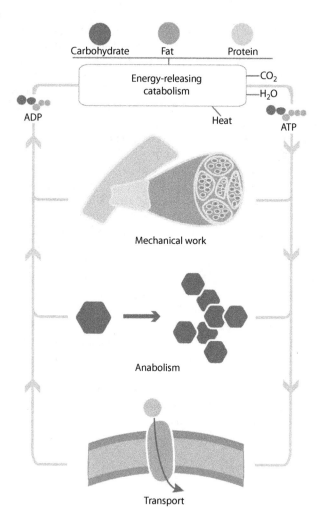

FIGURE 1.1 Overview of the relationship between macronutrients and energy produc-tion and its use. (Adapted from Gropper, S.A.S., J.L. Smith, and J.L. Groff. 2009. *Advanced Nutrition and Human Metabolism*, 5th ed. Australia: Wadsworth/Cengage Learning.)

water by 1°C. These are small units in reference to the body because a person's body contains much more than 1 g of water; in fact, approximately 60% of body weight is water (~40 kg!). Therefore, we refer to calories by using the kilocalorie. This unit is equivalent to 1000 calories and is the amount of heat required to raise 1 kg (1 L) of water by 1°C. A kilocalorie has many abbreviations: kcal, C, or calorie.

For our purposes, the most relevant unit for energy is the kilocalorie or the calo-rie. When reading a food label, it is easy to see that the number of calories supplied denotes relative nutrient content. In addition, exercise is often done with the desire to reach a goal for caloric expenditure. Therefore, we will be using calories throughout the rest of this chapter to discuss energy.

ENERGY BALANCE

In order to perform continuous work, the human body must be in energy balance and thus must possess adequate energy stores to support that work. Energy balance is the difference between the amount of energy placed into the body vs. the amount of energy used. In relation to the human body, energy balance is calculated in calories. Energy input is comprised of all calories consumed from eating or drinking. Energy output is made of the calories used by your body to do various daily tasks that range from breathing and pumping blood to running a mile. A negative energy balance occurs when a person burns more calories than he or she consumes through food or drink. Negative energy balance eventually results in a net loss of weight. Alternatively, a positive energy balance occurs if a person consumes more total calories than his or her body burns in a day, resulting in a net gain of weight—a problem we see in the general population resulting in obesity.

The amount of energy expended on a daily basis must be supplemented with the appropriate energy input. Usually, energy input is easy to monitor and calculate. It is comprised solely of the foods and drinks consumed, and is kept track of through the unit of calories. On the other hand, energy expenditure is more complicated to measure. It consists of many components that are not easily depicted by a food label or a formula.

For the purpose of exercise and nutrition, the amount of energy input required is dependent upon the total daily energy expenditure. For a given athlete, we must first know how much energy (or calories) he or she is expending and then estimate how many calories he or she will need to consume to result in an appropriate level of energy balance. Determination of an athlete's energy state can often lead to answers about many dietary questions or performance concerns. Thus, we are interested in total daily energy expenditure.

TOTAL DAILY ENERGY EXPENDITURE

We typically discuss the total energy expenditure (TEE) as the sum of all energy expenditures over a 24-h period. This metric is equivalent to the energy output of an individual. TEE is composed of several different aspects of human physiology and activities of daily life including the resting or basal metabolic rate, the thermic effect of eating, activities of daily living, and contributions from exercise and other physical activity (Figure 1.2).

TEE varies from person to person, making it difficult to estimate uniformly for any given individual. TEE is affected by many factors such as body weight, body composition, age, sex, genetics, lifestyle, and physical activity (Bernadot and Thompson 1999). In the following sections, we will discuss the different components of TEE and how to estimate each one.

Basal Metabolic Rate

In the majority of people, the largest contributor to TEE is the basal metabolic rate (BMR). The BMR accounts for 50% to 80% of the total daily energy expenditure (Carpenter et al. 1995; Reeves and Carpa 2003). BMR is the amount of energy that

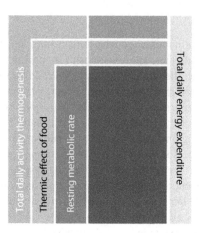

FIGURE 1.2 Schematic of the components of total daily energy expenditure. Basal metabolic rate can account for 50% to 70% of total daily energy expenditure. Thermic effect of food typically composes 10% of total daily energy expenditure.

is expended, or used, by the body purely to live and exist. Many internal body processes contribute to the BMR such as breathing, pumping of the heart to circulate blood, and thinking.

Another version of the BMR is the resting metabolic rate (RMR). This rate is almost the same as the BMR, but slightly higher because it accounts for waking rest, which requires slightly more calories than the pure basal rate; that is, the (RMR) is the energy required to lie quietly in bed. In general, the values can be considered equivalent because the RMR is only approximately 5% to 10% higher than the BMR for any given individual. For this reason, it is not necessary to differentiate between the two when referencing the total energy expenditure equation. However, it is necessary to select one term and stay consistent in your calculations. For uniformity, we will use BMR throughout this chapter.

There are many methods to determine the BMR, including using direct calorimetry (Dauncey 1980), indirect calorimetry (Reeves and Capra 2003), or the doubly labeled water method (Plasqui and Westerterp 2007). The three methods are considered to be within 3% of the actual BMR when performed under ideal conditions (Schoeller and van Santen 1982). Because these techniques may not be amenable to clinical settings, several equations have been developed to determine BMR that take into account an individual's age, sex, height, and weight. These equations are much easier to use than the aforementioned methods because they do not require time, money, or expensive machinery to conduct. However, these equations are much less accurate and must be understood as estimations rather than absolute values (Reeves and Capra 2003). Each of these equations may vary by up to 10% from the actual BMR of the tested individual (Henry 2005). However, the simplest way to calculate BMR is based solely on a person's weight. This is the least accurate method, but is the easiest to conduct and, in general, close enough to be useful. The BMR for a 24-h period is equal to 1 kcal burned per kilogram of body weight per hour (Forsum et al. 2006). BMR = 1 kcal/kg/h body weight/24 h or BMR over a 24-h period with the equation 10 kcal per pound of body weight (BMR = 10 kcal/lb body weight). These equations are rough estimates and should be understood as such.

BMR is affected by age, sex, nutritional state, genetic variations, and differences in the endocrine state (e.g., hyperthyroidism) (Institute of Medicine [U.S.] 2005). As people age, their BMR decreases (Figure 1.3). As a result, older adults often need to consume fewer calories per day than growing teenagers do. The main reason for the decline of BMR with age is that at young ages the body is constantly working to grow and develop, which requires large amounts of energy. Once net growth stops following puberty, the BMR decreases steadily. Also, as the body ages, muscle mass tends to decline (Roubenoff 2003). Muscle mass is another determinant for the BMR. At rest, muscle tissue uses more energy than fat tissue. Muscle mass relates to age and physical strength and is often improved through exercise. Fat-free mass (i.e., muscle mass) explains 70% to 80% of the variance in BMR (Institute of Medicine [U.S.] 2005). It is a common misbelief, however, that you can cause significant changes in your TEE by resistance exercise and increasing muscle mass; muscle typically contributes less than 20% to the BMR (Kaminsky 2006; Lazzer et al. 2010) and resistance training will increase resting metabolic rate but the metabolic rate per kilogram of muscle does not change. Even though organs like the brain, liver, and kidney contribute a fraction to overall body weight compared to muscle, the former organs are responsible for the vast majority of energy expenditure at rest (Lazzer et al. 2010). Sex is the final important factor affecting BMR. Intrinsically, females have a lower BMR than males do at every age because of the female body's ratio of fat mass, specifically essential fat, to muscle mass (Carpenter et al. 1995). It is also noteworthy that BMR in females does vary day-to-day as hormones that regulate menstruation peak and trough.

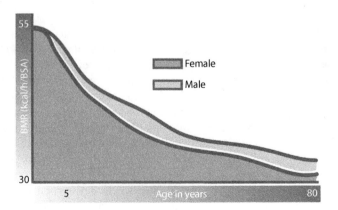

FIGURE 1.3 Relationship between age and basal metabolic rate. Although men and women have different basal metabolic rates, both decline over time. (Adapted from Mitchell, H.H. 1962. *Comparative Nutrition of Man and Domestic Animals*. New York: Academic Press.)

Thermic Effect of Food

In order to digest, absorb, transport, and store food that is consumed, the body must use energy. This use of energy is referred to as the thermic effect of food (TEF). The TEF accounts for about 10% of the TEE (de Jonge and Bray 1997; Stob et al. 2007). The TEF is variable depending on a person's activity level and the type of food consumed, but 10% is a common estimate. Individuals that are more active may burn more calories because of eating. In addition, the time of the meal relative to when exercise occurred may affect the TEF. However, there is no definitive evidence to prove these suggestions either way. Different sources of food will require different amounts of energy to process. In general, the magnitude of the TEF is 5% to 10% of calories ingested as carbohydrates, 0% to 3% as fats, and 20% to 30% as proteins; as you may note, the TEF for proteins is the greatest contribution (van Baak 2008). Fats require less energy to digest because they are almost exclusively sent directly for storage by the body in adipose tissue. Carbohydrates will burn some calories via breakdown and transport throughout the body. Proteins require the most energy for breakdown by enzymes and storage in muscle tissue. The TEF is often left out of TEE calculations because the value is negligible compared to the BMR, activities of daily living (ADL), and exercise/physical activity.

Activities of Daily Living

As mentioned earlier, most of the TEE is a function of BMR, which relative to the other components of TEE, cannot be manipulated by the individual. However, energy expended by ADL, exercise, and other physical activity can be manipulated. ADL are varied across the entire population. This term encompasses the majority of a person's lifestyle excluding specific physical exercise. It is obvious that occupations, leisure activities, and daily chores are different for everyone. During an 8-hour workday, a secretary will not use as much energy as a construction worker or a lumberjack. In addition, a person who weighs more will expend more energy to move, increasing the caloric expenditure for average daily behaviors compared to a person with less to carry.

For sedentary individuals, the ADL only contribute a minimal amount to the TEE compared to the BMR. Conversely, the ADL of a construction worker can be almost equal to the BMR. There are, of course, values in between as well. For example, a mildly active lifestyle could be a schoolteacher, who is on his or her feet most of the day but not working at a high pace. A moderate lifestyle could be a college student who must walk to and from class multiple times a day.

The lifestyle category is based on intensity of work level and duration on a daily basis. Lifestyle classification is subject to interpretation and should be considered as a relative measurement based on typical ideas of activity (Ainsworth et al. 2000). ADL lifestyle levels should not take into account time set aside as exercise. The contribution to TEE by exercise will be discussed in the next section. Calculating the contribution of a person's lifestyle to TEE is based on a percentage of the BMR that is then added to the TEE calculation. Table 1.1 depicts common multipliers. When adding up the separate components of TEE, start with the BMR and then multiply it by the BMR factor to determine the combined contribution from ADL and BMR.

TABLE 1.1

Estimating TEE from Approximations of Physical Activity

Lifestyle	BMR (%)	BMR Factor
Sedentary	10	1.1
Mildly active	15–20	1.15–1.2
Moderately active	30–40	1.3–1.4
Active	50–60	1.5–1.6
Very active	70–100	1.7–2

Source: Adapted from Williams, M.H. 2005. *Nutrition for Health, Fitness, and Sport*, 7th ed. Dubuque, IA: McGraw-Hill.

Note: To estimate TEE, calculate the individual's BMR and multiply by the appropriate BMR factor.

Exercise

Exercise is the most easily controlled and measured component of the TEE because it is voluntary. It should be obvious to anyone who has ever exercised that exercise requires energy and intense exercise can increase TEE 15 to 25 times (Kaminsky 2006). This can be verified by the production of heat by exercised muscle. Determining the caloric expenditure of different types of exercise can be tricky because it is based on intensity, duration, and, in part, the efficiency of movement.

The biggest determinant of the energy expended during exercise is the intensity. Different exercises expend different amounts of energy. Walking 1 mile at a moderate pace will not use as many calories as running the same distance. In addition, the weight of the individual makes a difference in the energy expenditure from exercise. To move a greater amount of weight requires more mechanical work output even at the same speed. Along the same lines, to move the same amount of weight at a faster pace requires more power (energy per unit time) because it results in a higher level of mechanical work output increasing the intensity and therefore caloric expenditure of the activity. Table 1.2 provides examples of how weight impacts the rate of calorie expenditure.

The amount of energy utilized is related to exercise intensity and is often measured by oxygen utilization. Oxygen is the major oxidizing substrate of metabolic processes, accepting electrons to produce usable energy. Oxygen molecules are inhaled through the lungs, transported to tissues by red blood cells, and then extracted by the tissue to use for energy production. The volume of oxygen consumed per unit time is referred to as VO_2. VO_2 typically is reported as milliliters or liters per minute and is often scaled to body weight (e.g., mL/kg/min). The VO_2 is a product of heart rate, stroke volume, and the arterio-venous difference (a-vO_2) in oxygen concentration; this latter metric is a measure of efficiency—the larger the a-vO_2, the more efficient the body is at extracting oxygen from the blood. The maximum rate of oxygen consumption that can be used for the production of energy during maximal physical exertion is referred to as VO_{2MAX} (Kaminsky 2006).

VO_{2MAX} is the maximal oxygen carrying capacity of the blood and is generally considered the best indicator of cardiorespiratory endurance and aerobic fitness. As

TABLE 1.2

Example of a Table of Activities to Estimate Caloric Cost per Activity

Activity	METs	kcal/min 120 lb	140 lb	160 lb	180 lb	200 lb
Showering	2	1.9	2.2	2.5	2.9	3.2
Dusting, taking out the trash	2.5	2.4	2.8	3.2	3.6	4.0
Walking the dog	3	2.9	3.3	3.8	4.3	4.8
Playing the drums	4	3.8	4.5	5.1	5.7	6.4
Mowing the lawn (power mower)	5.5	5.3	6.1	7.0	7.9	8.8
Bicycle (light effort)	6	5.7	6.7	7.6	8.6	9.5
Running (10 min/mile)	10	9.5	11.1	12.7	14.3	15.9

exercise intensity increases, so does oxygen consumption to help supply sufficient oxygen to obtain maximal ATP generation. However, a point is reached where exercise intensity cannot continue to increase without an increase in oxygen consumption. The point at which oxygen consumption plateaus defines the VO_{2MAX} or an individual's maximal aerobic capacity. During this time, heart rate remains relatively stable and the ratio of carbon dioxide produced to oxygen consumed will approach or exceed 1.0. Average values for VO_{2MAX} may be 32 to 43 mL/min/kg for a female aged 20 to 49 and 36 to 51 mL/min/kg for a male of the same age range. VO_{2MAX} is an indicator of an athlete's cardiorespiratory fitness level. A higher VO_{2MAX} indicates a higher tolerance for aerobic exercise and ability to reach higher intensities during exercise. At any given workload, an individual with a higher VO_{2MAX} will be consuming less oxygen than an individual with a lower VO_{2MAX} because of the physiologic adaptations associated with aerobic training. The impact of exercise intensity as a function of VO_{2MAX} on substrate utilization will be described in more detail later in this chapter.

Energy expenditure from exercise and physical activity can be assessed in a variety of ways. As with estimating BMR, direct calorimetry, indirect calorimetry, and doubly labeled water are standards in clinical research but may not be the most practical for a clinician or the average individual. Methods that are more practical include survey instruments, pedometers, accelerometers, or standardized tables of energy expenditure (Ainslie et al. 2003). Tables of the energy cost for various exercise and sport activities are available and vary widely and should be considered as crude approximations at best (see Table 1.2 for an example) (Maughan et al. 2000). The caloric expenditure depends on the body mass and fitness level of the individual and will have major influences on the energy associated with physical activity. Even aspects of biomechanical efficiency may lead to differences in energy expenditure. Our running and walking speeds are in a sense optimized for efficiency—if we are asked to run at an *uncomfortable* pace or change our mechanics (e.g., strike more mid-foot than hind-foot), the amount of energy used to exercise can change.

ENERGY STORAGE

Within plants and animals, energy exists in three main forms, called macronutrients. These macronutrients are carbohydrates, fats, and proteins (Gropper et al. 2009); it should be noted water is a fourth macronutrient and will be discussed later in the book in Chapter 10 on hydration. Breakdown of carbohydrates, fats, and proteins releases energy that can be utilized by cellular processes within the body. The digestive system utilizes various enzymes to separate the large macronutrient molecules into smaller molecules that can enter cells. Once inside cells, the nutrients flow through different energy production processes to release energy for cellular work.

As all calories consumed in the diet will originate from one of these three nutrients, it is possible to determine the daily caloric intake based solely on amounts of carbohydrate, fat, and protein ingested. Other nutrients like vitamins and minerals are very important in a daily diet, but do not provide direct energy for metabolism. They are useful, however, to support the process of energy metabolism and will be discussed in Chapter 12. The approximate amount of storage forms of energy can be found in Table 1.3.

Once ingested and appropriately processed, nutrients are stored in different ways inside the body. Carbohydrates can exist in several forms. Complex carbohydrates are converted to monomers such as glucose, which is an example of the simplest unit of a carbohydrate. Glucose can travel through the bloodstream to any cells that are in need of an energy source. Free glucose that is not used will then aggregate into

TABLE 1.3

Description of the Different Types of Carbohydrate and Fat Stores within the Body

	Grams	kcal
ATP/PCr	70	1
Phosphocreatine	80–90	4–5
Carbohydrate		
Liver glycogen	80–110	320–440
Muscle glycogen	250–375	1000–1500
Glucose in body fluids	10–15	40–60
Total	340–500	1360–2000
Fat		
Subcutaneous	7800–8900	70,200–80,000
Intramuscular	160–280	1440–2500
Total	7960–9180	71,640–82,620
Protein (muscle)	7500–12,000	30,000–48,000

Source: Maughan, R.J., IOC Medical Commission, and International Federation of Sports Medicine. 2000. *Nutrition in Sport, Encyclopaedia of Sports Medicine.* Osney Mead, Oxford: Blackwell Science; Williams, M.H. 2005. *Nutrition for Health, Fitness, and Sport,* 7th ed. Dubuque, IA: McGraw-Hill. With permission.

Note: Amounts are based on a 70-kg individual.

storage molecules called glycogen. Glycogen molecules are long chains of multiple glucose molecules that can be broken apart to release singular glucose molecules when needed. Glycogen is stored within muscle cells, which is useful because muscles are the most likely to need the glycogen during periods of work or exercise. Glycogen can also be found in the liver in much smaller quantities. Last, carbohydrates can be converted to fat tissue in the body if there is a surplus of glucose relative to energy needs or glycogen stores.

Ingested fat, once processed, is stored as adipose tissue throughout the body, especially subcutaneously. It is important to differentiate between the two types of fat stores—essential fat and nonessential fat—when it comes to energetics. Essential fat is stored in a variety of cells and is considered critical for metabolism, conduction of nerve impulses, cell structure, and protection from injury. Essential fat can represent 40% of total fat stores with the remaining 60% being storage fat or nonessential fat (Brooks et al. 2005). Storage fat is favored over essential fat when it comes to being used for energy production. Finally, small amounts of fat are converted to its component parts of free fatty acids and glycerol that circulate in the blood and are available to be used as energy.

Proteins can be used to make enzymes within the body, synthesize glucose, or be stored as muscle tissue. The amount of protein stored in the muscle can be quite significant. About 40% of the average individual's weight is due to muscle. That is larger than useable, nonessential storage fat, which may make up only 20% to 30% of an individual's body weight. However, we use very little protein to generate energy; thus, of all three energy storage sites, protein may be the least important for energy generation.

Previously, we discussed direct calorimetry as a way to measure calorie expenditure by the human body. It is possible to use the same method to determine calorie expenditure or equivalence of each macronutrient. To accomplish this, 1 g of each nutrient is combusted (or burned) inside a direct calorimeter. The heat given off by that nutrient can then be related to the calorie output. Direct calorimetry yields an energy value that is not under physiologic conditions; however, these values are good approximations of what occurs during the normal physiologic processes. The established values for nutrient and calorie equivalencies are

1 g carbohydrate = 4 kcal
1 g fat = 9 kcal
1 g protein = 4 kcal

ENERGY RELEASE OR CONSUMPTION IN CHEMICAL REACTIONS

We discussed the systemic view of energy metabolism and it is now time to delve into the cellular basics of energy production in the body. While most of the body's energy is tied up in maintaining chemical structures, free energy is required to do physical work. Under resting or sedentary conditions, most of the energy in the body is stored in chemical bonds and not free to participate in physical work. In order to release energy for physical use, molecular bonds must be broken and the energy stored in those bonds must be transferred to another usable form of energy. While this is a very simplistic view, it works as a good overall picture. However, in order to release energy, a small amount of energy is required to break that bond (Gropper et al. 2009). An analogous reference would be that it takes money to make money or it takes a spark to light a fire.

Chemical bonds exist within all of the macronutrients (carbohydrates, fats, and proteins) in order to hold together the subunit components of the larger molecules. These bonds have potential energy; that is, the energy we need to do work. Digestion serves to turn these larger molecules into smaller, more manageable ones. These are absorbed through the gastrointestinal tract, pass through the liver where they can undergo further biotransformation, and ultimately end up in systemic circulation where all tissues have access to these molecules. This digestive process of breaking down food and moving it across biologic membranes requires energy. Earlier we referred to this as TEF. When the foundational units of fat (e.g., palmitic acid), carbohydrate (e.g., glucose), or protein (e.g., lysine) are catabolized for energy, the by-products are carbon dioxide (CO_2) and water (H_2O); please note that in the case of proteins, there is an additional nitrogenous by-product such as urea. Following breakdown of macronutrients, usable energy is produced, which is referred to as free energy (ΔG or Gibb's free energy). The cell derives its energy from chemical reactions that are energy releasing or have a negative G-value ($-\Delta G$). A negative G-value indicates that a reaction will occur spontaneously to release energy after the initial investment of activation energy.

We can take a quick look at some relevant chemical reactions and their ΔG values (Table 1.4). The more negative the value, the more energy released. This energy can be coupled to other reactions to produce work. The second to last column in the table—the ratio of carbon dioxide to oxygen—will be discussed later in this chapter, but this ratio can tell us from a systems standpoint what the body is predominantly using as an energy source (i.e., fat, carbohydrate, or mixed diet). Before we move on, we want to discuss three energy carriers relevant to the capturing and use of energy from macronutrients.

TABLE 1.4
Examples of Various Chemical Reactions in the Body, Their Corresponding Value for Free Energy (ΔG), the Ratio of Carbon Dioxide Produced to Oxygen Consumed (i.e., Respiratory Quotient), and the Number of ATP Produced per Molecule

Molecule	Reaction	ΔG (kcal/mol)	CO_2/O_2	ATP Produced (Net)
ATP	$ATP + H_2O \rightarrow ADP + P_i$	−7.3	–	–
Creatine phosphate	$PCr + ADP \rightarrow Cr + ATP$	−10.3	–	1
Lactic acid	$C_3H_6O_3 + 3O_2 \rightarrow 3CO_2 + 3H_2O$	−326	1.0	2
Glucose	$C_{16}H_{12}O_6 + 6O_2 \rightarrow 6CO_2 + 6H_2O$	−686	1.0	36
Palmitic acid	$C_{16}H_{12}O_6 + 23O_2 \rightarrow 16CO_2 + 16H_2O$	−2338	0.7	101

ATP—Cellular Energy Currency

The released free energy is ultimately tied to the production of adenosine triphosphate (ATP), often referred to as the energy currency within the body. While ATP is found in all living tissue, it cannot be readily absorbed through the diet because either it degrades during processing or cooking of food or it is degraded within the gastrointestinal tract. Thus, we must make our ATP using the energy from the macronutrients we consume.

ATP is a small molecule consisting of a nucleoside component of DNA (adenine nucleic acid plus ribose sugar) covalently bound to three phosphate molecules. As depicted in Figure 1.4, the interphosphate bonds store large amounts of energy, especially the terminal (or delta) bond. Under normal conditions, adenosine diphosphate (ADP) coupled with an inorganic phosphate (P_i) is the preferred form of ATP in cells. ADP is the same as ATP minus the terminal phosphate linkage and is favored over ATP because it harbors less electrostatic repulsion by the phosphates, which are all negatively charged. In order to release the free energy of ATP, the unstable chemical bond holding the terminal phosphates together in ATP must be broken by input of a little bit of energy or help from an enzyme or both. The free energy of hydrolysis of ATP is affected by magnesium ions, which may be the basis for magnesium supplementation for performance enhancement. This phosphate bond within ATP represents the packaging of the firework. The bond itself does not appear to be active, but when a small amount of energy is supplied to break the bond, a significantly large release of energy occurs.

The way to release this energy is by hydrolysis, which means addition of water to break a bond. Water molecules, through the action of an enzyme such as ATPase, will break the bond between the two terminal phosphate molecules to release free energy. When this occurs in muscle cells, the free energy is used to help muscle fibers twitch by allowing the myosin head to release and engage further down the actin molecule (Figure 1.5). If many muscle cells release this energy at the same time, an entire muscle group, such as the quadriceps, will be propelled to contract.

Three cellular processes produce ATP within the body. They are ATP-PCr system, glycolysis, and oxidative phosphorylation. The ATP-PCr and glycolysis systems can occur in the relative absence of oxygen while the oxidative phosphorylation pathway requires oxygen to be present in sufficient amounts. Metabolic processes that do require the presence of oxygen are called aerobic processes; those that do not require the presence of oxygen are called anaerobic processes. While ATP can be produced under low and high oxygen environments, the amount of ATP produced is greater when oxygen is present. Another difference among these routes is the timing at which ATP is produced from the system (Figure 1.6). As will be discussed later in

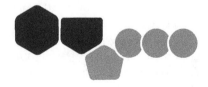

FIGURE 1.4 Stylized ATP molecule. Circles represent the high-energy phosphates.

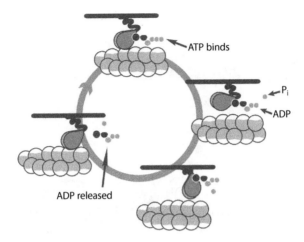

FIGURE 1.5 The role of ATP in muscle contraction. When ATP binds, the myosin head lifts off the actin molecule, flexes, the actin molecule slides, and the myosin head re-engages the actin filament.

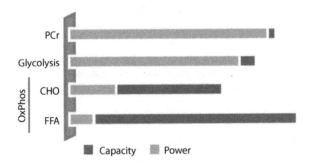

FIGURE 1.6 Schematic of time in exercise and rate of ATP production from various energy sources. Initial sources of ATP are from the most rapid producing sources like phosphocreatine (PCr) and glycolysis. The oxidative phosphorylation of carbohydrates and fats is required to sustain ATP production over time.

the chapter, the initial movement is supplied by anaerobic processes but sustaining movement relies heavily on aerobic processes.

Because of the differences in both speed of ATP production and capacity, these systems tend to be recruited in a temporal order to supply ATP. For example, the ATP-PCr system is utilized for immediate energy because it produces ATP very quickly and thus it is recruited first to meet ATP demands. Because this system has a low capacity, it cannot be used for a long duration. On the other hand, oxidative phosphorylation via the breakdown of carbohydrates or fats does not produce ATP as quickly. However, oxidative phosphorylation has a higher capacity for ATP production and can be used to support long duration activities. Figure 1.7 provides a schematic comparing the power vs. capacity of these systems when recruited. In the latter

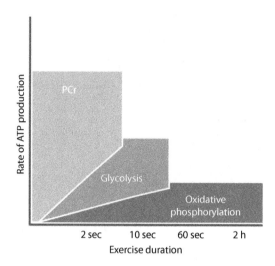

FIGURE 1.7 Comparison of various energy-producing pathways with respect to relative capacity and power (speed) of ATP production. CHO, carbohydrate; FFA, free fatty acids; OxPhos, oxidative phosphorylation; PCr, phosphocreatine. (Adapted from Williams, M.H. 2005. *Nutrition for Health, Fitness, and Sport*, 7th ed. Dubuque, IA: McGraw-Hill.)

cases of glycolysis or oxidative phosphorylation, ATP may not be directly formed from the chemical bonds within nutrients. ATP may be formed through intermediate *carriers* such nicotinamide adenine dinucleotide (NAD) and flavin adenine dinucleotide (FAD).

NAD and FAD—Electron Carriers

ATP is the product we associate with useable energy. Two other compounds, NAD and FAD, can be thought of as ATP intermediates because they carry energy in the form of electrons and protons that were captured from chemical bonds of nutrients. The energy stored within these molecules can be used to generate ATP through other biologic processes such as the electron transport chain. NAD is the oxidized form of NADH and FAD is the oxidized form of $FADH_2$. NAD consists of nicotinic acid (niacin or vitamin B_3) and has enough energy to produce approximately 3 ATP. FAD consists of a riboflavin moiety (vitamin B_2) and has enough stored energy to form 2 ATP.

NUTRIENT METABOLISM OVERVIEW

As discussed, ATP is the main currency for energy whereas glucose, free fatty acid, glycerol, and amino acids are the foundational units derived from food to generate ATP. Macronutrient stores consist of glucose derived from carbohydrates, free fatty acids, and glycerol from fat and amino acids from protein. Following production of sufficient ATP, it is stored as phosphocreatine. We will now discuss each component and how their pathways are similar or different. Figure 1.6 depicts the difference of when each system is utilized during exercise.

ATP-PCr System Overview

The ATP-PCr system can generate ATP the fastest (~10 mmol/kg dry muscle/sec), so it is generally thought to be the first utilized during physical activity. Immediately when beginning any movement, such as climbing a flight of stairs, the majority of the first 10 sec of work will be supplied by ATP stored within the cell. However, the cell does not store ATP per se; it stores the energy as phosphocreatine (PCr), a phosphorylated form of creatine.

PCr regenerates ATP molecules through substrate-level phosphorylation. Phosphorylation is the transfer of energy in two steps by breaking one phosphate bond and creating a new one on a different molecule. This decreases the free energy capability of the first molecule but increases the free energy capability of the second. At rest, PCr production occurs by breaking the terminal phosphate bond on ATP and creating a new bond with creatine, which is stored as phosphocreatine. PCr production occurs at rest when ATP is in surplus. During exercise, any free ATP is used for energy by breaking the terminal phosphate bond and forming ADP. In order to regenerate ATP quickly, PCr will transfer its phosphate molecule to ADP via substrate-level phosphorylation. The ATP-PCr system becomes exhausted when all immediate ATP and PCr molecules are used to produce energy. At this point, activity must stop or another source must serve as the source of ATP.

The formation of PCr is readily reversible and is catalyzed by the enzyme creatine kinase (Figure 1.8). Creatine kinase is found within both the cytosol of the cell and

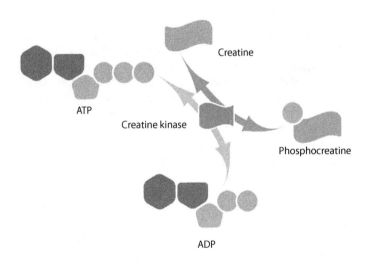

FIGURE 1.8 Schematic of the phosphocreatine reaction. The reaction is reversible. When energy is in surplus, formation of phosphocreatine and ADP is favored. When energy is required to do work, formation of creatine and ATP is favored.

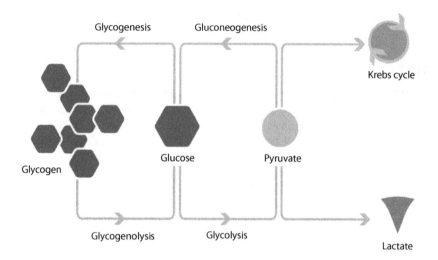

FIGURE 1.9 Schematic of the possible routes of glucose when ingested.

the mitochondria, although structurally creatine kinase is different between the two locations. In this reaction, ATP and creatine react to form an ADP and PCr. This system requires no oxygen because it releases energy solely from the breakage of ATP phosphate bonds.

Carbohydrate Overview

Most of the cells within the body can utilize multiple sources of nutrients for energy; the exceptions are red blood cells and the brain, as these cells require glucose to generate ATP. In fact, the brain consumes about 400 to 600 kcal of glucose per day, which accounts for nearly two-thirds of total glucose catabolism (Owen et al. 1967).

Within the cytosol of the cell, glucose in the cell can be stored as glycogen if energy is not required (i.e., glycogenesis). If glucose is needed, it can be supplied from the blood, glycogen breakdown (i.e., glycogenolysis), or formation of new glucose from non-glucose sources (i.e., gluconeogenesis) (Figure 1.9). To use glucose as energy, it is initially catabolized during glycolysis. In general, the 6-carbon glucose is split into two 3-carbon compounds. This splitting does require some input of ATP. These 3-carbon compounds ultimately end up as pyruvate, thus one glucose molecule yields two pyruvate.

Up to this point, no oxygen is required to convert glucose to pyruvate. If oxygen is limited, say during very high intensity exercise, energy can be obtained from pyruvate through its conversion to lactic acid via the enzyme lactate dehydrogenase. If sufficient amounts of oxygen are present, say during moderate intensity exercise, pyruvate will enter the mitochondria of the cell where it will be converted to acetyl CoA. During this process, pyruvate loses a carbon in the form of carbon dioxide to become a 2-carbon compound; the 2-carbon molecule then bonds with CoA, a pantothenic acid derivative (vitamin B_5). The newly formed acetyl CoA will enter the

Krebs cycle and the electron transport chain when energy is needed. Details of these processes will be discussed in the next section.

FAT OVERVIEW

Fats are typically found as triglycerides, which is a glycerol molecule joined to three chains of fatty acids. The first step in energy release is to cleave the fatty acids from glycerol. Glycerol, a 3-carbon compound, can be converted to pyruvate, also a 3-carbon compound. The next step in the process is similar to carbohydrate metabolism where pyruvate becomes acetyl CoA, and through the Krebs cycle and electron transport chain ATP is generated.

The fatty acids or free fatty acids are long carbon chains and catabolized usually through a process called beta-oxidation. Beta-oxidation forms 2-carbon compounds, which can be linked to CoA to form acetyl CoA. A small amount of energy is released and captured as NADH or $FADH_2$ each time a 2-carbon fragment is formed, but the vast majority of energy comes from the oxidation of this fragment during the oxidative phosphorylation. It is to be noted that these free fatty acids, which make up 95% of fat, cannot be used to produce glucose. Thus, fatty acids do not provide energy to red blood cells or the central nervous system.

While fatty acid catabolism may appear independent of glucose catabolism, they are linked. Fatty acid catabolism depends on glucose to maintain various intermediates within the Krebs cycle like oxaloacetate. Because of this linkage, it is thought that "fat burns in a carbohydrate flame" (McArdle et al. 2007). In extreme cases of glucose insufficiency such as starvation, uncontrolled diabetes, ketogenic diets, or prolonged exercise, the body will convert fat into ketone bodies because the 2-carbon compounds produced from beta-oxidation cannot be funneled through the Krebs cycle. The overproduction of ketone bodies can cause metabolic acidosis or a lowering of body pH.

PROTEIN OVERVIEW

Although protein catabolism to produce energy is small compared to carbohydrate and fat during sport and exercise, we will briefly discuss how protein and amino acids are used to derive ATP. Amino acids first undergo deamination; that is, they lose their nitrogen-containing amino group. Some amino acids are converted to pyruvate (e.g., alanine, glycine, serine), others are converted directly to acetyl CoA (e.g., isoleucine, leucine, tryptophan) or an acetyl CoA precursor acetoacetate (e.g, tyrosine, lysine). Others enter the Krebs cycle directly as intermediate compounds such as alpha-keto glutarate (e.g., arginine, histidine, proline), succinyl CoA (e.g., valine methionine, threonine), fumarate (e.g., phenylalanine, tyrosine) or oxaloacetate (e.g., aspirate, asparagine) (Gropper et al. 2009).

MECHANISMS OF ENERGY PRODUCTION

We have provided a brief overview of how macronutrients are used to generate ATP and a pathway that generates ATP directly. Now we can provide more detail about the pathways used by carbohydrates, fats, and proteins to generate ATP.

GLYCOLYSIS

In a previous section, we discussed substrate-level phosphorylation between PCr and ATP in the ATP-PCr system. Another form of substrate-level phosphorylation occurs in glycolysis when an ATP molecule transfers one phosphate to another molecule, specifically glucose. Loss of the phosphate molecule will decrease energy of the ATP, but increase the energy potential of glucose. Glucose is the starting point in glycolysis. As glucose is the only starting material for this process, carbohydrates are the only macronutrient source for glycolysis, but in order to be useful, the complex carbohydrates within the diet must be catabolized into glucose.

As mentioned, glycolysis requires the input of energy in order to retrieve the energy within the glucose molecule. This activation energy is accomplished through the consumption of two ATP molecules for every one glucose molecule. The result of glycolysis is the generation of four ATP molecules, which actually only produce a net gain of two ATP molecules available for cellular work (since it took two ATP to start the process).

Glycolysis is an anaerobic process and can sustain ATP output for up to 1 min. It is useful for running a 400-m race, which is not the pace of high-intensity exercise

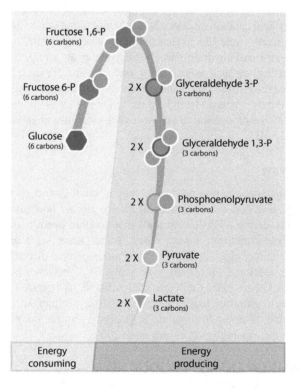

FIGURE 1.10 Schematic of glycosis. Left side of the diagram depicts intermediates that require energy to produce. Right side of the diagram depicts intermediates that produce energy. Note that not all intermediates are shown.

like a 40-yard dash that utilizes primarily PCr, but is a higher pace than a 1-mile race that would rely on oxidative phosphorylation. Glycolysis takes place in the cells' cytosol and converts glucose into two molecules of pyruvate. Pyruvate can continue in glycolysis and form lactic acid or be converted to another intermediate for entry into the Krebs cycle. Lactic acid is responsible for the burning sensation within the muscle during high intensity exercise. Lowering muscle pH caused by the accumulation of lactic acid, which interferes with muscle cross-bridging, ultimately halts exercise (Fitts 2008). Lactic acid is a limiting factor that will prevent the long-term utilization of glycolysis to produce energy during exercise. If sufficient oxygen is present, pyruvate will enter the Krebs cycle to produce much more ATP than glycolysis.

The pathway of lactate formation is found in Figure 1.10. One mol of ATP is used per glucose molecule for the first phosphorylation step (glucose to fructose 6-phosphate) and the second ATP is required to add a second phosphate group to fructose (fructose 6-phosphate to fructose 1,6 bisphosphate). The biphosphorylated fructose is cleaved to form two 3-carbon compounds. As you may notice, inorganic phosphates are added to these latter 3-carbon intermediates like glyceraldehyde 1,3 phosphate; this is accomplished by using an inorganic phosphate group and NAD. ATP is generated in the conversion of 1,3 bisphospho-glycerate to 3-phospho-glycerate; because there are two of these molecules, two ATP are generated. A second set of ATP is generated from the conversion of phosphoenolpyruvate to pyruvate. Finally, an NADH is consumed to convert pyruvate into lactate.

When oxygen concentration is limited, pyruvate is converted to lactic acid. The lactic acid produced within the muscle cannot be recycled. It is converted back to glucose within the muscle. Lactic acid is exported out of the muscle and the liver takes up the lactic acid and converts it into glucose via the Cori cycle. This process consumes ATP in order to produce glucose. This system is not efficient at clearing lactate during exercise and works more efficiently at rest (van Hall 2010). The only site that can utilize lactic acid for energy is cardiac tissue (Gertz et al. 1981).

OXIDATIVE PHOSPHORYLATION

At the end of glycolysis, we mentioned that pyruvate is formed and this compound has two fates—become lactic acid or be converted into an intermediate and enter the Krebs cycle. We will now discuss this latter situation. Substrate-level phosphorylation through PCr and in glycolysis is focused on small-scale energy transfer from one molecule to another, one phosphate bond at a time. The most prolific and sustainable form of phosphorylation to produce ATP from ADP is called oxidative phosphorylation. In order to produce large amounts of ATP that can be sustained over long periods of time, oxygen is required.

THE KREBS CYCLE

Oxidative phosphorylation can be thought of as two different processes that occur sequentially to produce ATP. Oxidation is the first step in the process. Oxidation reactions occur via oxygen addition, electron removal, and hydrogen ion liberation.

Prior to starting this process, pyruvate, from glycolysis, is converted into acetyl CoA and this takes place in the outer membrane of the mitochondria through the enzyme pyruvate dehydrogenase. Unlike glycolysis, glucose is not the only starting material for the Krebs cycle. The process of converting pyruvate to acetyl CoA does require coenzymes that contain prosthetic groups of magnesium, thiamine (as thiamine pyrophosphate), lipoic acid, FAD, and NAD. As some of these compounds contain B vitamins, supplementation has been theorized to increase exercise performance.

Oxidative phosphorylation produces ATP molecules from carbohydrate, fat, and protein sources. This is the only process that can utilize fats or proteins to produce energy. The formation of acetyl CoA is the final step before oxidation in the catabolism of fat. In this process, a free fatty acid undergoes beta-oxidation, which results in acetyl-CoA subunits that then enter the Krebs cycle (also known as the tricarboxylic acid [TCA] cycle). Conversely, various amino acids can enter the Krebs cycle at specific points in the cycle. For example, arginine enters the process in the period between the formation of citrate and succinate, but tyrosine enters at the fumarate step (Figure 1.11).

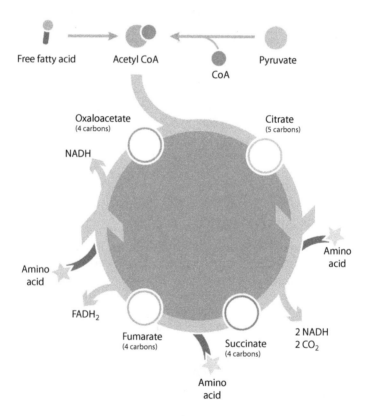

FIGURE 1.11 Overview of the Krebs cycle. Pyruvate, fatty acids, and selected amino acids can form acetyl-CoA. Throughout the cycle, amino acids can be used to produce energy. Note that not all intermediates are shown.

The Krebs cycle is a series of reactions that completely oxidize acetyl CoA. It is referred to as a cycle not because it generates acetyl CoA, but because a 4-carbon compound is cycled around and around. Maintaining this 4-carbon compound becomes important for physical performance and the need to maintain adequate carbohydrate supplies during exercise. While the Krebs cycle does not produce ATP directly, this process generates molecules capable of entering the electron transport system to yield ATP, NADH, and $FADH_2$.

The Electron Transport System (ETC)

The ETC consists of a series of proteins that serve as electron carriers within the inner membrane of the mitochondria. When electrons are passed protein to protein, a little bit of energy is released. While some of this energy is released as heat, the remaining energy is used to pump hydrogen ions against a concentration gradient; that is, from the low concentration of the inner mitochondrial space into the high concentration of intermembrane space. At the end of the chain, the final acceptor of these electrons is oxygen. Each oxygen atom of the oxygen molecule will accept two hydrogen ions and two electrons to form water as a by-product of metabolism. The passing of electrons generates a diffusion gradient, which allows passive diffusion of hydrogen ions back into the mitochondrial matrix through an ATP synthase to form ATP (Figure 1.12).

There are important micronutrients involved in the ETC to note as they have been implicated in exercise performance. CoQ_{10} (ubiquinone) is part of the electron

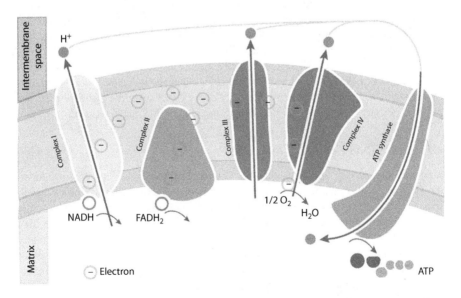

FIGURE 1.12 Overview of the electron transport chain. Hydrogen ions are pumped into the intermembrane space by the energy within NADH and $FADH_2$. The energy caused by the hydrogen ion gradient supplies energy to form ATP with the use of oxygen as a terminal electron acceptor.

transport chain that shuttles electrons from complex II to III. We draw your attention to CoQ_{10} because there has been research on supplementation in the active population to either enhance energetics or serve as an antioxidant (Mizuno et al. 2008).

Iron is the central piece within all the mitochondrial complexes with the exception of complex IV, which contains copper. Iron deficiency has been well studied in the active population because of its negative effects on oxygen carrying capacity (Beard and Tobin 2000; Lukaski 2004). It does appear copper status also is implicated in exercise and blood concentrations do change because of exercise (Clarkson and Haymes 1995).

OVERVIEW OF ENERGY USE DURING EXERCISE

This chapter started with a general discussion of metabolic rate and how our energy is used on a whole body scale. From the whole body aspect, we drilled down to the chemical aspect of how we derive energy from foodstuffs. We talked about how the phosphocreatine system and glycolysis can provide energy very quickly but in limited capacity. Then we moved to the Krebs cycle and oxidative phosphorylation, which use oxygen to derive more energy from our foodstuffs. We will now discuss how macronutrients supply fuel for exercise and what may determine the extent of their use.

When we transition from rest to being active, especially maximum activity, the blood flow to the muscle increases 15 times and the rate of energy turnover within the muscle can increase 1000-fold. The stimulus of the activation of metabolism is a high ADP to ATP ratio, which indicates available ATP is being used and more needs to be produced. However, there is a short 1 to 2 min lag time between the onset of exercise and the increase in oxygen supply (Maughan et al. 2000). It is during this time period that anaerobic systems like the phosphocreatine system and glycolysis can support early phases of exercise. Review Figure 1.6 to help understand the time lapse between metabolic systems. For the remainder of the chapter, we will return to the whole body aspect and provide a brief overview of substrate utilization during physical activity. This overview will be expanded upon in Chapters 2 and 4.

DETERMINING EXERCISE INTENSITY

First, we must revisit our discussion of exercise and exercise intensity. We introduced the term VO_{2MAX} as the metric to describe an athlete's cardiovascular fitness level. Exercise intensity is usually based on some fraction of this metric. For example, low intensity exercise may be defined at 50% of VO_{2MAX}, intense aerobic exercise may be 85% of VO_{2MAX}, and anaerobic exercise could be 110% of VO_{2MAX}. While many athletes do not have an opportunity to measure their VO_{2MAX}, there are several other methods to assess intensity. These include using heart rate, ratings of perceived exertion (RPE), or metabolic equivalent (MET).

The use of heart rate to monitor exercise intensity is a practical and reliable method. Heart rate has a linear relationship with VO_2, but the relationship depends on mode of exercise (Kaminsky 2006). The heart rate reserve method is based on the difference in the resting heart rate and the maximum heart rate, whereas the

%HR_{MAX} is based solely on the maximum heart rate. The best method to determine maximum heart rate is through exercise testing, but because this may not be practical, we can estimate it using the individual's age with HR_{MAX} equaling 220-age for relatively untrained individuals, but this may be debatable. Others have suggested more predictive equations (Robergs and Landwehr 2002). Using the heart rate method, a heart rate of <50% of HR_{MAX} is considered in the low intensity region, 55 to 70% of HR_{MAX} is moderate intensity, and >90% of HR_{MAX} is high intensity.

The RPE is a scale that was designed to associate perception with heart rate response. The RPE is historically a 20-point scale with a value of 7 relating to very, very light exercise and 19 being very, very hard. During exercise, the individual is asked to identify which value most reflects his or her current effort.

The MET is the amount of energy expended during 1-min rest. It is, in a sense, a measure of RMR. One MET is equivalent to 1.05 kcal/h/kg or 3.5 mL O_2/kg/min. There are tables of activities that list the activity and how many METs correspond to that activity. For example, jogging is 2 to 3 METs, but sprinting is >11 METs; obviously, sprinting is a higher intensity exercise. Table 1.5 converts between exercise intensities based on VO_{2MAX}, heart rate, RPE, and METs.

The American College of Sports Medicine (ACSM) also has a set of metabolic equations that convert an activity like walking, running, stepping, or cycling into an energy cost. As an example, if an athlete runs at 7 mph on a 2% grade for 10 min, we can estimate the amount of calories expended. The first step is to estimate the amount of oxygen consumed using the ACSM metabolic equation for running (Kaminsky 2006):

$$VO_2 = 3.5 + 0.2 \times \text{Speed} + 0.9 \times \text{Speed} \times \text{Fractional grade}$$

Note that the units for speed are in meters per minute, so 7 mph is 188 m/min. At this speed and incline, the athlete will use 44.4 mL/min/kg of oxygen. The next step is to convert the oxygen use to METs (1 MET = 3.5 mL/min/kg O_2); the athlete

---

TABLE 1.5
Converting between Different Metrics of Exercise Intensity

Intensity	VO_{2MAX} or HRR%	HR_{MAX}%	RPE	METs
Very light	<25	<30	<9	<2
Light	25–44	30–49	9–10	2–4
Moderate	45–59	50–69	11–12	4–6
Hard	60–84	70–89	13–16	6–8.5
Very hard	>84	>90	>16	>8.5
Maximal	100	100	20	10

Source: Kaminsky, L.A. 2006. *ACSM's Resource Manual for Guidelines for Exercise Testing and Prescription*, 5th ed. Baltimore: Lippincott Williams & Wilkins. With permission.

Note: VO_{2MAX} = maximal oxygen capacity, HRR% = heart rate reserve, HR_{MAX}% = percent maximal heart rate, RPE = rating of perceived exertion, METs = metabolic equivalents.

is working around 13 METs or, in more practical terms, 13 times more than RMR. If the athlete weighed 240 lb (or 109 kg), he or she would be consuming 4.8 L of oxygen per minute. A liter of oxygen consumed produces approximately 5 kcals of energy, so the athlete is expending 24 kcal per minute for 10 minutes of exercise, or 240 calories. Remember, gross caloric expenditure takes into account the normal calories consumed to function plus the calories from exercise. The list of metabolic equations can be found within the ACSM resource manual (Kaminsky 2006).

FUEL SOURCE SELECTION

Energy metabolism relates to both the intensity of exercise and its duration. The contribution of anaerobic energy sources (i.e., PCr, glycolysis) is inversely related to duration of exercise and positively related to exercise intensity. For example, if you look at Figure 1.6, you can see that for short duration activities (e.g., sprinting) systems like phosphocreatine and glycolysis may supply the majority of ATP. Longer duration activities would rely on oxidative phosphorylation because it can supply sufficient ATP.

Different exercise intensities influence the utilization of stores of energy as do different exercise durations. At rest, fat metabolism supplies the majority of ATP because it has a large capacity and the rate at which ATP is needed is slow. As exercise intensity increases, more and more calories start coming from carbohydrate sources. In Figure 1.13, this is demonstrated with two situations—someone exercising at 25% of his or her VO_{2MAX} and the same person at 85% of his or her VO_{2MAX}. As the exercise intensity increases, the contributions from muscle glycogen increase, accounting for a larger fraction of the ATP production. At the same time, the total amount of calories per unit time also increases.

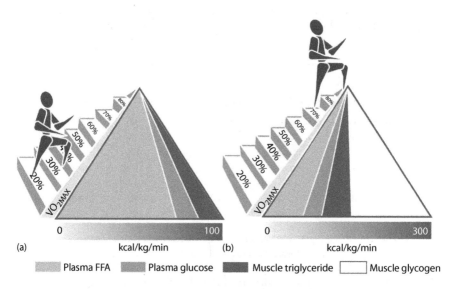

FIGURE 1.13 The relationship between exercise intensity and source of fuel for exercise. (a) 25% VO_{2MAX}; (b) 85% VO_{2MAX}. (Data from Romijn, J.A. et al. 1993. *Am J Physiol* 265(3 Pt 1):E380–E391.)

Determining what fuel source is being used goes back to some of the earlier equations looking at glucose or palmitate metabolism. We initially provided a ratio of carbon dioxide produced to the amount of oxygen consumed. For glucose, a ratio of 1.0 is found; that is, 1 mol of carbon dioxide is formed per mol of oxygen consumed. This ratio of 1.0 in general indicates carbohydrate is the predominant energy source. For palmitate, a ratio of 0.7 is found, indicating that for every 0.7 mol of carbon dioxide produced, 1 mol of oxygen is consumed. The ratio of 0.7 indicates predominant fat metabolism. Values in between 0.7 and 1.0 indicate mixed-fuel use. This ratio of carbon dioxide produced to oxygen consumed is referred to as the respiratory exchange ratio (RER) or respiratory quotient (RQ) (Table 1.6) (Figure 1.14). A value exceeding 1.0 indicates anaerobic use of energy because we are exhaling more carbon dioxide than our maximum ability to consume oxygen and may be exemplified in resistance training, which tends to be high intensity, short duration exercise (Lozano Almela et al. 2010; Ortego et al. 2009).

HIGH INTENSITY, SHORT DURATION EXERCISE

High intensity, short duration exercise typically means exercise that occurs in bouts of 5 to 60 sec at values of 85% of VO_{2MAX}. Both the PCr system and glycolysis will supply ATP for these types of activities, and the major determining factor, which will dictate the predominant pathway, will be duration. Very short activities (i.e., <5 sec) would emphasize PCr, but a 30-sec exercise would emphasize glycolysis. This is not to say aerobic pathways do not contribute ATP during short exercise durations, but they are minimal compared to anaerobic pathways. In later chapters, when we discuss dietary supplements, creatine will be discussed again as supplementation through the diet can augment the PCr system and assist in certain types of exercise.

TABLE 1.6

Summary of the Approximate Amount of Calories Available per Gram of Various Macronutrients and the Corresponding Respirator Quotient

Food	kcal/O$_2$	RQ	kcal/g
Carbohydrate	5.05	1.0	4.2
Fat	4.7	0.7	9.5
Protein	4.5	0.8	4.2
Mixed diet	4.82	0.82	–
Starvation	4.7	0.7	–

Source: Brooks, G.A., T.D. Fahey, and K.M. Baldwin. 2005. *Exercise Physiology: Human Bioenergetics and Its Applications*, 4th ed. Boston: McGraw-Hill. With permission.

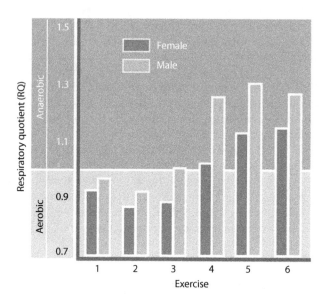

FIGURE 1.14 The relationship between respiratory quotient and resistance exercise for men and women. Numbers represent different strength exercises. (Adapted from Ortego, A.R. et al. 2009. *J Strength Cond Res* 23(3):932–938.)

Submaximal Exercise for Prolonged Periods

Both oxidative catabolism of carbohydrate and fat will contribute the majority of ATP during submaximal exercise ($VO_2 < 85\%$ VO_{2MAX}). The greatest amount of fat as a substrate occurs at 60% of VO_{2MAX} (Kaminsky 2006) (see Table 1.7 as an example). During prolonged exercise, there is a gradual shift from carbohydrate to

TABLE 1.7
Demonstration of the Relationship between METs, Total Calories Consumed in a 30-Min Time Period, and How Many Calories Are Approximately from the Catabolism of Fat

METs	Example Activity	kcal/kg/h	~% Fat Expended	Fat (kcal)	Total (kcal)
1	Resting, typing	1.2	80	34	42
2	Walking at a slow pace	2.4	70	59	88
3	Walking at an average pace, bowling	3.5	65	80	123
4	Walking at a fast pace, climbing stairs	5	55	96	175
5	Bicycling (10 mph)	6	45	95	210
7	Jogging	8.5	25	74	298
9	Running (8:30 min mile)	11	10	40	385

Note: Data are based on a 70-kg individual.

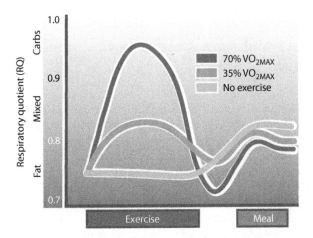

FIGURE 1.15 Changes in the respiratory quotient during prolonged exercise in overweight individuals. (Adapted from Pillard, F. et al. 2007. *Obesity (Silver Spring)* 15(9):2256–2262.)

fat catabolism, which may be explained by inhibitory effects of fats on the Krebs cycle (Kaminsky 2006).

During prolonged exercise, early time points rely more on carbohydrate as a fuel source (Figure 1.15). Over time, the RQ declines, indicating a migration to more fat as a fuel. During exercise, especially at higher intensities or longer duration, oxygen consumption may be a limiting factor. The preference of fuel source is balanced between two factors—the energy yield relative to oxygen used and the energy yield on a gram per gram basis. The preference for carbohydrate may be attributable to the fact that per oxygen molecule inhaled, carbohydrate offers approximately 6% more energy than fat (Brooks et al. 2005). As work is maintained, glycogen stores start to become a limiting factor, which helps explain the transition to more fat utilization. It has been estimated that glycogen can be depleted after 90 to 120 min of continuous exercise. On the other hand, on a gram per gram basis, fat offers more than two times the amount of energy that carbohydrates do. As individuals become more aerobically fit, their use of fat as a fuel during mild to moderate exercise is enhanced.

RECOVERY FROM EXERCISE

An increasing area of research is nutrition related to recovery from exercise. After exercise, oxygen uptake remains elevated for a few minutes. In general, the higher the intensity of exercise the higher the level of postexercise metabolism; the same is true for duration—the longer the duration of exercise the longer the postexercise metabolism window. There is evidence suggesting that metabolic rate may remain elevated for at least 12 h and possibly up to 24 h after very prolonged intense exercise (LaForgia et al. 2006). For athletes training hard, this elevation of metabolic rate postexercise will increase the difficulties in maintaining energy balance. It is unlikely, however, that active individuals who are exercising for health reasons will have such elevated metabolic rates for long periods. The enhanced metabolic state after exercise can be used to optimize recovery by adding the appropriate nutrients that replenish used energy stores such as carbohydrate or protein.

CONCLUSION

Exercise can be thought of on a continuum between power and endurance. Power indicates high intensity for short duration of time, whereas endurance is lower intensity but for longer duration. It is important to understand the athletes' activities to optimize their nutrition, not only what they consume but also when they consume it. Nutrient timing is an increasingly important aspect of nutrition to optimize the catabolic and anabolic processes associated with exercise.

Starting with the power end of the continuum, very high intensity exercise lasting only a few seconds—like a powerlift—relies on the phosphocreatine energy system; within seconds, this system can be depleted of its ATP-generating capacity. Nutritional interventions such as supplementation with creatine may augment the capacity of this system and is discussed in Chapter 5.

High intensity exercise, which can last a couple of minutes, is ultimately limited by the formation of lactic acid and the accumulation of hydrogen ions resulting in a decreased tissue pH. Nutritional strategies that focus on buffering the decrease in pH, such as beta alanine and sodium bicarbonate, may offer some performance benefit. In addition, ingestion of carbohydrate postexercise may facilitate recovery from this type of exercise and allow for higher performance during repeated bouts.

Continuing on, moderate intensity exercise requires the use of both fat and carbohydrate catabolism to supply sufficient ATP to sustain activity for longer periods of time (e.g., 60 min). Insufficient amounts of carbohydrate during exercise may ultimately result in an inability to continue to exercise; thus, strategies to increase muscle glycogen tend to be favored. Fat loading has shown equivocal evidence for helping in this type of scenario. As in the previous scenario, sufficient amount of carbohydrate or even carbohydrate-protein mixtures after exercise may facilitate recovery from this type of energy-depleting exercise. Carbohydrate and carbohydrate-protein mixtures for recovery are discussed in Chapter 3. In addition, hydration status also may impact performance and will be discussed in Chapter 11.

On the light intensity end of the continuum, fat oxidation is the primary energy source. Energy supply typically is not a rate-limiting variable unless there are insufficient carbohydrate supplies. As in the moderate intensity case, hydration status may be important and strategies to maintain optimal hydration therefore would be important. The contributions of vitamins and minerals are discussed in later Chapters 12.

REFERENCES

Ainslie, P., T. Reilly, and K. Westerterp. 2003. Estimating human energy expenditure: A review of techniques with particular reference to doubly labelled water. *Sports Med* 33(9):683–698.

Ainsworth, B.E., W.L. Haskell, M.C. Whitt et al. 2000. Compendium of physical activities: An update of activity codes and MET intensities. *Med Sci Sports Exerc* 32(9 Suppl):S498–S504.

Beard, J., and B. Tobin. 2000. Iron status and exercise. *Am J Clin Nutr* 72(2 Suppl):594S–597S.

Bernadot, D., and W.R. Thompson. 1999. Energy from food for physical activity: Enough and on time. *ACSM's Health Fit J* 3(4):14–18.

Brooks, G.A., T.D. Fahey, and K.M. Baldwin. 2005. *Exercise Physiology: Human Bioenergetics and Its Applications*, 4th ed. Boston: McGraw-Hill.

Carpenter, W.H., E.T. Poehlman, M. O'Connell, and M.I. Goran. 1995. Influence of body composition and resting metabolic rate on variation in total energy expenditure: A meta-analysis. *Am J Clin Nutr* 61(1):4–10.

Clarkson, P.M., and E.M. Haymes. 1995. Exercise and mineral status of athletes: Calcium, magnesium, phosphorus, and iron. *Med Sci Sports Exerc* 27(6):831–843.

Dauncey, M.J. 1980. Metabolic effects of altering the 24 h energy intake in man, using direct and indirect calorimetry. *Br J Nutr* 43(2):257–269.

de Jonge, L., and G.A. Bray. 1997. The thermic effect of food and obesity: A critical review. *Obes Res* 5(6):622–631.

Fitts, R.H. 2008. The cross-bridge cycle and skeletal muscle fatigue. *J Appl Physiol* 104(2):551–558.

Forsum, E., M. Lof, and D.A. Schoeller. 2006. Calculation of energy expenditure in women using the MET system. *Med Sci Sports Exerc* 38(8):1520–1525.

Gertz, E.W., J.A. Wisneski, R. Neese, J.D. Bristow, G.L. Searle, and J.T. Hanlon. 1981. Myocardial lactate metabolism: Evidence of lactate release during net chemical extraction in man. *Circulation* 63(6):1273–1279.

Gropper, S.A.S., J.L. Smith, and J.L. Groff. 2009. *Advanced Nutrition and Human Metabolism*, 5th ed. Australia: Wadsworth/Cengage Learning.

Henry, C.J. 2005. Basal metabolic rate studies in humans: Measurement and development of new equations. *Public Health Nutr* 8(7A):1133–1152.

Institute of Medicine (U.S.), Panel on Macronutrients, and Institute of Medicine (U.S.), Standing Committee on the Scientific Evaluation of Dietary Reference Intakes. 2005. *Dietary Reference Intakes for Energy, Carbohydrate, Fiber, Fat, Fatty Acids, Cholesterol, Protein, and Amino Acids*. Washington, DC: National Academies Press.

Kaminsky, L.A. 2006. *ACSM's Resource Manual for Guidelines for Exercise Testing and Prescription*, 5th ed. Baltimore: Lippincott Williams & Wilkins.

Knuttgen, H.G. 1995. Force, work, and power in athletic training. *Sports Sci* 8(4):1–6.

LaForgia, J., R.T. Withers, and C.J. Gore. 2006. Effects of exercise intensity and duration on the excess post-exercise oxygen consumption. *J Sports Sci* 24(12):1247–1264.

Lazzer, S., G. Bedogni, C.L. Lafortuna et al. 2010. Relationship between basal metabolic rate, gender, age, and body composition in 8,780 white obese subjects. *Obesity (Silver Spring)* 18(1):71–78.

Lozano Almela, M.L., V.D. Molina, M.A. Sanchez, P.J.B. Peinado, and F.J.C. Montero. 2010. Aerobic energy expenditure and intensity prediction during specific circuit weight training: A pilot study. *J Sport Exerc* 5(2):134–145.

Lukaski, H.C. 2004. Vitamin and mineral status: Effects on physical performance. *Nutrition* 20(7–8):632–644.

Maughan, R.J., IOC Medical Commission, and International Federation of Sports Medicine. 2000. *Nutrition in Sport, Encyclopaedia of Sports Medicine*. Osney Mead, Oxford: Blackwell Science.

McArdle, W.D., F.I. Katch, and V.L. Katch. 2007. *Exercise Physiology: Energy, Nutrition, and Human Performance*, 6th ed. Philadelphia, PA: Lippincott Williams & Wilkins.

Mitchell, H.H. 1962. *Comparative Nutrition of Man and Domestic Animals*. New York: Academic Press.

Mizuno, K., M. Tanaka, S. Nozaki et al. 2008. Antifatigue effects of coenzyme Q10 during physical fatigue. *Nutrition* 24(4):293–299.

Ortego, A.R., D.K. Dantzler, A. Zaloudek et al. 2009. Effects of gender on physiological responses to strenuous circuit resistance exercise and recovery. *J Strength Cond Res* 23(3):932–938.

Owen, O.E., A.P. Morgan, H.G. Kemp, J.M. Sullivan, M.G. Herrera, and G.F. Cahill, Jr. 1967. Brain metabolism during fasting. *J Clin Invest* 46(10):1589–1595.

Pillard, F., C. Moro, I. Harant et al. 2007. Lipid oxidation according to intensity and exercise duration in overweight men and women. *Obesity (Silver Spring)* 15(9):2256–2262.

Plasqui, G., and K.R. Westerterp. 2007. Physical activity assessment with accelerometers: An evaluation against doubly labeled water. *Obesity (Silver Spring)* 15(10):2371–2379.

Reeves, M.M., and S. Capra. 2003. Predicting energy requirements in the clinical setting: Are current methods evidence based? *Nutr Rev* 61(4):143–151.

Robergs, R.A., and R. Landwehr. 2002. The surprising history of the HR_{max} = 220-age equation. *J Exerc Physiol* 5(2).

Romijn, J.A., E.F. Coyle, L.S. Sidossis et al. 1993. Regulation of endogenous fat and carbohydrate metabolism in relation to exercise intensity and duration. *Am J Physiol* 265(3 Pt 1):E380–E391.

Roubenoff, R. 2003. Sarcopenia: Effects on body composition and function. *J Gerontol A Biol Sci Med Sci* 58(11):1012–1017.

Schoeller, D.A., and E. van Santen. 1982. Measurement of energy expenditure in humans by doubly labeled water method. *J Appl Physiol* 53(4):955–959.

Stob, N.R., C. Bell, M.A. van Baak, and D.R. Seals. 2007. Thermic effect of food and beta-adrenergic thermogenic responsiveness in habitually exercising and sedentary healthy adult humans. *J Appl Physiol* 103(2):616–622.

van Baak, M.A. 2008. Meal-induced activation of the sympathetic nervous system and its cardiovascular and thermogenic effects in man. *Physiol Behav* 94(2):178–186.

van Hall, G. 2010. Lactate kinetics in human tissues at rest and during exercise. *Acta Physiol (Oxf)* 199(4):499–508.

Williams, M.H. 2005. *Nutrition for Health, Fitness, and Sport*, 7th ed. Dubuque, IA: McGraw-Hill.

2 Nutrition for Endurance Athletes

Antonio Herbert Lancha, PhD
Luciana Oquendo Pereira Lancha, PhD, RD
Patrícia Lopes Campos-Ferraz, PhD
Rodrigo Branco Ferraz, MSc
School of Physical Education and Sports, Laboratory of
Nutrition Applied to Physical Activity and Metabolism,
University of São Paulo, São Paulo, Brazil

CONTENTS

HABITUAL INTAKE OF ELITE ENDURANCE ATHLETES

Endurance exercise sessions are defined as lasting more than 60 to 90 min; many endurance events may last from a few hours (marathon, Ironman, etc.) to a few days (orientation races, road race pro-cycling competitions such as Tour de France, Giro d'Italia, Race Across America, etc.), making it more difficult to achieve nutritional recommendations for these expedition-like competitions. During long-lasting moderate exercise, approximately equal amounts of fat and carbohydrate (CHO) are utilized by skeletal muscle to obtain energy; however, muscle glycogen reduction is associated with fatigue and reduced work capacity, as muscle tissue depends more on fat as an energy substrate in this situation, making blood glucose more important as energy fuel for contracting muscles in moderate to intense exercise (Genton et al. 2010; Melzer 2011; Melzer et al. 2013).

Furthermore, protein and energy requirements for endurance physical activities are also increased compared to sedentary counterparts and exercise, in general, is known to elicit appetite compensation mechanisms of different kinds (Hopkins et al. 2011).

The recent recommendations of CHO intake for endurance exercise are listed in Table 2.1.

TABLE 2.1

Recommendations of Carbohydrate Intake for Endurance Exercise

Pre-Exercise			Post-Exercise
3–4 h before	1 h before	Immediately before	First 30 min
4–5 g CHO/kg BW meal	1–2 g CHO/kg BW energy replenishing; liquid form	50–60 g CHO	1.5 g CHO/kg BW every 2 h until 6 h later

Source: American Dietetic Association et al. 2009. *J Am Diet Assoc* 109:509–527. With permission.

Note: Athletes undergoing intense training must have a CHO intake ranging from 7 to 10 g/kg BW or 60% TCI.

Elite endurance athletes from sport modalities in which the competition length usually lasts less than 12 h are thought to have most of their nutritional requirements fulfilled during this time. This seems to be true especially for male counterparts; in female athletes, however, mainly those competing in sports modalities in which body weight (BW) interferes with their performance, nutrition requirements of energy, CHOs, proteins, and some micronutrients probably are not being fully achieved. For example, elite Ethiopian distance male runners consume 8.1 to 10 g/kg BW of CHOs, 1.76 g/kg BW of protein (76% from vegetable sources and representing 12% of daily caloric intake), and 23.3% of the total caloric intake (TCI) from fat and adequate energy, while elite Kenyan male runners consume 10.4 g/kg BW of CHOs, 13.4% total caloric intake of fat, 1.2 g protein/kg BW (67% from vegetable sources and representing 10% TCI), and only 83% of total energy expenditure (Beis et al. 2011; Onywera et al. 2004). These two studies show that CHO and protein intake seem to be adequate in these elite athletes; however, energy intake in Kenyan counterparts is below the recommendations, with energy mainly coming from fat.

In female elite runners, studies have shown that dietary energy intake and other nutrients are well below current recommendations. A classic investigation by Deuster et al. (1986) in highly trained women indicated that 51 elite runners featured low dietetic intake of calcium, magnesium, zinc, and iron, although most of them could reach the recommend dietary allowances (RDAs) for those nutrients by taking supplements (Deuster et al. 1986).

In these athletes, energy intake was compatible with sedentary women's recommendation, as it was around 46 g/kg BW/day, but perhaps it might not have been adequate for women running 10 miles/day; furthermore, this study did not use a precise energy expenditure estimation method and under-reporting of dietary intake might have occurred, as described in other studies (Trabulsi and Schoeller 2001). Female elite long distance runners seem to be especially prone to various degrees of disordered eating and menstrual irregularities; both of them are important markers of the female athlete triad syndrome (De Souza et al. 2010; Torstveit and Sundgot-Borgen 2005).

As defined by Nattiv et al. (2007), the female athlete triad syndrome is a spectrum of eating behaviors that leads to low energy availability, low menstrual function, and bone density. The main treatment is increasing energy availability (Nattiv et al. 1994, 2007). It is important to note that the menstrual irregularities in female athletes seem to be related to a caloric deficit more than training volume or body fat (Loucks 2003; Scheid and De Souza 2010).

As opposed to other endurance sports, triathlons are composed of three modalities (swimming, biking, and running). Each has quite different demands on the athlete. Athletes are more likely to ingest solid food and liquids during the cycling part. The recent nutritional recommendations for endurance sports usually apply to triathlons as well.

A study from Cox et al. (2010) showed that what elite triathlon competitors consume before and during an Olympic-distance competition (lasting approximately 2 h) is quite different. Male and female athletes consume less than 26 g of CHO/h during the race, which is almost half of the recommended intake of 0.7 g/kg BW/h, mainly when the race was performed before noon. For a race performed later in the day, CHO intake was shown to be a little higher (Cox et al. 2010).

Most of the problems triathletes encounter during competitions are dehydration, gastrointestinal discomfort, CHO depletion, and hyperthermia, especially among slower competitors (Jeukendrup 2011). This is crucial when considering that many triathlon events occur in warm environments, which can affect many aspects of the competition, including the temperature of the liquids at aid stations going beyond the palatable level (Burdon et al. 2013).

Although nutrition has an important impact on performance in other sports like running or cycling, studies in triathletes fail to show a direct relationship between nutritional strategies during the race and final performance and, surprisingly, despite the increasing popularity of this sport, there is a limited quantity of studies in this population (Dolan et al. 2011).

Considering energy expenditure and intake in general, the longer the event, the more difficult it is to achieve nutritional recommendations. It has been shown that in cyclists competing in long professional road races, energy intake is well under their calculated energy expenditure, resulting in weight loss after some competitions. For example, García-Rovés et al. (1998) showed that professional road cyclists consumed an average of 80 kcal/kg BW during training, 12 g CHO/kg BW, 2.9 g protein/kg BW, and 2.3 g lipids/kg BW, which reaches and exceeds the recommendations (García-Rovés et al. 1998).

A classic study from Saris et al. (1989) showed that during the Tour de France, cyclists' energy expenditure accounted for approximately 8300 kcal/day. They consumed 5947 kcal on average during the race, which is only 49% of energy intake. Their macronutrient intake was distributed as 15% protein, 62% CHO (94 g/h of race), and 23% fat (Saris et al. 1989).

However, the same does not hold true for solo athletes during Race Across America (RAAM), where the estimated energy expenditure was 18,000 kcal/day, while the intake was approximately 10,000 kcal/day, resulting in a weight loss of almost 5 kg during 11 days (Knechtle et al. 2005). It is important to emphasize that elite cyclists exhibit a slightly different nutritional pattern during training periods for long competitions.

A study by García-Rovés et al. (2000) showed that protein intake during a race is reduced, compared to training periods; however, other nutrients like energy, CHO, and fat remained the same.

These data lead to the conclusion that it is possible to maintain energy intake in longer events if the daily journey lasts less than 6 h. Otherwise, like in the RAAM case, where a solo competitor can cycle for almost 22 h/day, energy intake is not supposed to match energy expenditure.

The main sources of CHOs and energy in the dietary intake of elite runners are usually sugar (20% TCI) and cooked rice (14% TCI) and in road race pro cyclists, maltodextrin (16% TCI), sweet cakes (15% TCI), and bread (11% TCI). Sweet cakes are also important sources of fat (27% TCI) along with margarine/butter (15%) (Onywera et al. 2004; Saris et al. 1989).

Taken together, the studies indicate that CHO and energy are usually matched during longer events (6 to 21 days) as long as they do not last more than 6 h/day in male athletes; however, in female counterparts, the risk of consuming fewer calories than needed has implications on bone health and hormones, resulting in a higher incidence of disordered eating or female athlete triad syndrome.

PERFORMANCE × CHO INTAKE PRIOR TO EXERCISE

A growing number of studies have been designed to test the hypotheses that training with low carbohydrate availability can ameliorate carbohydrate uptake before competition ("train low, compete high") (Burke 2007; Hawley and Burke 2010). This area of interest directly arises from some advances in our understanding of the molecular basis of training adaptation, and of how nutrient availability can modify the regulation of many contraction-induced events in skeletal muscle in response to exercise. Acutely manipulating substrate availability exerts great effects on muscle energy stores and patterns of fuel metabolism during exercise, as well as some processes activating gene expression and cell signaling (Burke et al. 2011). Accordingly, these manipulations, when repeated over weeks and months, have the potential to modulate numerous adaptive processes in muscle that ultimately drive the phenotype-specific characteristics observed in highly trained athletes. In this regard, "train low" has become a catchphrase in athletic circles as well as in the scientific literature to (incorrectly) describe a generic theme promoted as a replacement of the era of the high-CHO diet in sport.

However, there are many ways of achieving low CHO availability before, during, and after training sessions, which differ in the site targeted (i.e., intra- vs. extra-muscular), in the duration of exposure to reduced CHO availability, the number of tissues affected, as well as the frequency and timing of their incorporation into an athlete's training program. Although the optimal practical strategies to train low are not currently known, consuming additional caffeine, protein, and practicing CHO mouth rinsing before and/or during training may help to preserve the reduced training intensities that typically occur in the face of reduced CHO availability. Athletes should practice train-low workouts in conjunction with sessions undertaken with high-CHO availability so that their capacity to oxidize CHO is not blunted on race day.

THE IMPORTANCE OF MUSCLE CARBOHYDRATE ON PERFORMANCE

The amount of muscle CHO prior to exercise regulates many cellular events such as GLUT-4 translocation, rate of translation of post-exercise muscle IL-6 mRNA, and expression of enzymes related to CHO metabolism such as adenine mono phosphate kinase (AMPK), pyruvate dehydrogenase (PDH), and hexokinase. For example, low muscle CHO availability may enhance GLUT-4 translocation, AMPK, and glucolysis enzyme activity in order to restore glycogen stores more rapidly; inversely, CHO feeding during exercise can reduce post-exercise muscle IL-6 expression.

As muscle glycogen storage capacity is limited, it is advisable to maximize muscle glycogen stores before an event to ensure a better performance. Due to its importance, CHO must be provided during and after prolonged exercise as well (Castell et al. 2010). The mechanisms by which CHO may influence performance in prolonged exercise are blood glucose maintenance assuring high CHO oxidation, sparing muscle/liver glycogen stores, synthesizing glycogen in low-intensity exercise, and, finally, a central effect of CHO. It is a classic concept that endurance training affects skeletal muscle adaptations such as lower glycogen utilization and higher fat consumption compared to untrained individuals at the same exercise intensity. One of the various train-induced muscle adaptations responsible for that is an augment in muscle fiber I mitochondrial density (Hargreaves 2006). However, competitive athletes who push their limits to the top may experience very high demands of CHO oxidation in order to maintain their performance; thus, high CHO (50% to 70% daily caloric value) diets are usually consumed and prescribed for this population.

The first studies showing an ergogenic effect for CHO during exercise were performed in 1920 by Krogh and Lindhart (in Cox et al. 2010), who pointed out that subjects consuming high CHO diets classified the exercise as easy compared to subjects who consumed a high-fat diet. Since the 1960s, the link between CHOs and endurance sport has been extensively studied. To date, there is a strong body of evidence indicating the importance of CHO management on performance in long-lasting sport events, and some of this information will be discussed next.

CHO ingestion prior to exercise is crucial to performance, mainly to replenish muscle glycogen stores. A study was conducted with seven subjects who performed exercise (cycloergometer 50 W plus 20-W increment every 3 min) until exhaustion after muscle glycogen depletion in four different situations: below anaerobic threshold + 65% CHO pre-exercise meal, below anaerobic threshold + low CHO (10%) pre-exercise meal, above anaerobic threshold + 65% CHO pre-exercise meal, and above anaerobic threshold + low CHO (10%) pre-exercise meal. The outcomes were as follows: medium CHO pre-exercise meal significantly improved performance in intense exercise compared to a low-CHO regimen.

In 1985, Coyle and Coggan demonstrated that a CHO meal consumed 4 h before exercise elevated muscle glycogen concentration in 42% at the beginning of the practice. As CHO intake also has the capacity to enhance CHO oxidation (Pereira-Lancha et al. 2010) and reduce post-exercise free fatty acid release, athletes should be encouraged to maintain muscle glycogen stores in adequate levels prior to exercise or competition to ensure a better performance.

Elite triathlon athletes regularly involved in Olympic distance triathlons consumed 3 g CHO/kg BW before the competition (Cox et al. 2010), which seemed to have achieved the current recommendations. Hargreaves et al. (2004) indicated that a CHO meal containing 200 to 300 g CHO consumed 3 to 4 h before an exercise session was associated with an improvement in performance, whereas a CHO meal consumed 30 min prior to exercise could have adverse effects depending on the CHO glycemic index utilized. For example, eight cyclists who exercised moderately (65% VO_{2max}) until exhaustion were fed different glycemic index meals (1 g CHO/kg BW, 60 min before) and the results showed that when consuming low glycemic index food, performance was impaired but free fatty acids (FFA) release was enhanced during exercise, compared to a high glycemic index meal (Hargreaves et al. 2004; Stevenson et al. 2009).

Stevenson et al. were the ones who received the pre-test meal. A high glycemic index meal before exercise resulted in increased peak glucose levels and a low glycemic index meal resulted in increased fat oxidation (Stevenson et al. 2006).

Taken together, one could conclude that eating low glycemic foods before endurance exercise might be an interesting strategy for overweight or obese people exercising for health maintenance and fat loss, but not for athletes seeking superior performance.

CHO INTAKE DURING EXERCISE

In endurance activities, CHO intake also seems to be a determinant for performance. In these terms, nutritional supplements play an important role because they are designed to feature an optimum CHO transport rate, to be easily portable and nonperishable, and, finally, to have a reduced volume and weight. CHO bars and gels are very popular with endurance athletes and many studies have been conducted with these forms of CHO feeding during prolonged exercise. For more details, consult an excellent review by Cermak and Van Loon (2013).

One interesting strategy regarding performance and CHO ingestion during endurance exercise is mouth rinse with a 25 mL 6.4% maltodextrin solution by cyclists, taken each 12.5% of the distance completed, in which the athletes completed exercise in a significantly lower time compared to a control group. In this case, the cycling session lasted less than 1 h, and the authors attributed the improvement of performance by CHO mouth rinse to central mechanisms involving reward regions of the brain (Jeukendrup and Chambers 2010).

A few years ago, the hypothesis that a high daily CHO diet would blunt endurance training metabolic adaptations especially in untrained individuals gained strength in an article by Hansen et al. (2007). It was called "train high, compete low," and its rationale was amplifying training responses such as citrate synthase activation and fat oxidation, which increase in a low glycogen situation.

However, contradicting the former hypothesis, first in experimental models, it has been observed that trained rats who exercised in a high CHO availability condition had a higher increase in citrate synthase activity (Lancha et al. 1994) compared to a low CHO group. Nevertheless, in humans no differences in performance were noted in that specific situation (Cox et al. 2010).

Since CHO oxidation is augmented, and given the fact that muscle glucose transporters (GLUT-4) are activated with exercise, muscle glycogen reserves may not be sufficient to handle all CHOs needed during this activity; this makes CHO supplementation crucial to performance at the elite level (Pereira and Lancha 2004; Pereira-Lancha et al. 2010).

CHO INTAKE AFTER EXERCISE

To replenish glycogen stores after exercise, and to benefit from GLUT-4 activation, one must consume CHO after a workout. Athletes who consume CHOs in 10 g/kg BW/day after their practice, mostly using high glycemic index foods, had more rapid glycogen stores 24 h later when compared to low glycemic index food. Also, when a 4:1 CHO/protein ratio is achieved, muscle glycogen is restored more rapidly. This is due to a synergistic effect between CHO and protein: insulin released by CHO plus essential amino acids (EAAs) (e.g., leucine) act to restore glycogen stores and muscle protein synthesis.

PROTEINS AND AMINO ACIDS IN ENDURANCE EXERCISE

Endurance exercise is known for enhancing nitrogen release in urine and blood. Several studies show an increased protein turnover for active individuals. Endurance exercise recruits more oxidative muscle fibers than a resistance workout. Most of the published data shows an increased post-exercise fractional protein synthesis ranging from 22% to 85% in endurance sports sessions lasting more than 1 h (Poortmans et al. 2012).

Protein recommendations for active individuals or athletes range from 1.2 to 1.7 g/kg BW/day according to the American Dietetic Association (2009). It is remarkably increased when compared to sedentary individuals (dietary recommended intakes [DRIs] 0.8 g/kg BW/day or 8% to 12% of total calories). Endurance athletes maintain positive nitrogen balance when consuming approximately 1.2 to 1.6 g/BW.

Both quality and timing of protein ingestion seem to be important for muscle protein synthesis after exercise. Most studies focus on resistance training; however, they could be applied to endurance training regarding post-training muscle mass recuperation. Thus, there are a growing number of studies showing that a rapidly absorbed protein such as whey protein, administered after resistance training, is related to higher muscle protein synthesis. Whey protein seems to be more advantageous than others such as casein or soy protein due to a more rapid increase in muscle amino acid content. Twenty grams of whey protein, which contains approximately 8.6 g of EAAs, promotes a higher increase in protein synthesis not only in muscle but also in bone mass (Pasiakos 2012; Tang and Philips 2009).

Some authors relate this effect to the high amount of leucine featured in whey protein (Leenders and Van Loon 2011; Wall et al. 2013). Leucine has a special role in signal transduction and a potential role in inhibiting muscle proteolysis in humans, and the dose in which these effects are reported may be higher than those that promote maximal protein synthesis. Nevertheless, there are some fluctuations among the studies underlying this issue due to slightly different methodological approaches.

Branched chain amino acid (BCAA) supplementation has been studied for the last 20 years in endurance athletes, due to its potential role in delaying central fatigue. The three BCAAs are leucine, isoleucine, and valine, and they are metabolized primarily in muscle rather than in the liver, like most amino acids. BCAA and tryptophan are transported by the same transporter along the blood–brain barrier.

Thus, BCAA supplementation during prolonged exercise in theory could reduce free tryptophan availability to the blood–brain barrier, reducing serotonin production (a neurotransmitter responsible for fatigue), as will be discussed next. Although the connection between serotonin, chronic fatigue, and depression is well established in the clinical field, the correspondence to the sports arena does not seem to be valid. Many studies on BCAA supplementation in prolonged exercise failed to verify any improvement in performance of high-level athletes.

In a classic study by Blomstrand et al. (1991) where marathon runners were supplemented with 16 g BCAA, there was no improvement in running performance in faster athletes (<3 h 30 min) compared to slower athletes, although there was an improvement in cognition tests (Blomstrand et al. 1991). The same results were found when administering BCAA to glycogen-depleted cyclists in a crossover study; cognition tests showed improvement as well as fatigue perception, with no final performance improvements in the BCAA group, despite the prevention of BCAA/tryptophan alterations observed in the placebo group (Blomstrand et al. 1997). Taken together, these studies show that in trained individuals performing sub-maximal physical activity, the relation between BCAA and tryptophan on performance is not present, but the supplementation seems to reduce fatigue perception.

Although BCAAs seem not to improve performance in aerobic exercise, studies in experimental models show that BCAA supplementation in trained animals augments liver glycogen stores in resting state and in intense exercise. Leucine supplementation alone was shown to spare liver glycogen utilization in rats, improving resistance to fatigue (Campos-Ferraz et al. 2013). Furthermore, our group had already shown that BCAA supplementation in glycogen-depleted physically active humans ameliorated performance and enhanced fat oxidation (Gualano et al. 2011).

Taken together, these data demonstrate that BCAA supplementation may be useful for recreational athletes, not elite ones.

NEW RECOMMENDATIONS OF CHO INTAKE

CHOs during exercise are crucial for oxaloacetate generation, which can be utilized for acetyl-CoA oxidation, especially considering that glucose transport is taking place independently of insulin (Pereira and Lancha 2004). In this sense, if CHO is not available in adequate amounts in muscle tissue during vigorous exercise, glycogenic amino acid precursors are oxidized. The implications of these metabolic fates in the long term for performance are not clear.

To conclude, the importance of CHO fueling for optimal performance during top-level competitions is well established, and recent considerations about more specific recommendations are arising. The ultimate recommendations on CHO fueling are 30–60 g/CHO/h based on a maximal oxidation rate of CHO that did not consider the synergy between multiple CHO transporters. When multiple CHO transporters are considered (e.g., glucose and fructose), the maximal CHO rate during exercise can reach up to 105 g/h (Jeukendrup 2013).

REFERENCES

American Dietetic Association et al. 2009. Position of the American Dietetic Association, Dietitians of Canada, and the American College of Sports Medicine: Nutrition and athletic performance. *J Am Diet Assoc* 109:509–527.

Beis, L.Y., L. Willkomm, R. Ross et al. 2011. Food and macronutrient intake of elite Ethiopian distance runners. *J Int Soc Sports Nutr* 8:7. http://www.ncbi.nlm.nih.gov /pubmed/21595961.

Blomstrand, E., P. Hassmén, B. Ekblom, and E.A. Newsholme. 1991. Administration of branched-chain amino acids during sustained exercise—Effects on performance and on plasma concentration of some amino acids. *Eur J Appl Physiol Occup Physiol* 63(2):83–88. http://www.ncbi.nlm.nih.gov/pubmed/1748109.

Blomstrand, E., P. Hassmén, S. Ek, B. Ekblom, and E.A. Newsholme. 1997. Influence of ingesting a solution of branched-chain amino acids on perceived exertion during exercise. *Acta Physiol Scand* 159(1):41–49. http://www.ncbi.nlm.nih.gov/pubmed/9124069.

Burdon, C.A., N.A. Johnson, P.G. Chapman, A. Munir Che Muhamed, and H.T. O'Connor. 2013. Case study: Beverage temperature at aid stations in ironman triathlon. *Int J Sport Nutr Exerc Metab* 23(4):418–424. http://www.ncbi.nlm.nih.gov/pubmed/23295183.

Burke, L.M. 2007. New issues in training and nutrition: Train low, compete high? *Curr Sports Med Rep* 6(3):137–138.

Burke, L.M., J.A. Hawley, S.H. Wong, and A.E. Jeukendrup. 2011. Carbohydrates for training and competition. *J Sports Sci* 29(Suppl 1):S17–S27.

Campos-Ferraz, P.L., T. Bozza, H. Nicastro, and A.H. Lancha, Jr. 2013. Distinct effects of leucine or a mixture of the branched-chain amino acids (leucine, isoleucine, and valine) supplementation on resistance to fatigue, and muscle and liver-glycogen degradation, in trained rats. *Nutrition* 29(11–12):1388–1394. http://www.ncbi.nlm.nih.gov /pubmed/24103516.

Castell, L.M., L.M. Burke, S.J. Stear, and R.J. Maughan. 2010. BJSM reviews: A-Z of nutritional supplements: Dietary supplements, sports nutrition foods and ergogenic aids for health and performance part 8. *Br J Sports Med* 44(6):468–470. http://www.ncbi.nlm .nih.gov/pubmed/20495060.

Cermak, N.M., and L. Van Loon. 2013. The use of carbohydrates during exercise as an ergogenic aid. *Sports Med* 3(11):1139–1155.

Cox, G.R., R.J. Snow, and L.M. Burke. 2010. Race-day carbohydrate intakes of elite triathletes contesting olympic-distance triathlon events. *Int J Sport Nutr Exerc Metab* 20(4):299–306. http://www.ncbi.nlm.nih.gov/pubmed/20739718.

De Souza, M.J., R.J. Toombs, J.L. Scheid, E. O'Donnell, S.L. West, and N.I. Williams. 2010. High prevalence of subtle and severe menstrual disturbances in exercising women: Confirmation using daily hormone measures. *Hum Reprod* 25(2):491–503. http://www .ncbi.nlm.nih.gov/pubmed/19945961.

Deuster, P.A., S.B. Kyle, P.B. Moser, R.A. Vigersky, A. Singh, and E.B. Schoomaker. 1986. Nutritional survey of highly trained women runners. *Am J Clin Nutr* 44(6):954–962. http://www.ncbi.nlm.nih.gov/pubmed/3788842.

Dolan, S.H., M. Houston, and S.B. Martin. 2011. Survey results of the training, nutrition, and mental preparation of triathletes: Practical implications of findings. *J Sports Sci* 29(10):1019–1028. http://www.ncbi.nlm.nih.gov/pubmed/21623532.

García-Rovés, P.M., N. Terrados, S.F. Fernández, and A.M. Patterson. 1998. Macronutrients intake of top level cyclists during continuous competition—Change in the feeding pattern. *Int J Sports Med* 19(1):61–67. http://www.ncbi.nlm.nih.gov/pubmed/9506803.

García-Rovés, P.M., N. Terrados, S.F. Fernández, and A.M. Patterson. 2000. Comparison of dietary intake and eating behavior of professional road cyclists during training and competition. *Int J Sport Nutr Exerc Metab* 10(1):82–98. http://www.ncbi.nlm.nih.gov/pubmed/10939878.

Genton, L., K. Melzer, and C. Pichard. 2010. Energy and macronutrient requirements for physical fitness in exercising subjects. *Clin Nutr* 29(4):413–423.

Gualano, A.B., T. Bozza, P. Lopes De Campos et al. 2011. Branched-chain amino acids supplementation enhances exercise capacity and lipid oxidation during endurance exercise after muscle glycogen depletion. *J Sports Med Phys Fitness* 51(1):82–88.

Hansen, K.C., Z. Zhang, T. Gomez, A.K. Adams, and D.A. Schoeller. 2007. Exercise increases the proportion of fat utilization during short-term consumption of a high-fat diet. *Am J Clin Nutr* 85(1):109–116.

Hargreaves, M., J.A. Hawley, and A. Jeukendrup. 2004. Pre-exercise carbohydrate and fat ingestion: Effects on metabolism and performance. *J Sports Sci* 22(1):31–38. http://www.ncbi.nlm.nih.gov/pubmed/14971431.

Hawley, J.A., and L.M. Burke. 2010. Carbohydrate availability and training adaptation: Effects on cell metabolism. *Exerc Sport Sci Rev* 38(4):152–160.

Hopkins, M., A. Jeukendrup, N.A. King, and J.E. Blundell. 2011. The relationship between substrate metabolism, exercise and appetite control: Does glycogen availability influence the motivation to eat, energy intake or food choice? *Sports Med* 41(6):507–521. http://www.ncbi.nlm.nih.gov/pubmed/21615191.

Jeukendrup, A.E. 2011. Nutrition for endurance sports: Marathon, triathlon, and road cycling. *J Sports Sci* 29(Suppl 1):S91–S99. http://www.ncbi.nlm.nih.gov/pubmed/21916794.

Jeukendrup, A. 2013. The new carbohydrate intake recommendations. *Nestle Nutr Inst Workshop Ser* 75:63–71. http://www.ncbi.nlm.nih.gov/pubmed/23765351.

Jeukendrup, A.E., and E.S. Chambers. 2010. Oral carbohydrate sensing and exercise performance. *Curr Opin Clin Nutr Metab Care* 13(4):447–451. http://www.ncbi.nlm.nih.gov/pubmed/20453646.

Knechtle, B., A. Enggist, and T. Jehle. 2005. Energy turnover at the Race Across America (RAAM)—A case report. *Int J Sports Med* 26(6):499–503. http://www.ncbi.nlm.nih.gov/pubmed/16037895.

Lancha, A.H., M.B. Recco, and R. Curi. 1994. Pyruvate carboxylase activity in the heart and skeletal muscles of the rat. Evidence for a stimulating effect of exercise. *Biochem Mol Biol Int* 32(3):483–489. http://www.ncbi.nlm.nih.gov/pubmed/8032315.

Leenders, M., and L.J. Van Loon. 2011. Leucine as a pharmaconutrient to prevent and treat sarcopenia and type 2 diabetes. *Nutr Rev* 69(11):675–689.

Loucks, A.B. 2003. Energy availability, not body fatness, regulates reproductive function in women. *Exerc Sport Sci Rev* 31(3):144–148. http://www.ncbi.nlm.nih.gov/pubmed/12882481.

Melzer, K. 2011. Carbohydrate and fat utilization during rest and physical activity. *E Spen Eur E J Clin Nutr Metab* 6(2):e45–e52.

Melzer, K., L. Genton, and C. Pichard. 2013. Regulation of energy balance: Adjusting dietary intake to energy expenditure. *Nutr Clin Metabol* 27(3):134–138.

Nattiv, A., R. Agostini, B. Drinkwater, and K.K. Yeager. 1994. The female athlete triad. The inter-relatedness of disordered eating, amenorrhea, and osteoporosis. *Clin Sports Med* 13(2):405–418. http://www.ncbi.nlm.nih.gov/pubmed/8013041.

Nattiv, A., A.B. Loucks, M.M. Manore et al. 2007. American College of Sports Medicine position stand. The female athlete triad. *Med Sci Sports Exerc* 39(10):1867–1882. http://www.ncbi.nlm.nih.gov/pubmed/17909417.

Onywera, V.O., F.K. Kiplamai, M.K. Boit, and Y.P. Pitsiladis. 2004. Food and macronutrient intake of elite Kenyan distance runners. *Int J Sport Nutr Exerc Metab* 14(6):709–719. http://www.ncbi.nlm.nih.gov/pubmed/15657475.

Pasiakos, S.M. 2012. Exercise and amino acid anabolic cell signaling and the regulation of skeletal muscle mass. *Nutrients* 4(7):740–758.

Pereira, L.O., and A.H. Lancha. 2004. Effect of insulin and contraction up on glucose transport in skeletal muscle. *Prog Biophys Mol Biol* 84(1):1–27. http://www.ncbi.nlm.nih.gov/pubmed/14642866.

Pereira-Lancha, L.O., D.F. Coelho, P.L. de Campos-Ferraz, and A.H. Lancha, Jr. 2010. Body fat regulation: Is it a result of a simple energy balance or a high fat intake? *J Am Coll Nutr* 29(4):343–351. http://www.ncbi.nlm.nih.gov/pubmed/21041808.

Poortmans, J.R., A. Carpentier, L.O. Pereira-Lancha, and A. Lancha, Jr. 2012. Protein turnover, amino acid requirements and recommendations for athletes and active populations. *Braz J Med Biol Res* 45(10):875–890. http://www.ncbi.nlm.nih.gov/pubmed/22666780.

Saris, W.H., M.A. van Erp-Baart, F. Brouns, K.R. Westerterp, and F. ten Hoor. 1989. Study on food intake and energy expenditure during extreme sustained exercise: The Tour de France. *Int J Sports Med* 10(Suppl 1):S26–S31. http://www.ncbi.nlm.nih.gov/pubmed/2744926.

Scheid, J.L., and M.J. De Souza. 2010. Menstrual irregularities and energy deficiency in physically active women: The role of ghrelin, PYY and adipocytokines. *Med Sport Sci* 55:82–102. http://www.ncbi.nlm.nih.gov/pubmed/20956862.

Stevenson, E.J., C. Williams, L.E. Mash, B. Phillips, and M.L. Nute. 2006. Influence of high-carbohydrate mixed meals with different glycemic indexes on substrate utilization during subsequent exercise in women. *Am J Clin Nutr* 84(2):354–360. http://www.ncbi.nlm.nih.gov/pubmed/16895883.

Stevenson, E.J., P.E. Thelwall, K. Thomas, F. Smith, J. Brand-Miller, and M.I. Trenell. 2009. Dietary glycemic index influences lipid oxidation but not muscle or liver glycogen oxidation during exercise. *Am J Physiol Endocrinol Metab* 296(5):E1140–E1147. http://www.ncbi.nlm.nih.gov/pubmed/19223653.

Tang, J.E., and S.M. Philips. 2009. Maximizing muscle protein anabolism: The role of protein quality. *Curr Opin Clin Nutr Metab Care* 12(1):66–71.

Torstveit, M.K., and J. Sundgot-Borgen. 2005. Participation in leanness sports but not training volume is associated with menstrual dysfunction: A national survey of 1276 elite athletes and controls. *Br J Sports Med* 39(3):141–147. http://www.ncbi.nlm.nih.gov/pubmed/15728691.

Trabulsi, J., and D.A. Schoeller. 2001. Evaluation of dietary assessment instruments against doubly labeled water, a biomarker of habitual energy intake. *Am J Physiol Endocrinol Metab* 281(5):E891–E899. http://www.ncbi.nlm.nih.gov/pubmed/11595643.

Wall, B.T., H.M. Hamer, A. de Lange et al. 2013. Leucine co-ingestion improves post-prandial muscle protein accretion in elderly men. *Clin Nut* 32(3):412–419.

3 Dietary Supplements for Endurance Athletes

Melvin H. Williams, PhD, FACSM
Department of Human Movement Sciences,
Old Dominion University, Norfolk, Virginia

CONTENTS

INTRODUCTION

Endurance in sport may be defined in several ways. For example, anaerobic power endurance may be important for a 400-m dash and intermittent high-intensity endurance may be critical in team sports, such as football (soccer). Other chapters in this book, such as Chapters 5 and 6, provide proper nutritional strategies, including use of dietary supplements, for such athletic endeavors. This chapter will focus on aerobic endurance, or the ability to exercise continuously at submaximal intensity for prolonged periods of time. This definition includes such sports as race walking, cross-country running and skiing, road race cycling, distance swimming, triathlons, and similar sport endeavors. The energy demands of aerobic endurance exercise are presented in Chapter 1 and nutritional recommendations are presented in Chapter 2. This chapter will focus on dietary supplements.

Numerous dietary supplements are used by athletes for various reasons. The focus of this chapter is dietary supplements for performance enhancement and space limitations preclude an extensive discussion of each supplement. Since 2009, prominent exercise scientists in sport nutrition have written a series of articles, published in *The British Journal of Sports Medicine*, detailing the effects of numerous dietary supplements, sports nutrition foods, and ergogenic aids for health and performance. The title of each article is "A to Z of nutritional supplements: Dietary supplements, sports nutrition foods, and ergogenic aids for health and performance." These articles cover almost all supplements used by endurance athletes and may be of interest to the reader.

Success in aerobic endurance sports at the elite level of competition is dependent primarily on genetic endowment with physiological, psychological, and morphological traits specific to endurance performance. Respectively, these traits have been referred to as physical power, mental strength, and mechanical advantage. In addition to genetic endowment, elite athletes must also receive optimal sport-specific training to maximize those traits specific to their endurance sport. In endurance athletes, proper training will increase the ability of the muscles to use oxygen (physical power), prevent neural fatigue (mental strength), and maintain an optimal body weight (mechanical advantage).

In addition to genetic endowment and proper training, an appropriate diet, both in training and competition, is one of the key elements underlying success in endurance sports. Appropriate dietary strategies for endurance athletes relative to training, recovery, and competition are, as noted, presented in Chapter 2, while sound dietary practices for weight control are documented in Chapter 7.

However, elite athletes often attempt to go beyond appropriate training and nutritional recommendations and use numerous dietary supplements in attempts to maximize training, facilitate exercise recovery, promote health, and enhance performance. The use of dietary supplements is common among elite athletes. For example, two recent surveys revealed dietary supplement use by 87% of elite Canadian (Lun et al. 2012) and 73% of elite Finnish (Heikkinen et al. 2011) athletes. Dietary supplements are even popular with young athletes, being used by more than 63% of Japanese athletes participating in the 2010 Singapore Youth Olympic Games (Sato et al. 2012).

Elite endurance athletes may use dietary supplements for several reasons, including performance enhancement. When used for such purposes, they are often referred to as sports supplements. In their joint position stand on nutrition and athletic performance, the American Dietetic Association, Dietitians of Canada, and the American College of Sports Medicine (Rodriguez et al. 2009) highlighted the use of sports supplements relative to their efficacy, safety, and permissibility. In this regard, four categories of sports supplements were listed.

- Those not safe or permissible.
- Those not effective; research findings are negative.

- Those which may be effective; research findings are equivocal.
- Those considered to be effective; research findings are positive.

The use of dietary supplements by athletes may be recommended for various reasons. For example, malnourished athletes, such as endurance athletes with iron-deficiency anemia, may experience impaired oxygen metabolism, decreased aerobic capacity, and impaired aerobic endurance performance. In such athletes, iron supplementation may correct the deficiency and restore endurance performance to normal levels. Vitamin D and calcium supplements may be recommended for female athletes who may suffer some of the consequences, such as premature osteoporosis, of the Female Athlete Triad. However, the discussion in this chapter focuses on the effects of sport supplements in well-nourished athletes.

Relative to research procedures regarding the efficacy of performance-enhancing agents in sport, Burke (2008) has recommended studies using well-trained subjects and exercise tests that reflect actual practices in sport. However, Burke notes that there is a scarcity of studies involving elite performers and field-based studies. In recent years, there has been increased study of well-trained athletes in specific sport-related exercise tasks undertaken under controlled laboratory conditions. Whether the findings of these laboratory studies may be extrapolated to elite athletes in actual sport competition is questionable. However, if we can make a comparison to the use of other performance-enhancing substances in sport, such as the drug recombinant erythropoietin (rEPO), research findings in the laboratory (Ekblom and Berglund 1991), when compared to the recent United States Anti-Doping Agency (USADA) case against a multiple-year winner of the Tour de France who allegedly used rEPO (United States Anti-Doping Agency 2012), reflect a positive relationship between laboratory research and actual sport competition among elite endurance athletes.

SPORTS SUPPLEMENTS THAT ARE NOT SAFE OR PERMISSIBLE

The vast majority of commercial sports supplements, such as vitamins and minerals, are safe and permissible when used properly. However, as noted in Chapter 8, there may be safety issues with some supplements, particularly when consumed in excess. Moreover, use of some supplements may be prohibited by World Anti-Doping Agency (WADA) for various reasons.

For example, glycerol-containing supplements have been marketed to both endurance and strength athletes, and glycerol has been a component of some sport drinks. van Rosendal and others (2010) noted glycerol ingestion before, during, or following exercise is likely to improve the hydration state of the endurance athlete. The process involves consumption of approximately 1 g of glycerol with 20 to 25 mL of water per kilogram of body weight over the course of 1 h. Glycerol hyperhydration is designed to increase total body water and plasma volume, which could help prevent dehydration, improve temperature regulation while exercising in the heat, and enhance endurance performance. In a meta-analysis, Goulet and others (2007) reported that glycerol-induced hyperhydration was associated with a 2.6% improvement in endurance performance, mainly cycling. However, they also noted the dearth of data precluded more definitive conclusions regarding its ergogenic effects. Anecdotally, several elite U.S. marathon runners used glycerol in some of their best marathons run in the heat (Burfoot 2003).

However, glycerol administration may be considered a plasma expander designed to mask drug use and thus its use is prohibited by WADA. Moreover, excessive intake could cause nausea, vomiting, and headaches, and could contribute to development of hyponatremia.

Use of certain other supplements by athletes is prohibited by various sport-governing associations. Ephedrine, a stimulant found in some herbal supplements, has been alleged to enhance aerobic endurance performance, and is prohibited in competition by WADA. Various anabolic compounds designed to facilitate recovery in endurance athletes, such as androstenedione, androstenediole, and dehydroepiandrosterone (DHEA), are marketed as sports supplements and their use is also prohibited. Moreover, some supplements may contain banned substances as the result of accidental or intentional contamination during the manufacturing process. In one report, 25% of 58 sport supplements tested contained prohibited steroids or stimulants (Epstein and Dohrmann 2009). *Caveat emptor*, or "Let the buyer beware," is good advice for athletes considering the use of sports supplements, especially those purchased on the Internet.

Such sports supplements may be effective. For example, herbal pseudoephedrine may be found in some dietary supplements, such as Ma Huang, as well as over-the-counter nasal decongestants. Although research with pseudoephedrine supplementation is limited, several well-designed studies have demonstrated a performance-enhancing effect on endurance performance. When consumed 90 min prior to a 1500-m run, Hodges and others (2006) reported that pseudoephedrine (2.5 mg/kg body weight) improved performance by 2.1%, or about 6 sec. Pritchard-Peschek and others (2010) also reported that ingestion of 180 mg of pseudoephedrine 60 min prior to a cycling time trial improved performance by 5.1%. Both studies suggested the improved performance might have been associated with central nervous system stimulation and a beneficial psychological effect. However, one recent study reported no ergogenic effect of a 2.5-mg/kg dose of pseudoephedrine on 800-m track performance in female National Collegiate Athletic Association (NCAA) runners (Berry and Wagner 2012).

Use of pseudoephedrine was permitted at one time, but WADA reintroduced pseudoephedrine to its prohibited list in 2010, but only in competition. Similar supplements, including ephedrine, are prohibited by WADA, but only in competition. Athletes may use such supplements in attempts to enhance training, which could possibly lead to improved performance in competition.

Such sports supplements may also have serious health consequences. For example, in their text, Williams and others (2013) cited one report in which ephedra products accounted for 64% of all adverse reactions to herbs in the United States even though these products represented less than 1% of herbal product sales. They noted ephedra use has been associated with numerous health problems, including psychosis, severe depression, sleep disturbance, suicidal ideation, heart arrhythmias, and myocardial infarction. Ephedra use has also been associated with the deaths of several prominent professional athletes. In such cases, these health problems may have been associated with doses greater than those recommended.

SPORTS SUPPLEMENTS THAT ARE NOT EFFECTIVE

The vast majority of supplements marketed to endurance athletes have not been shown to enhance performance (Williams et al. 2013). Numerous supplements have been studied for their performance-enhancement potential, including substances associated with the three macronutrients (carbohydrate, fat, and protein), the micronutrients (vitamins and minerals), and various herbals, extracts, and constituents from natural foods. The following discussion lists those supplements that have not been determined to enhance aerobic endurance performance. Given space limitations, only one such supplement will be highlighted for discussion.

CARBOHYDRATE-RELATED SUPPLEMENTS

Carbohydrate stores in the body, as noted in Chapter 2, serve as the major energy source during aerobic endurance exercise and some dietary strategies may be recommended to enhance endurance performance. Moreover, as noted later, sports drinks with carbohydrate may enhance endurance performance under some conditions. However, numerous other carbohydrate metabolites have been studied for their performance-enhancing potential and the following have not been shown to be effective:

- Ribose
- Pyruvate
- DHAP (pyruvate and dihydroxyacetone)
- Lactate salts
- Multiple carbohydrate by-products

Ribose is a 5-carbon monosaccharide that comprises the sugar portion of adenosine found in adenosine triphosphate (ATP), the primary source of energy for muscle contraction. Most studies evaluated the effect of ribose supplementation on anaerobic exercise performance, but several studies evaluated its effect on endurance performance. In their text, Williams and others (2013) noted that 8 weeks of ribose supplementation had no ergogenic effect on 2000-m rowing performance, and concluded current data do not support an ergogenic effect of ribose supplementation.

FAT-RELATED SUPPLEMENTS

Fat may also serve as an energy source during exercise, but the body has sufficient stores to accommodate energy needs for most endurance events. Jeukendrup and Randell (2011) noted that the list of supplements that are claimed to increase or improve fat metabolism is long. However, they note that evidence is lacking relative to the efficacy of most products. The following fat-related metabolites or putative enhancers of fat metabolism have not been shown to enhance endurance performance:

- Medium-chain triglycerides (MCTs)
- Omega-3 fatty acids

- Conjugated linoleic acid
- Hydroxycitrate (HCA)
- Carnitine
- Phosphatidylserine

Williams and others (2013) note that MCTs have been suggested to be ergogenic because they are water soluble, they may be absorbed directly through the portal circulation and delivered directly to the liver, bypassing the chylomicron route in the lymph, and they may more readily enter the mitochondria in the muscle cells because they do not need carnitine. However, most studies have not shown any beneficial effects of MCT supplementation on endurance exercise performance, including the following exercise protocols in well-trained endurance cyclists and runners.

- 40-km cycling time trial after 2 h of submaximal cycling
- 100-km cycling time trial
- Treadmill run to exhaustion at 75% of VO_{2max}

PROTEIN-RELATED SUPPLEMENTS

Protein, although an important nutrient for endurance athletes, is not a major energy source during performance. Protein intake, either as a whole food such as milk or a supplement such as whey, may be an important consideration for recovery immediately following strenuous endurance exercise, but supplementation with the following numerous amino acids and protein-related metabolites has not been shown to enhance endurance performance (Williams 2005a):

- L-arginine
- L-citrulline
- Glutamine
- Branched chain amino acids (BCAA)
- Leucine, isoleucine, valine
- All other amino acids
- HMB (Beta-hydroxy-beta-methylbutyrate)

As noted later, nitrate supplementation has been theorized to enhance endurance performance by increasing nitric oxide (NO). Arginine supplementation has also been studied as a means to increase NO and enhance exercise performance. In a recent review of nitrate supplementation, Williams (2012) noted most dietary supplements marketed as a means to promote NO production contain L-arginine. In his review, Williams noted most studies report no ergogenic effect of L-arginine supplementation on various tests of aerobic endurance, and indicated that some research even suggests that L-arginine supplementation may impair endurance exercise performance. Williams further noted that underlying this lack of an ergogenic effect might be that while L-arginine supplementation may increase plasma levels of L-arginine, supplementation has rather consistently been shown to not increase NO or blood flow to the exercising muscle.

VITAMINS AND VITAMIN-LIKE SUBSTANCES

Vitamins and vitamin-like substances may play important roles in energy metabolism and other metabolic processes, but supplementation with the following has not been shown to improve performance (Williams 2004):

- Water-soluble vitamins
  - Thiamin (B_1)
  - Riboflavin (B_2)
  - Niacin
  - B_6 (pyridoxine)
  - B_{12} (cobalamin)
  - Folate
  - Pantothenic acid
  - Biotin
  - C (ascorbic acid)
  - B-vitamin complex
- Fat-soluble vitamins
  - A (retinol)
  - D (cholecalciferol)
  - E (tocopherol)
  - K (phylloquinone)
- Multivitamins
- Multivitamin/multimineral preparations
- Antioxidant vitamins
- Vitamin-like substances
  - Choline
  - Bee pollen
  - Coenzyme Q10
  - Quercetin
  - Carnitine

Vitamin B_{12} supplementation has been touted as a means to enhance endurance performance mainly because it plays an important role in the development of red blood cells (RBCs). Theoretically, an increase in RBC would improve oxygen delivery to the muscles during exercise. Vitamin B_{12} is not found in plant foods, and its absorption in the intestines is decreased in older individuals. Thus, an older, vegan athlete who does not consume vitamin-enriched foods could suffer a deficiency and benefit from supplementation. However, Williams and others (2013) noted that several well-controlled studies reached the general conclusion that vitamin B_{12} supplementation to well-nourished individuals does not help to increase metabolic function, such as VO_{2max}, or endurance performance.

MINERALS

Williams (2005b) notes that a mineral deficiency may impair performance. In particular, correcting an iron-deficiency anemia will improve aerobic endurance performance. Additionally, inadequate calcium intake may lead to premature osteo-porosis, particularly in female endurance athletes who may benefit from weight loss. However, with the possible exception of supplementation with phosphate salts and sodium, discussed next, Williams (2005b) indicates there is little evi-dence that supplementation with the following will enhance endurance perfor-mance in well-nourished athletes:

- Macrominerals
  - Calcium
  - Magnesium
  - Chloride
  - Potassium
- Trace minerals
  - Iron
  - Zinc
  - Copper
  - Chromium
  - Selenium
  - Manganese
  - Fluoride
  - Molybdenum
  - Iodine

In their text, Williams and others (2013) note that magnesium is involved in a number of physiological processes, some of which may be important for optimal oxygen metabolism. However, they cite a review and meta-analysis indicating that magnesium supplementation to physically active individuals with adequate magne-sium status does not enhance performance, including aerobic endurance.

HERBALS, EXTRACTS, CONSTITUENTS, AND RELATED SUPPLEMENTS

In his review, Williams (2006) noted numerous herbal supplements are marketed as ergogenic aids for athletes. Although ginseng has received some considerable research attention, there is a dearth of well-controlled research evaluating the efficacy of purported herbal ergogenics on human exercise or sport performance, including the following:

- Ginseng
  - Panax
  - Siberian
  - American
  - Ciwujia
- Capsicum
- Cordyseps sinensis
- Cytoseira canariensis
- Epigallocatechin-3-gallate (EGCG)

- Gamma oryzanol
- Ginkgo biloba
- Kava kava
- St. Johns wort
- Tribulus terrestris
- Yohimbine

Most of the research on herbals has focused on ginseng in its various forms. Although early research suggested ginseng could enhance endurance performance, the studies were poorly designed. For example, some studies did not have a control group. More recent research has employed sophisticated research designs, but in their meticulous review of research with the various forms of ginseng, Bahrke and others (2009) noted that despite attempts in recent investigations to improve on the scientific rigor used in examining the ergogenic properties of ginseng, many of the same methodological shortcomings observed in earlier studies persist, and enhanced physical performance after ginseng administration in well-designed investigations remains to be demonstrated. Most studies have found no ergogenic effect associated with the various forms of ginseng (Williams et al. 2013).

Other than essential nutrients, such as vitamins and minerals, foods contain numerous phytonutrients, also referred to as phytochemicals, that may influence physiological processes in the body. Many of these phytonutrients have been studied for their potential beneficial effects on health, and some have been theorized to have positive effects on physical and sport performance. As noted next, caffeine can be considered an effective sport supplement. Caffeine may be found in tea, but other substances present in green tea have been theorized to be ergogenic. In his review, Williams (2011) notes that green tea is rich in catechins and the most abundant green tea catechin (GTC) is epigallocatechin-3-gallate, or EGCG. One of the main hypothesized mechanisms of EGCG supplementation to enhance exercise performance is an increase in sympathetic nervous system activity, which could increase oxidation of fat during exercise. Most of the available research regarding the potential ergogenic effect of catechins during exercise, both in mice and humans, has focused on the increased oxidation of fat as an energy source during aerobic endurance tasks. Williams notes that research relative to the ergogenic effects of EGCG is somewhat limited, and that what is available may be confounded by supplementation protocols. In general, studies with mice, especially older mice, showed an increase in fat oxidation and improved endurance performance. Some studies with humans also provided evidence of increased fat oxidation following EGCG supplementation. However, in several studies evaluating the effects of EGCG supplementation on endurance exercise performance, including one study with well-trained athletes, no beneficial effect on cycling performance was reported. Based on current evidence, it is possible that EGCG can increase fat oxidation during exercise, but does not enhance performance.

SPORTS SUPPLEMENTS THAT MAY BE EFFECTIVE

Several sports supplements have been theorized to enhance endurance performance. However, the available research is somewhat inconsistent or limited, and thus sport scientists are generally undecided as to whether such supplements are effective. Thus, these supplements *may be* effective.

PHOSPHATE SALTS

As a component of various chemical compounds in the body, phosphates have multiple functions in human metabolism. One such compound is 2,3 biphosphoglycerate (2,3 BPG), which facilitates the release of oxygen from hemoglobin to the muscles. In their text, Williams and others (2013) highlight the results of four well-designed studies with highly trained endurance athletes conducted from 1984 to 1992. The supplementation protocols provided 3600 to 4000 mg of sodium phosphate daily for 3 to 5 days. In general, the investigators reported the following:

- Increased red blood cell 2,3 BPG
- Increased VO_{2max} 6 to 10%
- Increased treadmill run time to exhaustion
- Improved 40-k cycle ergometer time trial performance

However, other studies did not show an ergogenic effect associated with phosphate loading. A 1994 review noted a number of confounding variables in previous research and recommended more controlled research (Tremblay et al. 1994). However, equivocality continues. Two more recent studies involving 6 days of sodium phosphate loading to trained endurance athletes revealed diverse findings. Brewer and others (2012) concluded supplementation could have an additive effect on VO_{2peak} and possibly time trial performance, whereas West and others (2012) reported no effect on VO_{2peak}.

One difference among studies that Tremblay and others (1994) noted was the type of supplement being used, either calcium phosphate or sodium phosphate. Sodium phosphate was the supplement used in the four positive studies cited previously, and the sodium content may be an important consideration as per the following discussion.

SODIUM

Sodium, a mineral element, is important for many physiological functions in humans. In their text, Williams and others (2013) note one of those functions is to help maintain normal blood volume and blood pressure. The ingestion of a saline solution prior to exercise, known as sodium loading, has been theorized to expand the plasma volume and lead to cardiovascular responses that could benefit exercise performance. Williams and others cite several studies in which sodium loading, consumption of approximately 0.75 L of a high-sodium (164 mmol/L) solution, could elicit the following effects during endurance exercise under warm environmental conditions:

- Increased plasma volume
- Reduced thermoregulatory strain
- Reduced rating of perceive exertion (RPE) during exercise
- Greater run time to exhaustion on a treadmill
- Increased cycling time to exhaustion in warm conditions

However, Williams and others (2013) also cited evidence that consuming sodium tablets during exercise does not appear to enhance performance in Ironman-distance triathlon competition.

These results are interesting, but the number of studies is limited and additional research is needed to confirm a performance-enhancing effect of sodium loading.

SODIUM BICARBONATE

Sodium bicarbonate is an alkaline salt found naturally in humans. In the blood, it is a major component of the alkaline reserve that may help maintain an optimal pH by buffering various acids. Sodium bicarbonate is available as baking soda, a product not only used for baking, but also other household uses and personal care. Sodium bicarbonate may also be considered a dietary supplement and has been marketed on various Internet sites as a sports supplement. Its use in sports has been referred to as *soda loading* or *buffer boosting*.

One of the metabolic byproducts of prolonged intense anaerobic exercise, such as a 400-m track event, is lactic acid, the accumulation of which has been associated with fatigue. Sodium bicarbonate has been theorized to help buffer lactic acid and prevent premature fatigue in such exercise tasks, and has been studied for its performance-enhancing effect since the 1930s. In a recent meta-analysis of the effects of acute alkalosis and acidosis on exercise performance, Carr and others (2011a) noted that although individual responses may vary, their findings suggest the ingestion of 0.3 to 0.5 g of sodium bicarbonate per kilogram of body mass could improve mean power by 1.7% in high-intensity races of short duration, such as the 400-m dash, an event associated with anaerobic endurance.

Sodium bicarbonate supplementation has also been studied for its effects on aerobic endurance performance, but Williams and others (2013) noted the findings are equivocal relative to exercise tasks 4 min or longer. Studies reported enhanced performance in the following exercise tasks that, although primarily aerobic in nature, may have a significant anaerobic energy contribution at some point, such as a sprint near the finish.

- Cycle ergometer work output in a 4-min trial
- 1500-m track run
- 3000-m track run
- 5-k treadmill run
- 30-k cycling trial
- Maximal cycle ergometer work over 60 min

Conversely, a number of other studies reported no significant effect of sodium bicarbonate supplementation on other aerobic endurance tests, such as the following:

- Run to exhaustion at 110% of the anaerobic threshold following 30 min of running at the lactate threshold
- 1500-m track run
- 30-min cycling time trial

In their review, Spriet and others (2008) noted that although the use of sodium bicarbonate as a sports supplement is legal, the incidence of negative side effects is high. Nausea, gastrointestinal distress, and diarrhea may be common problems.

β-Alanine

Beta-alanine (β-alanine) is a naturally occurring amino acid that can be taken up by muscle cells and combined with histidine to form carnosine. One function of carnosine is to help buffer lactic acid, which, similar to sodium bicarbonate, may be theorized to help prevent premature fatigue in intense, anaerobic exercise lasting several minutes.

Hobson and others (2012), in a meta-analysis of 15 studies, indicated that in line with the purported mechanisms for an ergogenic effect of β-alanine supplementation (median dose, 179 g), exercise lasting 1 to 4 min was improved when compared to placebo. However, exercise lasting 3 to 4 min could also have a significant aerobic component. Moreover, these investigators also noted that β-alanine supplementation improved performance in exercise tasks lasting more than 4 min, although the significance of the data was not as strong as for the shorter time frame. The median effect of β-alanine supplementation was a 2.85% improvement in the outcome of an exercise measure, when a median total of 179 g of β-alanine is supplemented. However, in their review, Hoffman and others (2012) noted that the benefits of β-alanine ingestion and endurance exercise performance appear to be inconclusive.

Excessive intake, more than 800 mg in a single dose, may increase risk of parathesia, or the sensation of numbness or tingling on the skin.

Nitrates

Nitrates are natural inorganic components of plant foods, mostly in vegetables. Excellent sources include celery, Chinese cabbage, spinach, lettuce, kohlrabi, leek, and red beetroot. Most studies evaluating the performance-enhancing effects of nitrate supplementation have used beetroot juice as the source. Beetroot is the term used in England for the vegetable known in the United States as the red beet. Doses used in studies approximate 300 to 500 mg of nitrate, an amount found in about 500 mL of beetroot juice. Supplementation protocols were either acute, about 2.5 h prior to exercise, or more prolonged such as daily doses for 5 to 6 days.

In recent reviews, Williams (2012, 2013) summarized the hypothesized ergogenic effect of nitrate supplementation. In brief, after ingestion, dietary nitrate is processed in the gastrointestinal tract, enters the circulation, and is eventually processed in the salivary glands to nitrite, which eventually enters the systemic circulation. The nitrite then may be further reduced in the blood vessels, heart, skeletal, and other tissues to form bioactive nitric acid (NO). Williams (2012) notes that NO may affect various physiological functions important to exercise performance. In particular, NO is a potent vasodilator and may regulate several skeletal muscle functions, such as force production, blood flow, mitochondrial respiration, and glucose homeostasis.

In his review, Williams (2012) notes that NO is also produced naturally in the body during exercise, and may be a major factor supporting physiological processes in the body that lead to improvement in exercise performance with proper training. Although a vigorous exercise training program may be a very effective means to increase NO production and enhance sport performance, surveys indicate that NO supplements are increasingly popular among athletes and may be considered sports supplements.

Various substances have been used to increase production of NO in humans, including drugs such as nitroglycerin and amyl nitrate and inorganic nitrate and nitrite salts. However, their use is not recommended. Dietary supplements, particularly food sources of nitrates, have also been studied as a means to increase NO and enhance exercise performance, and such protocols constitute the majority of current research studies.

Various study protocols have been used to evaluate the ergogenic effect of nitrate supplementation, including various placebos such as nitrate-depleted beetroot juice; various time frames of supplementation, including acute (several hours) and chronic (several days) before testing; various dosages; multiple dependent variables; varying levels of exercise intensity; and specific exercise tasks. Most aerobic endurance exercise tests involved cycling or treadmill running; although the two exercise tasks are different, one could assume that enhanced performance in one would be applicable to the other. The following represent some of the key findings in an overall review of these studies:

- Increase of plasma nitrite concentration. Plasma nitrite is a marker for NO, so this finding suggests NO is increased with nitrate supplementation.
- Reduced oxygen cost of exercise. This is one of the most consistent findings. Six studies reported reduced oxygen consumption for a given exercise task, suggesting an improvement in oxygen efficiency.
- Increased exercise time to exhaustion. Subjects involved in both cycling and treadmill running improved exercise time to exhaustion.
- Improved performance in sport-specific tests. Several studies used sport-specific time trials, mainly cycling, and nitrate supplementation enhanced performance in such trials.
- Improved performance by well-trained athletes. Many studies used physically untrained subjects, but several used trained cyclists in a sport-specific protocol and reported improved performance following beetroot supplementation.

Collectively, these data suggest dietary nitrate supplementation may be an effective sport supplement and, in general, are supported in a recent review by Jones and others (2013).

However, not all data are supportive. Peacock and others (2012) reported nitrate supplementation had no effect on performance in a 5-k running time trial in 10 highly trained male endurance athletes—cross-country skiers. The study was conducted in the off-season when the skiers were running as a major component of their training program. The time trial was performed indoors and the 5-k performance times approximated 16:40. However, this study evaluated the effect of a single acute dose of potassium nitrate (614 mg nitrate) 2.5 h prior to the time trial. Christensen and others (2013) studied the effect of beetroot juice supplementation on the endurance and repeated sprint capacity in 10 elite endurance cyclists. Although the beetroot juice increased plasma nitrate and nitrite levels compared with placebo, the time trial performances were similar, as were average power outputs. They concluded that intake of beetroot juice had no effect on performance in elite cyclists.

SPORTS SUPPLEMENTS CONSIDERED EFFECTIVE

Carbohydrate, as blood glucose and glycogen stored in the muscle and liver, is the main energy source for aerobic endurance athletes. Research has shown that carbohydrate supplementation may enhance prolonged aerobic endurance performance. For example, in their review, Coombes and Hamilton (2000) concluded the commercially available sports drinks, whose main ingredients are water and carbohydrate, are one of the few nutritional food products that may enhance sport performance in exercise tasks where performance may be impaired by dehydration and depleted endogenous carbohydrate reserves.

As noted previously, several other sports supplements may enhance aerobic endurance performance, and possibly some, such as glycerol, nitrates, and sodium bicarbonate, might fit into this category and be considered effective. However, only one sport supplement appears to fit this category, and that supplement is caffeine. In their review of nutrition for distance events, Burke and others (2007) noted while caffeine is an ergogenic aid of possible value to distance athletes, most other supplements are of minimal benefit.

CAFFEINE

Caffeine, an alkaloid that appears naturally in many plants, may be classified as a drug, a stimulant found in several over-the-counter products; as a food ingredient, found naturally in coffee and tea; and as a dietary supplement, often marketed as guarana and kola nut, other natural sources of caffeine. Some sports supplements referred to as performance candy, such as Buzz Bites, contain caffeine.

Caffeine has been studied for its performance-enhancing effects since the late 1890s and has been popular with athletes for nearly a century. In 1939, Boje recommended that pure caffeine preparations be banned in athletic competition and the International Olympic Committee eventually banned its use in 1972. However, because caffeine is so common in many beverages consumed by athletes, it was removed from the prohibited list by WADA in 2004. However, it remains on the WADA monitoring list.

Caffeine may exert a positive ergogenic effect on a variety of exercise performance tasks. However, Williams and others (2013) indicated most research has focused on aerobic endurance performance, and numerous studies, reviews, meta-analyses, and position statements by sports-related associations support its efficacy as an ergogenic aid. Williams and others noted caffeine supplementation could enhance performance in a variety of aerobic endurance tasks, including the following:

- 15-min cycling performance following 135 min of sustained cycling
- Cycling to exhaustion at 80% VO_{2max}
- 2000-m rowing time
- Run time to exhaustion at 85% VO_{2max}
- 8-k run time

Other reviews, particularly two meta-analyses, support the performance-enhancing effect of caffeine supplementation. In their meta-analysis, Doherty and Smith (2004) reported that caffeine supplementation enhanced exercise performance by 12.3%, and even more so in endurance exercise tasks. In particular, time-to-exhaustion protocols improved test outcome more than short-term exercise. However, as noted previously, time-to-exhaustion protocols are not representative of typical sports performance. Following this review in 2004, more studies began to employ the time-trial as the exercise protocol. Five years later, in one of the more specific reviews relative to the effect of caffeine supplementation on aerobic endurance exercise, Ganio and others (2009) restricted their analysis to studies employing only a time-trial endurance test. They analyzed 21 high-quality studies using time trials of 5 min or more. Although variable among studies, the mean improvement in performance with caffeine ingestion was 3.2%. They concluded caffeine ingestion could be an effective ergogenic aid for endurance athletes when taken before or during exercise in moderate quantities (3 to 6 mg/kg body mass). They also noted abstaining from caffeine at least 7 days before use would give the greatest chance of optimizing the ergogenic effect.

Mechanism

Caffeine, as a stimulant, might be expected to increase work capacity. In the 1970s, one of the prominent theories underlying its performance-enhancing mechanism relative to aerobic endurance was an increase in fatty acid metabolism. An increase in fatty acid oxidation during exercise could spare the use of muscle glycogen, thus prolonging cycle or run time to exhaustion. However, this mechanism would not be applicable to shorter-term aerobic endurance events, such as a 5-k run. Graham and others (2008) eventually noted there is very little evidence to support the hypothesis that caffeine has ergogenic effects as a result of enhanced fat oxidation.

Davis and Green (2009) indicated a more favorable hypothesis seems to be that caffeine stimulates the central nervous system, noting that caffeine acts antagonistically on adenosine receptors, thereby inhibiting the negative effects adenosine induces on neurotransmission, arousal, and pain perception. In support of this possible psychological effect, Doherty and Smith (2005) performed a meta-analysis on 21 studies and reported that in comparison to placebo, caffeine reduced the RPE during exercise by 5.6%. Their regression analysis indicated the RPE obtained during exercise could account for approximately 29% of the variance in the improvement in exercise performance. The results demonstrate that caffeine reduces RPE during exercise and this may partly explain the subsequent ergogenic effects of caffeine on performance. However, Davis and Green (2009) note that the exact mechanisms behind caffeine's action remain to be elucidated.

Caffeine Combined with Other Supplements

Caffeine has also been combined with other performance-enhancing substances, including sodium bicarbonate, creatine, and carbohydrate, to determine if there would be an additive effect.

Carr and others (2011b) reported that caffeine supplementation to well-trained rowers improved 2000-m rowing ergometer performance by about 2%, but when combined with sodium bicarbonate, the resultant gastrointestinal symptoms may prevent performance enhancement. They recommend further investigation of ingestion protocols that minimize side effects.

Tarnopolsky (2010) notes that although caffeine and creatine appear to be ergogenic aids, they do so in a sport-specific context, and there is no rationale for their simultaneous use in sport.

Both carbohydrate and caffeine can improve endurance performance, so Conger and others (2011) conducted a systematic literature review coupled with meta-analysis of 21 studies to ascertain whether caffeine ingested with carbohydrate improves endurance performance more than carbohydrate alone. The overall effect size was 0.26, indicating that the carbohydrate/caffeine combination provides a small but significant improvement in performance compared to carbohydrate alone.

Recommended Supplementation Protocol

Caffeine appears to be an effective ergogenic aid for aerobic endurance exercise performance. The recommended dose, approximately 5 mg per kilogram body weight consumed 60 to 90 min prior to exercise, is considered to be safe and permissible in athletic competition. However, studies involving the performance-enhancing effect of caffeine have revealed large interindividual responses to caffeine, suggesting that individual characteristics should be considered when using it for performance enhancement. Indeed, individuals in some studies experienced adverse reactions to caffeine and impairment in exercise performance.

CONCLUSION

More than 50,000 dietary supplements are listed in the Natural Medicines Comprehensive Database, and many of these supplements are targeted to physically active individuals, including elite athletes. In a recent issue of a popular worldwide magazine for endurance runners, a full-page advertisement promoted a supplement designed to provide athletes with an *endurance edge*. The accompanying verbiage suggests the product contains nitrates, which, as discussed previously, *may* enhance aerobic endurance by increasing nitric oxide levels in the body. However, perusal of the list of ingredients on the website reveals no evidence of actual nitrate content. L-Arginine is listed, but as noted previously is ineffective in increasing markers of nitric oxide production. Moreover, as do all such supplements, the label contains the disclaimer, "These statements have not been evaluated by the Food and Drug Administration."

As noted previously, the vast majority of sport supplements marketed to endurance athletes are not effective. Some may also be dangerous, and their use may be associated with various health problems. The use of some in sport is prohibited by WADA and may lead to banishment from competition for several years, as happened recently to an Olympic gold medal winner who purchased a performance-enhancing substance at a convenience store. Several websites provide relevant information on various sports supplements. In the United States, www.supplement411.org is a website sponsored by the USADA that provides information on high-risk supplements. The website www.supplementsafetynow.com is also sponsored by the USADA along with numerous sport-governing associations, such as the National Football League, the National Basketball Association, and the National Collegiate Athletic

Association. Its mission is to protect citizens whose health may be threatened by the consumption of dangerous over-the-counter products disguised as "healthy" supplements.

However, some sport supplements possess the potential to provide an ergogenic effect for endurance athletes. For example, research with nitrate supplementation provides support for an enhanced utilization of oxygen during exercise and some evidence of improved endurance in well-trained athletes performing laboratory-based time trials. Moreover, the form of nitrate supplementation, such as juice extracts from nitrate-containing vegetables, may confer some health benefits. Dietary nitrates may, via their vasodilative effects, help reduce blood pressure, and may be one of the reasons the vegetable-laden Dietary Approaches to Stop Hypertension (DASH) diet is an effective means to help reduce high blood pressure. More research is needed to ascertain the performance-enhancing effects of nitrate supplementation, as well as the other dietary supplements whose use *may* enhance aerobic endurance performance.

Caffeine appears to have a solid base of evidence supporting its ability to enhance aerobic endurance performance. When consumed in recommended doses, it appears to be a safe, effective, and permissible supplement. However, individual responses to caffeine may vary, and athletes who consider the use of caffeine as an ergogenic aid should experiment with its use in training prior to using it for competition. The same advice may be applied relative to the use of any purported sports supplement.

REFERENCES

Bahrke, M.S., W.P. Morgan, and A. Stegner. 2009. Is ginseng an ergogenic aid? *Int J Sport Nutr Exerc Metab* 19:298–322.

Berry, C., and D.R. Wagner. 2012. Effect of pseudoephedrine on 800-m-run times of female collegiate track athletes. *Int J Sports Physiol Perform* 7:237–241.

Boje, O.D. 1939. Doping: A study of the means employed to raise the level of performance in sport. *Bull Health Org League Nat* 8:439–469.

Brewer, C.P., B. Dawson, K.E. Wallman, and K.J. Guelfi. 2012. Effect of repeated sodium phosphate loading on cycling time trial performance and VO_{2peak}. *Int J Sport Nutr Exerc Metab* October 30. Epub ahead of print.

Burfoot, A. 2003. Drink to your health. *Runner's World* 38(7):52–59.

Burke, L.M. 2008. Caffeine and sports performance. *Appl Physiol Nutr Metab* 33:1319–1334.

Burke, L.M., G. Millet, M.A. Tarnopolsky, and International Association of Athletics Federations. 2007. Nutrition for distance events. *J Sports Sci* 25(Suppl 1):S29–S38.

Carr, A.J., W.G. Hopkins, and C.J. Gore. 2011a. Effects of acute alkalosis and acidosis on performance: A meta-analysis. *Sports Med* 41:801–814.

Carr, A.J., C.J. Gore, and B. Dawson. 2011b. Induced alkalosis and caffeine supplementation: Effects on 2000-m rowing performance. *Int J Sport Nutr Exerc Metab* 21:357–364.

Christensen, P.M., M. Nyberg, and J. Bangsbo. 2013. Influence of nitrate supplementation on VO(2) kinetics and endurance of elite cyclists. *Scand J Med Sci Sports* 23:e21–e31.

Conger, S.A., G.L. Warren, M.A. Hardy, and M.L. Millard-Stafford. 2011. Does caffeine added to carbohydrate provide additional ergogenic benefit for endurance? *Int J Sport Nutr Exerc Metab* 21:71–84.

Coombes, J., and K. Hamilton. 2000. The effectiveness of commercially available sports drinks. *Sports Med* 29:181.

Davis, J.K., and J.M. Green. 2009. Caffeine and anaerobic performance: Ergogenic value and mechanisms of action. *Sports Med* 39:813–832.

Doherty, M., and P.M. Smith. 2004. Effects of caffeine ingestion on exercise testing: A meta-analysis. *Int J Sport Nutr Exerc Metab* 14:626–646.

Doherty, M., and P.M. Smith. 2005. Effects of caffeine ingestion on rating of perceived exertion during and after exercise: A meta-analysis. *Scand J Med Sci Sports* 15:69–78.

Ekblom, B., and B. Berglund. 1991. Effect of erythropoietin administration on maximal aerobic power. *Scand J Med Sci Sports* 1:88–93.

Epstein, D., and G. Dohrmann. 2009. What you don't know might kill you. *Sports Illustrated* 110(30):54–60.

Ganio, M.S., J.F. Klau, D.J. Casa, L.E. Armstrong, and C.M. Maresh. 2009. Effect of caffeine on sport-specific endurance performance: A systematic review. *J Strength Cond Res* 23:315–324.

Goulet, E.D., M. Aubertin-Leheudre, G.E. Plante, and I.J. Dionne. 2007. A meta-analysis of the effects of glycerol-induced hyperhydration on fluid retention and endurance performance. *Int J Sport Nutr Exerc Metab* 17:391–410.

Graham, T.E., D.S. Battram, F. Dela, A. El-Sohemy, and F.S. Thong. 2008. Does caffeine alter muscle carbohydrate and fat metabolism during exercise? *Appl Physiol Nutr Metab* 33:1311–1318.

Heikkinen, A., A. Alaranta, I. Helenius, and T. Vasankari. 2011. Dietary supplementation habits and perceptions of supplement use among elite Finnish athletes. *Int J Sport Nutr Exerc Metab* 21:271–279.

Hobson, R.M., B. Saunders, G. Ball, R.C. Harris, and C. Sale. 2012. Effects of β-alanine supplementation on exercise performance: A meta-analysis. *Amino Acids* 43:25–37.

Hodges, K., S. Hancock, K. Currell, B. Hamilton, and A.E. Jeukendrup. 2006. Pseudoephedrine enhances performance in 1500-m runners. *Med Sci Sports Exerc* 38:329–333.

Hoffman, J.R., N.S. Emerson, and J.R. Stout. 2012. β-Alanine supplementation. *Curr Sports Med Rep* 11:189–195.

Jeukendrup, A.E., and R. Randell. 2011. Fat burners: Nutrition supplements that increase fat metabolism. *Obes Rev* 12:841–851.

Jones, A.M., S.J. Bailey, and A. Vanhatalo. 2013. Dietary nitrate and O(2) consumption during exercise. *Med Sport Sci* 59:29–35.

Lun, V., K.A. Erdman, T.S. Fung, and R.A. Reimer. 2012. Dietary supplementation practices in Canadian high-performance athletes. *Int J Sport Nutr Exerc Metab* 22:31–37.

Peacock, O., A.E. Tjønna, P. James et al. 2012. Dietary nitrate does not enhance running performance in elite cross-country skiers. *Med Sci Sports Exerc* 44:2213–2219.

Pritchard-Peschek, K.R., D.G. Jenkins, M.A. Osborne, and G.J. Slater. 2010. Pseudoephedrine ingestion and cycling time-trial performance. *Int J Sport Nutr Exer Metab* 20:132–138.

Rodriguez, N.R., N.M. DiMarco, S. Langley et al. 2009. American Dietetic Association, Dietitians of Canada, and the American College of Sports Medicine: Nutrition and athletic performance. *J Am Diet Assoc* 109:509–527.

Sato, A., A. Kamei, E. Kamihigashi et al. 2012. Use of supplements by young elite Japanese athletes participating in the 2010 youth Olympic games in Singapore. *Clin J Sport Med* 22:418–423.

Spriet, L.L., C.G. Perry, and J.L. Talanian. 2008. Legal pre-event nutritional supplements to assist energy metabolism. *Essays Biochem* 44:27–43.

Tarnopolsky, M.A. 2010. Caffeine and creatine use in sport. *Ann Nutr Metab* 57(Suppl 2):1–8.

Tremblay, M.S., S.D. Galloway, and J.R. Sexsmith. 1994. Ergogenic effects of phosphate loading: Physiological fact or methodological fiction? *Can J Appl Physiol* 19:1–11.

United States Anti-Doping Agency. 2012. Report on proceedings under the world anti-doping code and the USADA protocol. http://d3epuodzu3wuis.cloudfront.net/Reasoned Decision.pdf. Accessed November 1, 2012.

van Rosendal, S.P., M.A. Osborne, R.G. Fassett, and J.S. Coombes. 2010. Guidelines for glycerol use in hyperhydration and rehydration associated with exercise. *Sports Med* 40:113–129.

West, J.S., T. Ayton, K.E. Wallman, and K.J. Guelfi. 2012. The effect of six days of sodium phosphate supplementation on appetite, energy intake and aerobic capacity in trained men and women. *Int J Sport Nutr Exerc Metab* 22:422–429.

Williams, M.H. 2004. Dietary supplements and sports performance: Introduction and vitamins. *J Int Soc Sports Nutr* 1:1–6.

Williams, M.H. 2005a. Dietary supplements and sports performance: Amino acids. *J Int Soc Sports Nutr* 2:63–67.

Williams, M.H. 2005b. Dietary supplements and sports performance: Minerals. *J Int Soc Sports Nutr* 2:43–49.

Williams, M.H. 2006. Dietary supplements and sports performance: Herbals. *J Int Soc Sports Nutr* 3:1–6.

Williams, M.H. 2011. Sports supplements: Efficacy, safety, permissibility. Green tea extracts, green tea catechins, and epigallocatechin-3-gallate (EGCG). http://static.abbottnutrition .com/cms/easa/media/williams-egcg.pdf. Accessed November 3, 2012.

Williams, M.H. 2012. Nitrate supplementation and endurance performance. *Marathon & Beyond* 16(5):114–128.

Williams, M.H. 2013. Nitrate supplementation—Can it help you *beet* your PR? *RRCA Club Running* Spring/Summer, 10–12.

Williams, M.H., D.E. Anderson, and E.S. Rawson. 2013. *Nutrition for Health, Fitness, and Sport.* New York: McGraw-Hill.

4 Nutrition for Strength Power Athletes

Caoileann H. Murphy, MSc, RD
Stuart M. Phillips, PhD, FACSM, FACN
Department of Kinesiology, McMaster University,
Hamilton, Ontario, Canada

CONTENTS

INTRODUCTION

Strength and power are important characteristics in the performance of many sports. This is most apparent in lifting events (i.e., Olympic lifting, powerlifting) and throwing events (i.e., javelin, discus, shot put, and hammer). The ability to generate explosive muscle power is also critical to success in sprints (100 to 200 m) and jumping events, as well as intermittent passages of play in team sports like rugby and American football. Bodybuilders strive to develop and enlarge their musculature for competitive exhibition. Due to the potent nature of resistance exercise in promoting strength gains, hypertrophy, and, in certain circumstances, increases in muscle power, athletes competing in these events will typically include some form of resistance exercise into their overall training program. Sport-specific training varies markedly between the different types of athletes and is generally sequenced so as not to interfere with resistance training. While resistance training plays a supportive role in team sports and track and field events, it is the major training focus in lifting events and bodybuilding. Given the vast heterogeneity in sport-specific training programs of strength-power athletes and their consequent metabolic implications, this chapter will focus on the major nutritional issues underpinning resistance training. The sports of Olympic lifting, powerlifting, and bodybuilding will also be addressed given the emphasis on resistance exercise in the overall training program for these athletes.

WHAT ARE THE FUNCTIONAL DEMANDS OF TRAINING AND COMPETITION?

Resistance training when performed as a small component of the overall training program or as its major focus is usually a planned and sequenced activity. Components of the program are carefully planned within each session, microcycle, and longer training macrocycle (Burke 2007). The outcomes of resistance training that lead to an increase in muscle size or strength include neural adaptations and positive net muscle protein balance, with the contribution of these factors varying according to the stage of the resistance training program. The primary goal of training in powerlifters and Olympic lifters is to enhance strength and power, respectively. Traditional powerlifting training typically involves high-force, low-velocity exercises with mastery usually touted as requiring a decrease in repetition range and increased volume. Periodization of training in Olympic lifters typically involves a transition from high-volume, high-force, low-velocity movements, characteristic of traditional powerlifting, to more explosive, low-repetition training in preparation for competition. The emphasis on higher velocity "explosive" Olympic lifts results in greater improvements in power and strength over more traditional strength-based lifting, derived mainly from neural rather than hypertrophy adaptations, and is increasingly being included in the training of powerlifters (Slater and Phillips 2011). While gains in muscle mass can occur during any phase of training in a traditional powerlifting program, the initial phase of the macrocycle represents the most favorable time for skeletal muscle gains in Olympic lifters (Slater and Phillips 2011). As hypertrophy represents the primary goal of training in bodybuilders, their training programs are usually of greater volume than those of Olympic and powerlifters, incorporating higher repetition ranges with multiple sets per muscle group and short rest periods between sets.

Competition demands of a number of strength-requiring sports are typically characterized by explosive single efforts, with significant recovery between each effort. Thus, the phosphagen energy systems (adenosine triphosphate and phosphocreatine) supply the main fuel source. However, resistance training involving repetitive lifts requires a high rate of energy supply from both the phosphagen energy systems and glycogenolysis. Possible causes of fatigue during resistance exercise include a decline in intramuscular pH, depletion of phosphagen energy system stores, and impaired energy production from glycogenolysis (Slater and Phillips 2011).

WHAT DO STRENGTH-POWER ATHLETES EAT?

While there are a reasonable number of reports on the dietary intakes of national- and international-level male lifters, throwers, and bodybuilders, the majority of these are over 20 years old and data on the dietary practices of contemporary athletes and elite performers is lacking. Considering the enthusiasm with which strength athletes appear to embrace new scientific findings, as well as fads, it is unfortunate that data that is more recent does not exist (Burke 2007). In addition, studies on female strength-power athletes are less common reflecting perhaps the lower numbers of females involved in these sports. Nevertheless, available data indicate that during normal training phases, these athletes have high absolute energy intakes. This is unsurprising given the muscularity of these athletes and the association between muscle mass and resting energy expenditure, which when added to their exercising energy expenditure would yield a high daily total. However, when expressed relative to body mass, the energy intakes of strength-power athletes are generally similar to those reported for athletes in other sports (Slater and Phillips 2011). Data from national- and international-level competitors suggest that energy intakes tend to fall short of the current strength athlete guidelines of ~185–210 g kg^{-1} d^{-1} body mass, with intakes of approximately 150–180 g kg^{-1} d^{-1} reported in males and 110–150 g kg^{-1} d^{-1} in females (Faber et al. 1986, 1990). The limited number of dietary intake surveys conducted in elite athletes suggests slightly higher energy intakes of 210–240 g kg^{-1} d^{-1} (Chen et al. 1989; Tarnopolsky et al. 1988), although further work is needed to confirm this in modern world-class strength athletes. Alternatively, it has been suggested that the apparent failure of several groups of strength-power athletes to meet energy intake guidelines may be a reflection of the fact that taller and/or more muscular individuals have lower resting energy requirements relative to body mass (Slater and Phillips 2011). Thus, consideration may need to be given to the lower relative energy requirements of larger athletes when determining the adequacy of energy intakes (Slater and Phillips 2011).

Dietary intake data typically show carbohydrate intakes of 3–5 g kg^{-1} d^{-1} in lifters and throwers (Chen et al. 1989; Faber et al. 1990), while bodybuilders appear to consume carbohydrate intakes equivalent to 4–7 g kg^{-1} d^{-1} independent of sex (Kim et al. 2011; Tarnopolsky et al. 1988). The dietary fat intake of lifters and throwers is generally higher than recommended for healthy individuals, usually accounting for ~40% of total dietary intake (Chen et al. 1989; Faber et al. 1990). In contrast, in bodybuilders the majority of dietary surveys report fat intakes closer to 30% of dietary intake (Tarnopolsky et al. 1988), presumably to account for the slightly higher carbohydrate intakes in this group. As expected, protein intakes in strength-power athletes are high with average intakes exceeding 2 g kg^{-1} d^{-1} (Chen et al. 1989; Tarnopolsky et al. 1988), although individual studies have reported mean intakes as high as 4.3 g kg^{-1} d^{-1} (Kim et al. 2011).

It has become increasingly recognized that simply assessing total daily protein intakes of strength-power athletes will not address if protein intake has been optimized to support gains in muscle mass and strength (Slater and Phillips 2011). Indeed, the per meal dose, protein source, timing of consumption, and daily distribution pattern of protein intake are now recognized as key factors influencing adaptations to resistance training. Unfortunately, few studies have examined these aspects of protein consumption in strength-power athletes, making it difficult to determine compliance with current nutritional guidelines not merely in terms of total protein intake but of important modifiers of adaptive responses via protein doses, timing, source, and pattern of intake. Future studies are required to assess the nutritional intakes and eating patterns of contemporary, elite athletes, with emphasis on the timing of nutrient intake in relation to training.

WHAT SHOULD STRENGTH-POWER ATHLETES EAT?

Training nutrition has a number of important roles for the elite strength-power athlete: improving work capacity acutely (i.e., enhancing the training stimulus) by fueling individual training sessions, promoting recovery between training sessions not only of the muscle but also of connective tissues, supporting body composition and weight category goals and enhancing metabolic and physiological training adaptations, including skeletal muscle hypertrophy.

Strength-power athletes are notorious for high protein intakes. Indeed, historical references to high protein diets date as far back as ancient Greece and the legendary wrestler, Milo of Kroton. It is now generally accepted in the sports nutrition literature that strength-athletes require, or at least can benefit from, protein intakes above the current recommended daily allowance (RDA) of 0.8 g kg^{-1} d^{-1} for the general population. The RDA, which was determined based on the inherently flawed nitrogen balance method and set at a level to prevent deficiency in 98% of the population, is unlikely to reflect the protein intakes required to optimize all aspects of muscle mass, muscle function, and muscle metabolic processes in resistance-training athletes (Phillips et al. 2007). In support of this thesis, a recent meta-analysis concluded that consuming higher protein (either through protein supplementation or a higher protein diet providing >1.2 g kg^{-1} d^{-1}) during prolonged resistance exercise training resulted in significantly greater gains in fat-free mass (~1.0 kg), muscle fiber cross-sectional area (~50%), and strength (~20% for single repetition maximum in the leg press) compared to training without additional protein in young subjects (Cermak et al. 2012). Importantly, these findings were evident despite the fact that, before the intervention, all groups were consuming protein at a level higher than the RDA (~1.2 g kg^{-1} d^{-1}) indicating that ingesting protein above this level promoted greater adaptations to resistance exercise training. Of note, resistance-trained groups were shown to be even more responsive to higher protein intake than their untrained counterparts were, with protein supplementation/high protein diets resulting in a four-fold larger increase in fat-free mass relative to the lower protein conditions. These findings suggest that in strength-power athletes, high protein intake is important in maximizing anabolic responses to training.

In addition to the factors directly related to promoting maximal adaptations to resistance exercise training, the optimal level of protein intake for strength-power athletes should also maintain optimal function of all protein-requiring processes in the body such as the metabolic pathways in which amino acids act as intermediates, immune function, and the production of plasma proteins (Phillips et al. 2007). While it would be extremely difficult to measure the amount of protein required to optimize the functioning of all of these pathways, when we consider that the nature of exercise is such that there is an upregulation of protein-requiring processes, it appears unlikely that the minimal level of protein required by sedentary individuals would provide for the ideal intake in strength athletes (Phillips et al. 2007).

A number of studies have employed the nitrogen balance method in an attempt to determine protein requirements in strength athletes. Data from these studies indicates that the protein needs of athletes can be as high as twice the RDA (Tarnopolsky et al. 1988). While the nitrogen balance method is the method on which the RDA for protein is based, there are a number of serious technical limitations associated with it such as the implausibly high nitrogen balance typically observed with high protein intakes, and increased economy of nitrogen use with low protein intakes (Phillips et al. 2007). Furthermore, the relevance of being in "nitrogen balance" (i.e., satisfying the minimal requirement) to an elite level athlete who wishes to optimize the adaptive response to training, as well as support the optimal function of all physiological protein-requiring processes in the body, is questionable. Thus, alternative approaches have been used. Utilizing isotopically labeled tracers, it was reported that consumption of a "low" protein diet (0.86 g kg^{-1} d^{-1}) by a group of strength-trained athletes resulted in an accommodated state in which whole body protein synthesis was reduced compared with medium (1.4 g kg^{-1} d^{-1}) and high (2.4 g kg^{-1} d^{-1}) protein diets (Tarnopolsky et al. 1992). No difference in whole body protein synthesis was observed between the medium and high protein diets; however, leucine oxidation was increased on the high protein diet, demonstrating that this protein intake was providing amino acids in excess of the rate at which they could be incorporated into muscle or used for other amino acid requiring processes. It is worth noting that these results do not demonstrate that 1.4 g kg^{-1} d^{-1} was required to saturate the need for dietary protein, but merely that 0.86 g kg^{-1} d^{-1} resulted in an adapted state and was insufficient to promote maximal rates of protein synthesis. The measurement of whole body protein synthesis does not necessarily reflect the rates of protein synthesis within individual tissues such as muscle; thus, it is unclear from this study what body proteins were being made at a submaximal rate at 0.86 g kg^{-1} d^{-1}, but if muscle protein synthesis was negatively affected, then clearly these findings would be of relevance to strength athletes.

The optimal intake of protein for strength athletes is difficult to define; however, general guidelines recommend athletes undertaking strength training to ingest up to 1.6–1.7 g kg^{-1} d^{-1} (Slater and Phillips 2011). There is also evidence that an intense period of resistance training reduces protein turnover and improves net protein retention (Hartman et al. 2006). It has been postulated that these data mean that the minimal dietary protein requirements of experienced strength athletes may be lower than the recommended guideline (Slater and Phillips 2011). On the other hand, others have argued that these data do not necessarily indicate that resistance training lowers protein requirements. It has been suggested that weightlifting provides such a potent anabolic stimulus that it may cause a shift in the hierarchy of amino acid requiring processes toward muscle protein synthesis. This could mean a greater proportion of circulating amino acids are taken up by skeletal muscle in both the fasted and fed states, potentially at the adaptive "expense" of other amino acid requiring processes (Phillips 2006).

While there is ongoing debate within the scientific literature regarding the protein requirements of strength athletes, it appears that this may be unnecessary as the majority of these athletes are habitually consuming intakes high enough to promote full function of the multitude of physiological processes that require dietary protein (Phillips 2006). The extremely high protein intakes reported in some groups of strength athletes (Kim et al. 2011) has led to the safety of such high intakes to be questioned. While exceeding the upper range for protein intake guidelines likely provides no further benefit, merely promoting increased amino acid catabolism and protein oxidation (Moore et al. 2009), the health risks of high protein intake seem to be minimal for otherwise healthy athletes (Phillips 2012). It is worth noting, however, that the body adapts to relatively high protein loads by increasing the capacity for amino acid catabolism. Thus, it is likely that the habitual consumption of a high protein diet means the athlete is "forced" to continue consuming greater protein intakes so that fed state gains can balance fasted state losses. Indeed, at least anecdotally, elite strength-trained athletes who eat extremely high protein intakes up to qualifying competitions report losing substantial amounts of muscle mass when they subsequently reduce their protein intake. Thus, in these situations, athletes should wean themselves off extremely high intakes in order to avoid such losses. Another potential problem with excessive protein intakes is that they may interfere with the ability of some athletes to achieve optimal intakes of other macronutrients, particularly carbohydrate, without exceeding their energy requirements (Phillips 2012). This is more likely to be a problem in athletes with lower energy intakes, such as females, and those involved in sprinting, throwing events, or team sports as training likely poses a greater challenge to glycogen stores than strength athletes who solely perform resistance exercise. Therefore, in these athletes a "more is better" approach to dietary protein may hinder other dietary goals within the wider sports nutrition strategy, potentially resulting in impaired training adaptations and/or limiting the ability to train effectively.

When it comes to the role of dietary protein in supporting optimum training adaptations in athletes, the total protein content of their diet may not be the most important factor to consider. A rapidly growing body of evidence shows that the quantity per meal, source (plant vs. animal), and timing of an athlete's protein intake in relation to the training stimulus, as well as the distribution of protein throughout the day have critically important influences on the overall anabolic response, such that hypertrophy may be quite different despite identical total protein intakes.

TIMING AND THE RATIONALE FOR PROTEIN CONSUMPTION AROUND RESISTANCE TRAINING

Changes in muscle mass result from changes in net muscle protein balance (i.e., the rate of muscle protein synthesis minus the rate of breakdown), with the magnitude and duration of the positive periods of net muscle protein balance determining the extent of muscle hypertrophy (Phillips et al. 2007). A session of resistance exercise stimulates increased rates of both muscle protein synthesis (MPS) and muscle protein breakdown (MPB) for up to 48 h (Phillips et al. 1997). Although resistance exercise stimulates MPS to a greater extent than MPB, the net muscle protein balance only becomes positive when amino acids are ingested (Churchward-Venne et al. 2012). This is primarily accomplished through the synergistic effect of amino acid intake and resistance exercise on MPS and forms the rationale for the recommendation to consume protein in close temporal proximity to the performance of resistance exercise.

When is the optimal time to consume protein with respect to training bouts? Some studies have shown that pre-exercise consumption of protein can enhance MPS, while others have shown no effect (Phillips and Van Loon 2011). Thus, it is currently unclear whether pre-exercise protein feeding can increase MPS and long-term gains in muscle mass. It has been hypothesized that the pre-exercise consumption of a large dose (>20 g) of a leucine-rich, slowly digested, high quality protein might support a robust MPS response if it allows the resultant increase in aminoacidemia to coincide with the post-exercise period (Burke et al. 2012). While this could benefit athletes who struggle to consume adequate protein after a resistance session due to issues related to poor appetite or access to food, further work is needed to determine the efficacy of this potential strategy. Consumption of protein during exercise may accelerate MPS rates and possibly suppress muscle protein breakdown either during the rest intervals between sets or after the exercise bout, potentially contributing to an enhanced anabolic response. However, few studies have examined peri-workout protein ingestion with resistance exercise with the exception of a study from Beelen et al. (2008), who showed that the co-ingestion of protein (0.15 g kg^{-1} h^{-1}) and carbohydrate (0.15 g kg^{-1} h^{-1}) did enhance MPS during a 2-h resistance training session and early into recovery, but this did not extend into the overnight fasting period. However, in an 8-week resistance training study, ingesting whey protein immediately before the start of exercise (0.15 g kg^{-1}) and after each training set (0.006 g kg^{-1}) had no greater effect on muscle mass or strength than did a placebo in previously untrained men (Weisgarber et al. 2012). While it is possible that the relatively small amount of protein consumed after each set (~0.5 g) was too low to produce significant muscle hypertrophy, further work needs to be conducted, especially in well-trained populations, to examine whether there may be any anabolic advantage to consuming protein during exercise for elite strength athletes.

It is unequivocal that immediate post-exercise amino acid provision is an effective nutrition-based strategy to enhance MPS above rates observed with exercise alone (Churchward-Venne et al. 2012). Sport nutrition guidelines emphasize the importance of early post-exercise protein consumption as it has been suggested that a window of anabolic opportunity exists in the early post-exercise period during which protein must be consumed in order for a synergistic effect with exercise to occur. This relates to the fact that exercise-induced increases in rates of MPS are greatest immediately after exercise (~100% to 150% above basal rates), and thus the synergistic effects of exercise and feeding on MPS are likely greatest during this time period (Churchward-Venne et al. 2012). However, recently there has been some debate over the critical nature of consuming protein immediately after exercise. Resistance exercise increases MPS for up to ~48 h (Phillips et al. 1997), indicating that consumption of dietary protein at any point within the two days following a resistance training session would likely stimulate synergistic effects on MPS similar to those observed when amino acids are provided immediately after resistance exercise. In support of this, consumption of 15 g of whey protein 24 h after a single session of resistance exercise has been shown to stimulate greater MPS than the same dose provided at rest (Burd et al. 2011). Nevertheless, the synergistic enhancement of resistance exercise-induced elevations in MPS by protein provision is likely greatest immediately post-exercise and fades over time (Churchward-Venne et al. 2012). Thus, a simple message for strength training athletes is that protein ingestion should begin early after exercise (i.e., immediately to 2 h post-exercise) to promote recovery and possibly enhance adaptation (Phillips and Van Loon 2011).

PROTEIN QUANTITY

A classic saturable dose-response relationship has been shown to exist between protein intake and the rate of MPS following resistance exercise (Moore et al. 2009; Witard et al. 2014). Moore et al. (2009) fed isolated egg protein to young, resistance-trained males in graded quantities from 0 to 40 g immediately after a session of resistance exercise performed in the fasted state. MPS showed a dose-dependent increase from 0 to 20 g; however, doubling protein intake to 40 g did not further enhance MPS and stimulated a marked increase in whole-body leucine oxidation rates. Corroborating these data, Witard et al. (2014) recently showed that a 20-g dose of whey protein is sufficient to maximally stimulate MPS after a bout of resistance exercise performed following the consumption of a high protein breakfast, with larger doses failing to further augment post-exercise MPS and, instead, stimulating amino acid oxidation and catabolism. Taken together, these data indicate that the optimum amount of protein to consume to maximize the anabolic response after resistance exercise is approximately 20 to 25 g (8 to 10 g essential amino acids [EAA]) of high-quality protein in larger men (~85 kg). Consuming greater quantities appears to offer no further benefit in terms of MPS and results in the oxidation of the excess amino acids, which reflects greater oxidative fate of protein when the goal is to enhance gains in muscle mass. Although studies have yet to clearly establish whether the optimal quantity of protein to consume to maximally stimulate MPS after resistance exercise varies between athletes of different body weights, based on the available evidence from acute studies, a body weight corrected dose of 0.25 to 0.3 g kg^{-1} appears to be an effective amount.

PROTEIN SOURCE

Different dietary protein sources, even among those considered to be of high quality, have been shown to differ in their capacity to stimulate MPS (Figure 4.1) and promote gains in muscle mass over time in combination with resistance training (Phillips and Van Loon 2011). For example, the consumption of fat-free fluid milk following a bout of resistance exercise resulted in greater net muscle protein accretion in the hours following the exercise session compared to an isonitrogenous and isoenergetic soy beverage in young men (Wilkinson et al. 2007). When studied chronically over 12 weeks of resistance training, the repeated post-exercise consumption of fat-free milk promoted greater gains in lean body mass than did the soy beverage (Hartman et al. 2006). In addition, studies comparing the two main proteins in milk (whey and casein) have demonstrated that the whey protein fraction promotes a superior MPS response and results in greater gains in strength and muscle mass when supplemented over several weeks of resistance training (Tang and Phillips 2009). While the reasons why some high quality protein sources produce greater muscle protein accretion than others do are not entirely clear at present, it

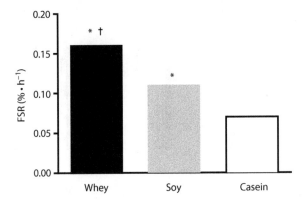

FIGURE 4.1 Mixed muscle protein fractional synthetic rate (FSR) after ingestion of 20 g of whey hydrolysate, casein, or soy protein following resistance exercise. †, Whey consumption resulted in significantly greater FSR compared to both casein and soy; *, soy ingestion resulted in significantly greater FSR than casein. (Redrawn from Tang, J.E. et al. 2009. *J Appl Physiol* 107(3):987–992. With permission.)

appears to be related to the divergent characteristics of the aminoacidemia caused by different protein sources.

An increase in plasma amino acid concentrations is a potent stimulator of MPS (Tang and Phillips 2009). Studies have shown that the achievement of a rapid and pronounced plasma concentration of EAA, particularly leucine, is associated with increased rates of MPS and anabolic cell-signaling, both at rest and following resistance exercise compared to a slow rate of appearance of these amino acids (West et al. 2011). Amino acid delivery into plasma after the consumption of a dietary protein source reflects the rate of digestion and absorption, along with its amino acid composition. While the amino acid profiles of whey and casein are relatively similar, their rate of digestion varies markedly. Whey is acid-soluble and is quickly digested, resulting in a rapid, pronounced, but transient increase in postprandial plasma EAA/leucine concentrations (Tang and Phillips 2009). Casein, on the other hand, effectively "clots" when exposed to stomach acid, slowing the rate of gastric emptying, resulting in a much more moderate but sustained rise in plasma amino acids. The superior capacity of whey to stimulate MPS over that of soy is not due to differing digestion/absorption kinetics as soy is also rapidly digested. However, the leucine content of soy compared to whey is lower, which results in a lower peak leucinemia and hence lower stimulation of MPS following the ingestion of soy vs. whey (Tang et al. 2009). The differences between whey, casein, and soy protein in terms of EAA content and blood leucine response to ingestion are illustrated in Figures 4.2 and 4.3, respectively.

While the EAA are primarily responsible for stimulating MPS, the branched chain amino acid (BCAA) leucine appears to have a particularly important role as a key metabolic regulator of MPS through activation of the mTOR pathway (Atherton et al. 2010a). When considering protein feeding strategies that will optimize the MPS response following resistance exercise, a protein source with high leucine content

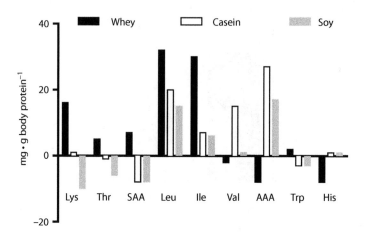

FIGURE 4.2 Differences between human body protein essential amino acid (EAA) content (FAO Expert Consultation 2013) and that of the whey, casein, and soy. The EAA content was taken from the values reported by Tang et al. (2009) for commercially available whey hydrolysate, micellar casein, and isolated soy protein. All values are in mg amino acids g^{-1} protein. AAA, aromatic amino acids; His, histidine; Ile, isoleucine; Leu, leucine; Lys, lysine; SAA, sulphur amino acids; Thr, threonine; Trp, tryptophan; Val, valine. (Adapted from Tang, J.E., and S.M. Phillips. 2009. *Curr Opin Clin Nutr Metab Care* 12(1):66–71.)

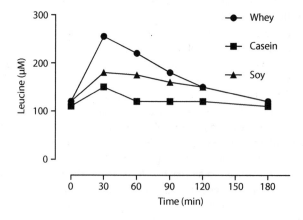

FIGURE 4.3 Blood leucine concentration after ingestion of 20 g of whey hydrolysate, casein, or soy protein. Whey consumption results in a rapid increase in blood leucine concentration, which is of greater amplitude and is considerably more rapid compared to casein and soy ingestion. (Redrawn from Tang, J.E. et al. 2009. *J Appl Physiol* 107(3):987–992. With permission.)

and rapid digestion kinetics, in order to promote a rapid leucinemia spike, would be an effective option (Churchward-Venne et al. 2012). A recent study characterizing the plasma amino acid responses to the ingestion of 20 g of protein from a range of commonly consumed protein-rich foods reported that skimmed milk produced a significantly higher and faster peak leucine concentration than all other foods or liquids (soy milk, beef steak, egg, liquid meal supplement) (Burke et al. 2012). Peak values for EAAs, BCAA, and leucine after a soy beverage consumption tended to be lower than for the other protein sources, perhaps reflecting the lower leucine/BCAA content of soy. In addition, ingestion of liquid forms of protein achieved peak plasma amino acid concentrations twice as quickly as solid protein-rich foods (~50 min vs. ~100 min), suggesting that the form of the food may be an important determinant of post-prandial aminoacidemia. Nonetheless, more research is needed to determine the physiological relevance of food form in the regulation of MPS after resistance exercise.

In summary, current evidence suggests the type/source of protein consumed after resistance exercise influences the magnitude of the acute muscle protein synthetic response and, when practiced over time, the same acute protein turnover responses translate into longer-term phenotypic responses affecting training adaptations. The more effective protein source should have a high leucine content and rapid digestion kinetics in order to promote a rapid leucinemia spike and contain a full complement of EAA to support and sustain the protein synthetic response; proteins such as whey protein and bovine skimmed milk have been tested and fall into this category.

DISTRIBUTION OF DAILY PROTEIN INTAKE

The importance of the distribution of daily protein intake has received some attention as a potential strategy to augment muscle protein accretion. A strong rationale for considering protein distribution throughout the day comes from acute studies showing that ~8 to 10 g of EAA is sufficient to induce a maximal stimulation of MPS both at rest and after resistance exercise. Since it appears that only dietary EAA are required to maximally stimulate muscle protein synthesis, it has been suggested a balanced pattern of protein intake with consumption of 8 to 10 g of EAA at each meal would maximally and efficiently stimulate MPS on numerous occasions throughout the day. From a practical standpoint, 8 to 10 g of EAA translates into approximately 20 to 25 g of high-quality protein, which can be obtained from moderate servings of a number of protein-rich foods as shown in Table 4.1. While there is little data available on the meal-to-meal protein intakes of strength-power athletes specifically, typical eating patterns in many Western societies would consist of a skewed pattern of protein intake in which ~50% of daily protein intake is consumed at a late-day dinner-time meal and small amounts are consumed at breakfast and pre-bed. At least theoretically, consuming protein in this skewed fashion would result in a full stimulation of MPS, but also a high oxidation and catabolism of amino acids over and above the maximally stimulatory protein dose of 0.25–0.3 g protein/kg/meal, in response to the dinner meal while protein doses consumed at breakfast and pre-bed may be insufficient to maximally stimulate MPS. As mentioned previously, resistance exercise increases the sensitivity of MPS rates to dietary amino acid provision for up to 48 h after the exercise session. Thus, consuming protein in this skewed pattern may hamper adaptations to training. Providing some support for this hypothesis, it was observed that both whole body (Moore et al. 2012) and muscle (Areta et al. 2013) protein synthesis tended to be greater when 80 g of whey protein was consumed as four 20-g doses every 3 h compared to the same amount consumed

TABLE 4.1

Quantities of Some Common Foods Providing 10 g of Essential Amino Acids (EAA)

Food	Quantity Providing 10 g EAA	% Leucine (of EAA Content)
Chicken breast, baked	80 g	18
Beef, lean, roasted	100 g	21
Tuna, tinned in water, drained	95 g	19
Milk, skimmed	650 mL	21
Eggs, poached	180 g (3–4 large eggs)	19
Yogurt, plain, nonfat	360 g	21
Cheese, cheddar, reduced fat	95 g	20
Cottage cheese	170 g	21

Note: % Leucine represents proportion of EAA content accounted for by leucine. EAA/leucine content determined using Nutrition Data via USDA National Nutrient Database for Standard Reference, Release 25.

as either two large (40 g) doses every 6 h, or eight small (10 g) doses every 1.5 h over the 12-h recovery period following a session of resistance exercise. In the future, it will be important to assess whether these acute protein synthetic benefits translate into a superior adaptive response to prolonged resistance training.

It is worth noting that the muscle becomes refractory to persistent aminoacidemia (Atherton et al. 2010b), indicating the protein-containing meals should be spaced out throughout the day. In the absence of any data to provide a rationale for greater meal frequencies, 3 to 4 feedings daily seems an appropriate recommendation. A potentially important and perhaps underappreciated opportunity for strength athletes to consume a protein-rich meal is before bed. It has recently been demonstrated that the ingestion of a larger protein dose (40 g of casein) immediately before bed resulted in a greater stimulation of MPS overnight (Res et al. 2012), suggesting this may be a viable feeding strategy to optimize MPS during the otherwise fasted 8- to 10-h fast period that typically accompanies sleep. Such a pre-sleep meal would likely also facilitate recovery as it would allow repair/remodeling of proteins during the overnight period. Considering the prolonged duration of the overnight fast, larger protein doses, such as those used in the study by Res and colleagues, may be optimal in the pre-bed meal.

In summary, strength athletes should aim to consume protein in a balanced manner throughout the day, with the ingestion of ~25 g (or 0.25 to 0.3 g/kg) of high quality protein in 3 to 4 protein feedings evenly spaced throughout the day. It is notable that the available studies determining the optimal dose of protein required to maximally stimulate MPS have been conducted using either isolated protein supplements or single protein-rich foods (i.e., beef). When protein-containing foods are consumed in the context of a mixed meal, the co-ingestion of substantial amounts of other nutrients such as fat and fiber may affect rates of digestion and subsequent aminoacidemia (Burke et al. 2012). Given the role of the pattern of aminoacidemia in influencing the MPS response, further studies will have to confirm the ideal quantity of protein athletes should consume at each mixed meal to optimize the MPS response, which is likely higher than that for isolated protein sources.

CARBOHYDRATE NEEDS

Glycogenolysis plays an important role in the production of energy during repetitive lifts in resistance training. Various studies have reported that a single resistance training session results in a 24% to 40% decrease in muscle glycogen content from relevant muscles (Slater and Phillips 2011). The extent of depletion is affected by characteristics of the training session including duration, volume, and intensity, with higher repetition, moderate-load sessions such as those undertaken during the hypertrophy phases of training programs resulting in the largest reductions in muscle glycogen stores (Slater and Phillips 2011). These results have led to the idea that carbohydrate is a potentially limiting substrate during resistance exercise workouts (Burke 2007). In support of this thesis, some studies have reported reductions in isometric strength, isokinetic force production, and workload capacity during resistance training sessions performed with compromised muscle glycogen stores (Jacobs et al. 1981), although this is not a universal finding (Mitchell et al. 1997). The variation between methods used to induce glycogen depletion between studies may, at least in part, account for the inconsistency between studies as different protocols used various combinations of exercise and dietary carbohydrate restriction. However, the current literature supports the opinion that pre-exercise muscle glycogen stores do not appear to affect brief resistance training capacity (Slater and Phillips 2011). Furthermore, when the volume and intensity of resistance exercise is matched, commencing resistance exercise with low muscle glycogen does not appear to impair the MPS response in the early recovery period (Camera et al. 2012). On the other hand, it is possible that inadequate glycogen levels will impair performance in any training session or competitive event that relies on rapid and repeated glycogen breakdown (Slater and Phillips 2011). Overall, the literature fails to provide sufficient evidence to make definitive guidelines about total carbohydrate intake for strength athletes and longitudinal studies are required to systematically investigate the influence of various levels of intake on the outcomes of a resistance training program. Because resistance training forms only one aspect of the overall training program for sprinters and throwers, and resistance exercise-induced skeletal damage impairs glycogen resynthesis, it would seem reasonable to encourage strength-athletes to consume a moderate carbohydrate intake (Slater and Phillips 2011). While carbohydrate recommendations of 6 g kg^{-1} d^{-1} for strength athletes exist in the literature, this may not be suitable for all athletes such as larger individuals with lower relative energy expenditure or females in whom high carbohydrate intakes may compromise intakes of other nutrients within a smaller energy requirement. Thus, current experts recommend daily carbohydrate intakes of 4–7 g kg^{-1} d^{-1} for strength athletes depending on their phase of training (Slater and Phillips 2011). One exception to this might be if significant reductions in body fat need to be achieved during the lead up to a strength athlete's competitive season. In this situation, there is some evidence to support carbohydrate intakes below the range recommended above (Phillips and Van Loon 2011). This is discussed further in this chapter. Finally, perhaps even more important than total carbohydrate intake, strength-power athletes should consume carbohydrate strategically around training sessions to promote optimal carbohydrate availability at key time points for glycogen restoration (Slater and Phillips 2011).

CARBOHYDRATE AFTER RESISTANCE EXERCISE

The importance of post-exercise carbohydrate ingestion to restore muscle glycogen stores is well accepted in endurance and team sports. Considering that resistance training usually accounts for only one component of the overall training program for many strength athletes, carbohydrate should be routinely ingested after resistance training to replete glycogen levels and enhance recovery (Slater and Phillips 2011). This may be especially critical when the recovery period between resistance workouts is limited. For example, Haff and colleagues showed that carbohydrate intake during and after a resistance training session enhanced performance in a second bout of resistance exercise undertaken after a 4-h recovery period, allowing participants to complete more work in the subsequent training session (Haff et al. 1999). Co-ingesting protein with carbohydrate after resistance exercise lowers the carbohydrate intake required to replenish muscle glycogen stores. For example, the intake of 0.8 g kg^{-1} h^{-1} carbohydrate plus 0.2–0.4 g kg^{-1} h^{-1} protein results in similar rates of muscle glycogen resynthesis over 5 h of recovery as 1.2 g kg^{-1} h^{-1} carbohydrate alone following intermittent exercise, with a similar response evident after resistance exercise (Beelen et al. 2010). This reduction in post-exercise carbohydrate requirements is advantageous for strength athletes working off a tighter energy budget such as females and those aiming to reduce body fat levels.

As discussed previously, the ingestion of protein after resistance exercise stimulates muscle protein synthesis, inhibits protein breakdown, and allows for net muscle protein accretion. Carbohydrate ingestion during recovery attenuates the exercise-induced increase in protein breakdown but does not affect protein synthesis rates. This means that post-exercise intake of carbohydrate alone improves net muscle protein balance, but in order for the net balance to become positive (and for muscle protein accretion to occur) protein must be ingested (Churchward-Venne et al. 2012). In light of the inhibitory effect of carbohydrate consumption on muscle protein breakdown, a number of studies have investigated whether the co-ingestion of protein and carbohydrate after resistance exercise could enhance net muscle protein accretion over and above that of protein alone. Staples and colleagues (2011) reported that the addition of 50 g of carbohydrate to a 25-g dose of whey protein after an acute bout of resistance exercise resulted in similar rates of muscle protein synthesis and breakdown as compared to the ingestion of 25 g of whey protein alone in young men. These findings, which are corroborated by the results of a number of other studies, indicate that when protein intake is sufficient, carbohydrate does not further enhance post-exercise muscle protein turnover (Phillips and Van Loon 2011).

HYDRATION

In order to allow for the most intense training possible, strength athletes should be encouraged to undertake resistance training in a state of euhydration. This is supported by evidence showing that when resistance training is commenced in a hypohydrated state (reduction in body weight of ~2.5% to 3%), there is a reduction in workload capacity (Kraft et al. 2012). While it may be argued that 2.5% to 3% hypohydration is unlikely to occur in an athlete undertaking a typical resistance training session, it must be acknowledged that resistance exercise forms only one component of the training program for many strength athletes. Furthermore, a substantial number of athletes, even those competing at an elite level, have been shown to arrive at training in a state of hypohydration (Maughan et al. 2004). Therefore, strength athletes should be advised to follow general hydration guidelines for all athletes (Shirreffs and Sawka 2011). This means making use of fluids during training and implementing rehydration strategies after exercise. When viewed from an integrated perspective, consumption of a liquid form of protein and carbohydrate after resistance training would provide a convenient way for strength athletes to achieve the four goals of recovery—rehydration, restoration of metabolized glycogen, restoration/repair of damaged proteins, and remodeling proteins (Phillips and Van Loon 2011). This may be particularly relevant in athletes who struggle to consume sufficient food intake post-exercise for practical or physiological reasons. Bovine fluid milk represents an excellent option for strength athletes when consumed as a post-exercise recovery drink. Consumption of milk in the immediate period after resistance exercise has been shown to augment lean mass gain over several weeks and, from a rehydration perspective, has also been shown to be equivalent or better than water and isotonic sports drinks for the restoration of fluid balance (Watson et al. 2008). While the quantity of milk required to provide ~20 g of protein (~600 mL skimmed milk provides ~30 g of carbohydrate; see Table 4.1) may not deliver sufficient carbohydrate for strength athletes in whom glycogen repletion is a priority, flavored versions of milk (i.e., chocolate), which contain added carbohydrate as a simple sugar, can be used (600 mL skimmed chocolate milk: ~20 g protein, ~70 g carbohydrate). Therefore, milk, and its flavored varieties, would be a cost-effective alternative to supplements to enhance recovery (Phillips and Van Loon 2011).

NUTRITION TO MANIPULATE BODY COMPOSITION

While the expression of strength has a significant neural component, it is also closely associated with skeletal muscle mass. Thus, muscle mass is an important determinant of performance in strength-power sports and achieving and/or maintaining gains in muscle mass represents an important goal for many of these athletes. An athlete's ability to achieve gains in lean body mass is influenced by characteristics of the resistance training program, training experience, gender, genetics, and, to some degree, nutrition (Burke 2007). Nutritional tactics proposed to support lean body mass gains include being in a positive energy balance, protein-related strategies discussed previously, and the strategic timing of carbohydrate intake around workouts.

A positive energy balance promotes an increase in body mass partitioned into lean body mass and body fat. Even in the absence of a training stimulus, overfeeding is associated with a gain in lean body mass provided that a moderate to high protein intake is consumed (Bray et al. 2012). Regrettably, most studies of caloric overfeeding have been undertaken with sedentary participants and the interaction between overfeeding and resistance exercise on body composition has not been well characterized. The magnitude of the positive energy balance needed to maximize gains in lean body mass is an area of contention. This relates to the fact that a gain in fat mass is usually undesirable for strength and power athletes, many of whom need to maximize the ratio of strength or power to body mass (Slater and Phillips 2011). Ideally, added energy to promote positive energy balance should support gains in lean mass while minimizing gains in body fat; however, this is a hard point to define. While further study is required to determine the optimal increase in energy intake to achieve this goal, a practical target of ~500 kcal d^{-1} over requirements has been suggested by sports nutrition experts (Burke 2007). In the absence of resistance exercise, such a daily increase would theoretically result in an increase in fat mass of ~0.4 kg wk^{-1} (~1 lb wk^{-1}); however, some lean mass would also be gained (Bray et al. 2012). When calculating the increase in energy intake required, the athlete should also take into account the energy costs of additional training sessions performed to promote muscle gains. Hence, surfeit energy intakes should be equivalent to cover the energy cost of the increased training load and sufficient to promote gains in lean mass. Changes in body composition should be monitored over a sustained period and energy intake adjusted if weight gain is insufficient or if body weight gain as fat mass exceeds acceptable levels. Evidence from sedentary populations indicates that the changes in body composition induced by several weeks of positive energy balance are influenced by the protein content of the diet (Bray et al. 2012). In this study, higher protein intakes (15% to 25% of energy) were associated with greater lean body mass accrual without additional fat mass gain compared to diets lower in protein (5%) energy (Bray et al. 2012). Further work is required in resistance trained athletes to determine if protein intakes higher than 25%, which are often consumed by resistance-trained athletes, are even more effective during periods of positive energy balance in facilitating greater gains in lean body mass and muscle function while attenuating the rise in body fat. In addition, some evidence exists to suggest that longer duration weight gain periods and nutrition counseling may be advantageous in supporting lean mass gains while minimizing the impact on body fat in elite athletes (Garthe et al. 2011a).

A strategy that strength and power athletes may use to increase total energy intake is by consuming carbohydrate before, during, and after the workout. This will help the athlete to achieve a positive energy balance and, as discussed under carbohydrate needs previously, may promote better training during prolonged workouts. The consumption of protein after workouts, with attention to dose, source, and daily timing pattern, would also be a key strategy for athletes to enhance adaptations to training and promote hypertrophy over time as we have detailed under protein needs.

REDUCING BODY FAT

Olympic lifting and powerlifting are weight division sports, meaning that moderately low body fat levels are required in these athletes to optimize their power-to-body mass ratio. In bodybuilding, low body fat levels are desired during competitive periods to enhance aesthetic appearance. Thus, achieving reductions in body fat represents a common body composition target for many of these athletes. Attempts to reduce body fat through dieting (i.e., intentional weight loss through induction of a negative energy balance) are frequently accompanied by reduction in muscle mass (Weinheimer et al. 2010). Although the performance implications of a decrease in skeletal muscle are unknown in bodybuilders, given the aesthetic component and subjective nature of the competition, the loss of skeletal muscle mass in lifters may compromise strength and therefore performance (Slater and Phillips 2011). To avoid this situation, nutritional strategies should be employed to decrease fat mass while preserving muscle. A large body of evidence shows that higher protein intakes, at the expense of carbohydrates, can enhance both the preservation of muscle mass and the loss of fat mass during periods of energy restriction (Wycherley et al. 2012). Moreover, it appears that a synergism exists between resistance exercise training and high protein intakes during weight loss, resulting in an even greater ratio of fat-to-lean mass loss when the two strategies are combined (Mettler et al. 2010). In a systematic review and pseudo-meta-analysis, Helms and colleagues (2014) recently evaluated the effects of dietary protein intake on body composition in energy-restricted, resistance-trained, lean athletes in an attempt to develop protein intake recommendations for these athletes. However, highlighting the lack of available research in this area, of the six studies included in the review, only two actually compared well-matched groups of athletes consuming different protein intakes (Mettler et al. 2010; Walberg et al. 1988). In the absence of sufficient data necessary to make a truly evidence-based recommendation, protein intakes of ~1.8–2.7 g kg^{-1} d^{-1} (or ~2.3–3.1 g kg^{-1} fat-free mass) have been proposed (Helms et al. 2014; Phillips and Van Loon 2011). In addition, a meta-analysis of randomized controlled trials (Abargouei et al. 2012) showed that hypoenergetic diets that contained a high quantity of dairy foods result in a significantly greater weight loss, fat mass reduction, and lean mass retention/gain compared to conventional calorie-restricted diets, suggesting that strength athletes may benefit from high dairy consumption. A number of bioactive components in dairy foods may contribute to this effect. For example, the amino acid leucine, which is highly enriched in milk proteins, is a potent stimulus for muscle protein synthesis and may be critically important for the muscle-sparing effect. The enhancement of fat loss may involve potential antiadipogenic and prolipolytic effects of leucine and calcium, increased fecal fat excretion, a decrease in fat absorption, and an increase in fat oxidation. Other mechanisms that may account for the efficacy of high protein diets include thermogenic and satiety-promoting effects, which are greater than are those of carbohydrate and fat (Phillips and Van Loon 2011).

The rate of weight loss (and therefore severity of energy deficit) has also been shown to influence changes in body composition and strength performance in elite athletes (Garthe et al. 2011b). Therefore, strength power athletes should allow sufficient time to achieve weight/fat loss goals, aiming for a slow rate of weight loss of approximately 0.5 kg wk^{-1} via a moderate energy deficit of ~500 kcal d^{-1} (although there will be individual differences). In order to manage recovery goals within a tight energy budget, athletes should be encouraged to time their meals so that one of the planned meals during the day coincides with the immediate post-exercise recovery period, rather than consuming an extra recovery meal (Sundgot-Borgen and Garthe 2011).

While a slow controlled loss of weight for competition or training purposes represents an ideal situation, in practice athletes and sports dietitians/nutritionists may not always have extended periods of time available to modify body composition. Mettler and colleagues (2010) reported that consuming protein at the upper end of the acceptable macronutrient distribution ranges (AMDR) outlined by the U.S./Canadian dietary guidelines committee (i.e., 35% of dietary energy from protein) during a 2-week period of marked energy restriction (40% reduction in energy intake) resulted in the preservation of lean mass and the loss of ~1.2 kg fat mass in resistance-trained athletes. This was in contrast to a control group consuming 15% energy from protein (~1 g kg^{-1} d^{-1}) that lost similar body fat but also experienced a significant reduction in lean body mass. Of note, the preservation of lean body mass in the high protein group resulted in less absolute weight loss compared to the standard protein control group, which may need to be considered when devising nutritional plans for athletes in whom the primary goal is simply to "make weight" rather than optimizing fat-to-muscle mass ratio.

In another study, 30 days of a ketogenic diet (~22.0 g d^{-1} carbohydrate, 2.8 g kg^{-1} d^{-1} protein) combined with normal training resulted in a ~1.9 kg loss of fat mass with no loss of lean body mass and no decrements in explosive strength performance in elite male gymnasts (Paoli et al. 2012). The authors of this study reported that, at first, some athletes complained that they were unable to complete workouts, but these effects were transient and disappeared after the first week of the ketogenic diet allowing all of the athletes to train as they normally would. The authors attributed this to a keto-adaptation period of ~7 days that is required for full metabolic adjustment to the diet. As such, a ketogenic diet may not be ideal as a very short-term strategy (several days) to induce body fat/weight loss without impairing performance. In the same vein, athletes who intermittently consume carbohydrates during a ketogenic diet may reduce their ability to train effectively (Paoli et al. 2012). Thus, when adequate time is available (~30 days), very low carbohydrate ketogenic diets may be a potential nutritional strategy to achieve substantial reductions in body fat without impairing strength performance. However, further work is required to confirm the efficacy of these diets in strength power athletes and to determine the optimal dietary protocol.

In summary, in order to reduce body fat levels while preserving muscle mass in strength athletes, they should be encouraged to consume higher protein intakes ~1.8–2.7 g kg^{-1} d^{-1} (~2.3–3.1 g kg^{-1} fat free mass) that would form up to 35% of an athlete's total energy intake, while continuing to incorporate the strategies related to protein dose, source, and timing around training, which have been shown to enhance muscle hypertrophy. Ideally, athletes should assume a moderate energy restriction (energy deficit of ~500 kcal d^{-1}) to allow gradual reductions in body fat/weight (~0.5 kg wk^{-1}). However, when more rapid reductions are required, combining a more severe energy restriction with protein intakes toward the higher end of the range recommended above may help to reduce the loss of skeletal muscle. Reducing carbohydrate to ~40% of energy (with an emphasis on low GI sources) may facilitate fat loss (Phillips and Van Loon 2011). This usually means reducing carbohydrate to 3–4 g kg^{-1} d^{-1}; however, the decision regarding the level of carbohydrate restriction should be dictated by how much training performance may be compromised by consuming lower than recommended carbohydrates (Phillips and Van Loon 2011). Consuming carbohydrate strategically around workouts would help to ensure adequate carbohydrate availability to support intense training and may potentially help to compensate for low total carbohydrate intake over the day. Severe energy restriction (<30 kcal kg^{-1} d fat-free mass) should be avoided as it is associated with menstrual dysfunction, hormonal imbalance, and detrimental effects on bone mineral density (Sundgot-Borgen and Garthe 2011). Although most of the research into the consequences of low energy availability has been conducted in females, some studies indicate that males are also at risk of adverse consequences including loss of lean mass and possibly performance decrements but also metabolically based problems (Sundgot-Borgen and Garthe 2011).

COMPETITION NUTRITION

There is little evidence that acute nutritional strategies can enhance competition performance in lifters and throwers (Slater and Phillips 2011). During competition, these athletes are provided with a designated number of opportunities to achieve a maximal weight or distance, with significant recovery between each effort. Therefore, muscle fuel reserves are unlikely to limit performance. In contrast to the throwing events, Olympic weightlifting, powerlifting, and bodybuilding are weight-category sports. While sufficient time should be allocated to achieve the specified weight-category, in practice strength athletes remain vulnerable to rapid weight loss tactics to "make weight" such as acute food/fluid restriction, resulting in a state of glycogen depletion and hypohydration (Slater and Phillips 2011). Although these tactics are usually associated with performance decrements in sports requiring a significant contribution from aerobic and/or anaerobic energy metabolism, activities requiring high power output and absolute strength characteristic of lifting competitions are less likely to be influenced by acute weight loss (Slater and Phillips 2011). Furthermore, the weigh-in is usually performed 2 h before a weightlifting competition, giving athletes time to at least partially recover from any acute weight loss strategies. Nevertheless, strength athletes should be strongly discouraged from using extreme weight loss methods that place their health at risk. In the 24 to 48 h before competition weigh-in, acute weight loss strategies that may be safe and appropriate include the use of low residue, low volume diets, and moderate fluid restriction. In combination, these strategies can safely induce a 2% to 3% reduction in body mass. However, acute weight loss strategies should always be undertaken under the supervision of a sports dietitian/sports medicine professional and should be trialed in training to ensure they are well tolerated by the athlete (Slater and Phillips 2011).

REFERENCES

Abargouei, A.S., M. Janghorbani, M. Salehi-Marzijarani, and A. Esmaillzadeh. 2012. Effect of dairy consumption on weight and body composition in adults: A systematic review and meta-analysis of randomized controlled clinical trials. *Int J Obes (Lond)* 36(12):1485–1493.
Areta, J.L., L.M. Burke, M.L. Ross et al. 2013. Timing and distribution of protein ingestion during prolonged recovery from resistance exercise alters myofibrillar protein synthesis. *J Physiol* 591(9):2319–2331.

Atherton, P.J., K. Smith, T. Etheridge, D. Rankin, and M.J. Rennie. 2010a. Distinct ana-
    bolic signalling responses to amino acids in C2C12 skeletal muscle cells. *Amino Acids*
    38(5):1533–1539.
Atherton, P.J., T. Etheridge, P.W. Watt et al. 2010b. Muscle full effect after oral protein: Time-
    dependent concordance and discordance between human muscle protein synthesis and
    mTORC1 signaling. *Am J Clin Nutr* 92(5):1080–1088.
Beelen, M., R. Koopman, A.P. Gijsen et al. 2008. Protein coingestion stimulates muscle
    protein synthesis during resistance-type exercise. *Am J Physiol Endocrinol Metab*
    295(1):E70–E77.
Beelen, M., L.M. Burke, M.J. Gibala, and L.J. van Loon. 2010. Nutritional strategies to pro-
    mote postexercise recovery. *Int J Sport Nutr Exerc Metab* 20(6):515–532.
Bray, G.A., S.R. Smith, L. de Jonge et al. 2012. Effect of dietary protein content on weight
    gain, energy expenditure, and body composition during overeating: A randomized con-
    trolled trial. *JAMA* 307(1):47–55.
Burd, N.A., D.W. West, D.R. Moore et al. 2011. Enhanced amino acid sensitivity of myofi-
    brillar protein synthesis persists for up to 24 h after resistance exercise in young men.
    J Nutr 141(4):568–573.
Burke, L. 2007. Strength and power sports. In *Practical Sports Nutrition*. M.S. Bahrke, J.
    Park, L. Alexander, and J. Anderson (eds.). Champaign, IL: Human Kinetics.
Burke, L.M., J.A. Winter, D. Cameron-Smith, M. Enslen, M. Farnfield, and J. Decombaz.
    2012. Effect of intake of different dietary protein sources on plasma amino acid profiles
    at rest and after exercise. *Int J Sport Nutr Exerc Metab* 22(6):452–462.
Camera, D.M., D.W. West, N.A. Burd et al. 2012. Low muscle glycogen concentration does not
    suppress the anabolic response to resistance exercise. *J Appl Physiol* 113(2):206–214.
Cermak, N.M., P.T. Res, L.C. de Groot, W.H. Saris, and L.J. van Loon. 2012. Protein supple-
    mentation augments the adaptive response of skeletal muscle to resistance-type exer-
    cise training: A meta-analysis. *Am J Clin Nutr* 96(6):1454–1464.
Chen, J.D., J.F. Wang, K.J. Li et al. 1989. Nutritional problems and measures in elite and
    amateur athletes. *Am J Clin Nutr* 49(5 Suppl):1084–1089.
Churchward-Venne, T.A., N.A. Burd, and S.M. Phillips. 2012. Nutritional regulation of mus-
    cle protein synthesis with resistance exercise: Strategies to enhance anabolism. *Nutr
    Metab (Lond)* 9(1):40.
Faber, M., A.J. Benade, and M. van Eck. 1986. Dietary intake, anthropometric measure-
    ments, and blood lipid values in weight training athletes (body builders). *Int J Sports
    Med* 7(6):342–346.
Faber, M., A.J. Spinnler-Benade, and A. Daubitzer. 1990. Dietary intake, anthropometric
    measurements and plasma lipid levels in throwing field athletes. *Int J Sports Med*
    11(2):140–145.
FAO Expert Consultation. 2013. Dietary protein quality evaluation in human nutrition. http://
    www.fao.org/ag/humannutrition/35978-02317b979a686a57aa4593304ffc17f06.pdf.
Garthe, I., T. Raastad, and J. Sundgot-Borgen. 2011a. Long-term effect of nutritional counsel-
    ling on desired gain in body mass and lean body mass in elite athletes. *Appl Physiol
    Nutr Metab* 36(4):547–554.
Garthe, I., T. Raastad, P.E. Refsnes, A. Koivisto, and J. Sundgot-Borgen. 2011b. Effect of two
    different weight-loss rates on body composition and strength and power-related perfor-
    mance in elite athletes. *Int J Sport Nutr Exerc Metab* 21(2):97–104.
Haff, G.G., M.H. Stone, B.J. Warren et al. 1999. The effect of carbohydrate supplementation
    on multiple sessions and bouts of resistance exercise. *J Strength Cond Res* 13(2):111–117.
Hartman, J.W., D.R. Moore, and S.M. Phillips. 2006. Resistance training reduces whole-body
    protein turnover and improves net protein retention in untrained young males. *Appl
    Physiol Nutr Metab* 31(5):557–564.

Helms, E.R., C. Zinn, D.S. Rowlands, and S.R. Brown. 2014. A systematic review of dietary protein during caloric restriction in resistance trained lean athletes: A case for higher intakes. *Int J Sport Nutr Exerc Metab* 24(2):127–38.

Jacobs, I., P. Kaiser, and P. Tesch. 1981. Muscle strength and fatigue after selective glycogen depletion in human skeletal muscle fibers. *Eur J Appl Physiol Occup Physiol* 46(1):47–53.

Kim, H., S. Lee, and R. Choue. 2011. Metabolic responses to high protein diet in Korean elite bodybuilders with high-intensity resistance exercise. *J Int Soc Sports Nutr* 8:10.

Kraft, J.A., J.M. Green, P.A. Bishop, M.T. Richardson, Y.H. Neggers, and J.D. Leeper. 2012. The influence of hydration on anaerobic performance: A review. *Res Q Exerc Sport* 83(2):282–292.

Maughan, R.J., S.J. Merson, N.P. Broad, and S.M. Shirreffs. 2004. Fluid and electrolyte intake and loss in elite soccer players during training. *Int J Sport Nutr Exerc Metab* 14(3):333–346.

Mettler, S., N. Mitchell, and K.D. Tipton. 2010. Increased protein intake reduces lean body mass loss during weight loss in athletes. *Med Sci Sports Exerc* 42(2):326–337.

Mitchell, J.B., P.C. DiLauro, F.X. Pizza, and D.L. Cavender. 1997. The effect of preexercise carbohydrate status on resistance exercise performance. *Int J Sport Nutr* 7(3):185–196.

Moore, D.R., M.J. Robinson, J.L. Fry et al. 2009. Ingested protein dose response of muscle and albumin protein synthesis after resistance exercise in young men. *Am J Clin Nutr* 89(1):161–168.

Moore, D.R., J. Areta, V.G. Coffey et al. 2012. Daytime pattern of post-exercise protein intake affects whole-body protein turnover in resistance-trained males. *Nutr Metab (Lond)* 9(1):91.

Paoli, A., K. Grimaldi, D. D'Agostino et al. 2012. Ketogenic diet does not affect strength performance in elite artistic gymnasts. *J Int Soc Sports Nutr* 9(1):34.

Phillips, S.M. 2006. Dietary protein for athletes: From requirements to metabolic advantage. *Appl Physiol Nutr Metab* 31(6):647–654.

Phillips, S.M. 2012. Dietary protein requirements and adaptive advantages in athletes. *Br J Nutr* 108(Suppl 2):S158–S167.

Phillips, S.M., K.D. Tipton, A. Aarsland, S.E. Wolf, and R.R. Wolfe. 1997. Mixed muscle protein synthesis and breakdown after resistance exercise in humans. *Am J Physiol* 273(1 Pt 1):E99–E107.

Phillips, S.M., D.R. Moore, and J.E. Tang. 2007. A critical examination of dietary protein requirements, benefits, and excesses in athletes. *Int J Sport Nutr Exerc Metab* 17(Suppl):S58–S76.

Phillips, S.M., and L.J. Van Loon. 2011. Dietary protein for athletes: From requirements to optimum adaptation. *J Sports Sci* 29(Suppl 1):S29–S38.

Res, P.T., B. Groen, B. Pennings et al. 2012. Protein ingestion before sleep improves post-exercise overnight recovery. *Med Sci Sports Exerc* 44(8):1560–1569.

Shirreffs, S.M., and M.N. Sawka. 2011. Fluid and electrolyte needs for training, competition, and recovery. *J Sports Sci* 29(Suppl 1):S39–S46.

Slater, G., and S.M. Phillips. 2011. Nutrition guidelines for strength sports: Sprinting, weightlifting, throwing events, and bodybuilding. *J Sports Sci* 29(Suppl 1):S67–S77.

Staples, A.W., N.A. Burd, D.W. West et al. 2011. Carbohydrate does not augment exercise-induced protein accretion versus protein alone. *Med Sci Sports Exerc* 43(7):1154–1161.

Sundgot-Borgen, J., and I. Garthe. 2011. Elite athletes in aesthetic and Olympic weight-class sports and the challenge of body weight and body compositions. *J Sports Sci* 29(Suppl 1): S101–S114.

Tang, J.E., and S.M. Phillips. 2009. Maximizing muscle protein anabolism: The role of protein quality. *Curr Opin Clin Nutr Metab Care* 12(1):66–71.

Tang, J.E., D.R. Moore, G.W. Kujbida et al. 2009. Ingestion of whey hydrolysate, casein, or soy protein isolate: Effects on mixed muscle protein synthesis at rest and following resistance exercise in young men. *J Appl Physiol* 107(3):987–992.

Tarnopolsky, M.A., J.D. MacDougall, and S.A. Atkinson. 1988. Influence of protein intake and training status on nitrogen balance and lean body mass. *J Appl Physiol* 64(1):187–193.

Tarnopolsky, M.A., S.A. Atkinson, J.D. MacDougall, A. Chesley, S. Phillips, and H.P. Schwarcz. 1992. Evaluation of protein requirements for trained strength athletes. *J Appl Physiol* 73(5):1986–1995.

Walberg, J.L., M.K. Leidy, D.J. Sturgill et al. 1988. Macronutrient content of a hypoenergy diet affects nitrogen retention and muscle function in weight lifters. *Int J Sports Med* 9(4):261–266.

Watson, P., T.D. Love, R.J. Maughan, and S.M. Shirreffs. 2008. A comparison of the effects of milk and a carbohydrate-electrolyte drink on the restoration of fluid balance and exercise capacity in a hot, humid environment. *Eur J Appl Physiol* 104(4):633–642.

Weinheimer, E.M., L.P. Sands, and W.W. Campbell. 2010. A systematic review of the separate and combined effects of energy restriction and exercise on fat-free mass in middle-aged and older adults: Implications for sarcopenic obesity. *Nutr Rev* 68(7):375–388.

Weisgarber, K.D., D.G. Candow, and E.S. Vogt. 2012. Whey protein before and during resistance exercise has no effect on muscle mass and strength in untrained young adults. *Int J Sport Nutr Exerc Metab* 22(6):463–469.

West, D.W., N.A. Burd, V.G. Coffey et al. 2011. Rapid aminoacidemia enhances myofibrillar protein synthesis and anabolic intramuscular signaling responses after resistance exercise. *Am J Clin Nutr* 94(3):795–803.

Wilkinson, S.B., M.A. Tarnopolsky, M.J. Macdonald, J.R. Macdonald, D. Armstrong, and S.M. Phillips. 2007. Consumption of fluid skim milk promotes greater muscle protein accretion after resistance exercise than does consumption of an isonitrogenous and isoenergetic soy-protein beverage. *Am J Clin Nutr* 85(4):1031–1040.

Witard, O.C., S.R. Jackman, L. Breen, K. Smith, A. Selby, and K.D. Tipton. 2014. Myofibrillar muscle protein synthesis rates subsequent to a meal in response to increasing doses of whey protein at rest and after resistance exercise. *Am J Clin Nutr* 99(1):86–95.

Wycherley, T.P., L.J. Moran, P.M. Clifton, M. Noakes, and G.D. Brinkworth. 2012. Effects of energy-restricted high-protein, low-fat compared with standard-protein, low-fat diets: A meta-analysis of randomized controlled trials. *Am J Clin Nutr* 96(6):1281–1298.

5 Dietary Supplements for Strength Power Athletes

Eric S. Rawson, PhD, FACSM
Charles E. Brightbill, MS
Cortney N. Steele, MS
Department of Exercise Science, Bloomsburg
University, Bloomsburg, Pennsylvania

CONTENTS

INTRODUCTION

Strength power athletes, weightlifters, bodybuilders, throwers, etc., are often characterized as a group of individuals who consume an inordinate amount of dietary supplements in an attempt to augment sports performance. A related stereotype is that this group of athletes, if they believe it will improve their performance, will consume dietary supplements regardless of safety. In some cases, both of these stereotypes might be correct, which is of concern. In addition, strength and power are not exclusively a type of athlete but characteristics necessary for success in many sports. Thus, any dietary supplements alleged to improve exercise performance where strength and power are contributing factors to success are candidates for use and abuse by a large number of athletes. This chapter describes the dietary supplement intake behaviors of strength power athletes, and acts as a resource on the safety and efficacy of dietary supplements that may enhance strength and power performance during competition or training.

For a dietary supplement to be valuable for a strength power athlete, or to enhance strength and power in an athlete with other primary sporting objectives, it must enhance performance of high-intensity exercise or improve training adaptations. Additionally, the benefit-to-risk ratio must be acceptable and the supplement must not contain any ingredients banned by sporting organizations. Where possible, this review will focus on data derived from human studies. Although studies that employ animal models offer unique perspectives, species differences in response to dietary supplements can confuse the interpretation of available research. We hope to provide the most practical recommendations possible, and so will focus on clinical trials.

DIETARY SUPPLEMENT BEHAVIORS
OF STRENGTH POWER ATHLETES

Although it may sound like an easy undertaking, determining the dietary supplement behaviors of strength power athletes, or any athletes, can be very difficult. Athletes may not know what they are ingesting, due to mislabeled products (ingredients not listed, substitutions, adulterations) (Newmaster et al. 2013), multi-ingredient products, or products that are administered by coaches without appropriate athlete education. In addition, there are approximately 29,000 dietary supplements available on the U.S. market, and new products arrive regularly. Further, surveys can be fraught with issues such as recall bias that can lead to erroneous results. Designing the survey that captures all available and commonly ingested dietary supplements is a challenge. An additional challenge is how to classify the athletes by training status (e.g., Olympian vs. elite vs. collegiate vs. recreational) and how to include those who exercise intensely and may be elite, but do not participate in an organized or easily documented sport (e.g., professional footballers vs. competitive bodybuilders vs. military warfighters vs. health club members). This review is not meant to summarize the use of all dietary supplements by athletes or by strength power athletes. Only a small number of dietary supplements may be beneficial for strength power athletes, or for athletes for whom strength and power is an important component of their performance or training. These include creatine monohydrate, sodium bicarbonate, β-alanine, protein and amino acids, β-hydroxy β-methyl butyrate (HMB), caffeine, and carbohydrate. This review will focus on these compounds.

Reportedly, dietary supplement use in the general population is as high as 50% in the United States; supplement use appears to be higher in elite athletes. In a review, Maughan et al. (2007) cited data from the International Association of Athletics Federations that suggests dietary supplement use by athletes is about 86% (range 77% to 89%). About 53% used non-vitamin/mineral supplements that could potentially have an ergogenic effect on strength and power performance, such as creatine, protein, and caffeine (Maughan et al. 2007). No obvious differences in dietary supplement use were evident between elite strength power (e.g., 89% of jumpers) and endurance athletes (89% of race walkers). Across all categories of Canadian Olympians, 69% and 74% used some type of dietary supplements at the Atlanta and Sydney Olympic Games, respectively (Huang et al. 2006). Huang et al. (2006) reported that the use of nutritional (non-vitamin/mineral) dietary supplements at these Olympic Games was 39% and 43%. Creatine was the most commonly used non-vitamin/mineral supplement consumed in 1996 (14%), which decreased to 12% in 2000. Conversely, protein and amino acid use increased from 3% to 13% and 7% to 15%, respectively, from 1996 to 2000. The authors observed that dietary supplement use was higher in individual vs. team sport athletes, regardless of the nature of the sport, which is something that should be addressed in future studies.

Heikkinen and colleagues (2011) reported a decrease in dietary supplement use between 2002 and 2009 in a large sample of Finnish Olympians. Total dietary supplement use decreased from 82% to 73%, and non-vitamin/mineral dietary supplement use decreased similarly from 60% to 52%. Consumption of dietary supplements related to strength and power performance decreased significantly or tended to decrease, including protein (47% to 33%), carbohydrates (24% to 16%), and creatine (16% to 8%). Only amino acid ingestion increased (4% to 7%). In speed and power athletes, creatine use was 35% in 2002, decreasing to 19% in 2009. Team sport athletes ingested less creatine at both time points (11% and 6%). Lun et al. (2012) reported similar supplement use (87%) between a large sample of high performance Canadian athletes (n = 440; 76% national/international level) and a subset of power athletes (91%). Interestingly, dietary supplement use in endurance athletes within this sample was also similar (91%). Power athletes reported taking dietary supplements to increase lean mass or strength (16%) and to enhance recovery (18%). Less than half (40%) of power athletes reported attendance at some type of dietary supplement workshop, indicating a lack of formal education on the use of sports supplements.

Froiland et al. (2004) reported on dietary supplement use in 203 non-endurance sport Division I collegiate athletes. Eighty-nine percent were current or former supplement users, with energy drinks (74%), protein (48%), creatine (37%), caffeine (11%), and HMB (8%) use reported. About 43% took supplements to improve strength and power and about 43% for weight or muscle gain. Goston and Correia (2010) reported dietary supplement intake in 1102 health club members from 50 gyms in Belo Horizonte, Brazil. Most participants performed strength training (83%), and about half of them (46%) exercised to improve muscle strength or mass. Only 36% of all gym members reported supplement use (28% of women; 45% of men), but 58% of users ingested supplements related to strength and power development (i.e., creatine, protein/amino acids, HMB). When analyzed individually, use of these supplements seemed low compared to competitive athletes (8% creatine, 6% branched chain amino acids [BCAAs], 1% HMB).

The prevalence of dietary supplement use in elite athletes appears higher than the general population. Elite athletes commonly ingest dietary supplements to increase strength/power or gain lean mass/weight. As dietary supplement adulteration, substitution, and contamination is a real problem (see Chapter 8), strength and power athletes should be made aware of the benefit-to-risk ratio of dietary supplement use. The following section summarizes published data on the small number of dietary supplements that may be beneficial for strength power athletes, or for athletes for whom strength and power are important components of their performance or training. Additionally, risk of adverse events documented through research is discussed.

CREATINE MONOHYDRATE

Creatine is a non-essential nutrient that is produced in the body (≈1 to 2 g/d) and consumed in the diet through the consumption of meat, poultry, and fish (3 to 4 g creatine/kg meat). About 95% of creatine is stored in skeletal muscle (124.4 mmol/kg dry muscle [dm] total creatine; 49 mmol/kg dm free creatine; 75.5 mmol/kg dm phosphorylcreatine) (Harris et al. 1974), where it is used to sustain adenosine triphosphate (ATP) levels during times of high energy need. The creatine kinase energy system, where phosphorylcreatine donates its phosphate to adenosine diphosphate (ADP) to remake ATP, can maintain ATP levels for about 8 to 10 sec at maximal exercise intensity. Muscle creatine is degraded non-enzymatically to creatinine and excreted in the urine.

In 1993, Harris et al. (1992) published a seminal paper describing increased muscle creatine levels following creatine monohydrate ingestion. These data have been validated many times over the years using either the muscle biopsy technique or nuclear magnetic resonance spectroscopy. On average, creatine monohydrate supplementation results in about a 20% increase in muscle creatine. Increased muscle creatine levels can be achieved with a short-term high-dose protocol (about 20 g/d for about 5 d) or a longer-term lower-dose protocol (about 3 g/d for about 30 d), and muscle creatine uptake can be enhanced in the presence of exercise, insulin, carbohydrate, or combined carbohydrate and protein (reviewed by Gualano et al. 2012). It appears that elevated muscle creatine levels can be maintained indefinitely with a small daily dose (2 to 5 g), but this cannot be confirmed as there are few studies lasting longer than several weeks. Both high- and low-dose protocols result in an increase in the performance of brief high-intensity exercise, particularly when there are repeated bouts (Gualano et al. 2012; Rawson et al. 2011).

The effects of creatine monohydrate supplementation on exercise performance have been investigated in hundreds of studies and have been extensively reviewed (Branch 2003; Gualano et al. 2012; Rawson and Volek 2003; Volek and Rawson 2004). In a meta-analysis, Branch (2003) concluded that creatine monohydrate supplementation improves the performance of brief (<30 sec), high-intensity exercise, especially when there are repeated bouts. Whether creatine monohydrate can benefit a strength power athlete depends on training/competition exercise intensity and duration. The magnitude of the effect of creatine monohydrate supplementation on sports performance is small in absolute terms, but significant to an elite athlete; for example, a decrease of 0.9 sec in a 100-m sprint or a 1.8 sec decrease in two successive 100-m swims (Gualano et al. 2012). Table 5.1 depicts the effects of creatine supplementation on performance as a function of exercise intensity and time.

In a review, Rawson and Persky (2007) highlighted the mechanisms through which creatine monohydrate supplementation potentially exerts an ergogenic effect. These include adaptations that occur before (increased muscle phosphorylcreatine and glycogen), during (increased phosphorylcreatine resynthesis rate), and after (reduced inflammation/muscle damage, increased expression of growth factors, lower protein degradation) exercise, potentially causing a spontaneous increase in training volume. In fact, the greatest benefit of creatine monohydrate supplementation for the strength power athlete is, perhaps, improved performance during strength and conditioning outside of competition. In a narrative review, Rawson and Volek (2003) reported a greater increase in strength and resistance exercise performance when creatine supplementation was combined with resistance training, compared to resistance training and placebo ingestion (see Figures 5.1 and 5.2).

The safety of creatine monohydrate ingestion has been well addressed and better studied than most sports dietary supplements (Gualano et al. 2012; Lopez et al. 2009; Persky and Rawson 2007). It appears that when recommended doses are ingested,

TABLE 5.1
Effects of Creatine Supplementation on Performance as a Function of Exercise Intensity and Duration

Variable	Effect
ATP-PCr system (≤300 s)	
Arm ergometry	↔
Bicycle ergometry	↑
Isokinetic torque production	↑
Isometric force production	↑
Isotonic strength	↑
Jumping	↑
Sprint running	↑
Speed skating	↑
Swimming	↑
Glycolysis (30–150 s)	
Bicycle ergometry	↑
Isokinetic torque production	↔
Isometric force production	↑
Isotonic strength	↑
Jumping	↔
Kayaking	↔
Sprint running	↔
Swimming	↔
Oxidative phosphorylation (>150 s)	
Bicycle ergometry	↑
Isokinetic torque production	↔
Isotonic strength	↔
Kayaking	↔
Sprint running	↔
Swimming	↔/↓
Rowing	↔

Source: Adapted from Gualano, B. et al. 2012. *Amino Acids* 43(2):519–529 and based on the meta-analysis from Branch, J.D. 2003. *Int J Sport Nutr Exerc Metab* 13(2):198–226.

Note: ↔ no effect, ↑ improvement, ↓ impairment.

creatine monohydrate is safe in terms of muscular, cardiovascular, renal, hepatic, and thermoregulatory function. Of greater importance is the proliferation of "novel" creatine supplement products sold under the premise of increased absorption, greater muscle uptake, and larger improvements in exercise performance relative to creatine monohydrate (Jäger et al. 2011). There appear to be no data to support such claims, which is not surprising as the absorption of creatine monohydrate is approximately 100%. More worrisome is the fact that unlike creatine monohydrate, safety data are

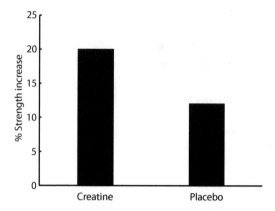

FIGURE 5.1 Effects of creatine supplementation and concurrent resistance training on maximal strength (1-, 3-, and 10-RM). (Adapted from Rawson, E.S., and J.S. Volek. 2003. *J Strength Cond Res* 17(4):822–831.)

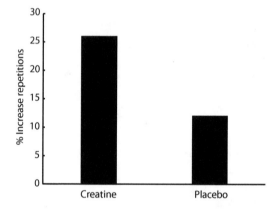

FIGURE 5.2 Effects of creatine supplementation on resistance exercise performance (repetitions at a given percentage of maximal strength). (Adapted from Rawson, E.S., and J.S. Volek. 2003. *J Strength Cond Res* 17(4):822–831.)

scant or completely unavailable for these products. In fact, some of these products contain little creatine, or appear to be pro-creatinine, and do not increase muscle creatine levels (Giese and Lecher 2009; Harris et al. 2004). If a strength and power athlete chooses to use creatine supplements, there is no reason for him or her to use a non-creatine monohydrate product.

BUFFERS

The effects of sodium bicarbonate ($NaHCO_3$) supplementation on exercise performance have been well studied and reviewed in both meta-analytic (Carr et al. 2011;

Matson and Tran 1993; Peart et al. 2012) and narrative (Jones 2014) formats. Intense exercise increases H^+ accumulation, potentially reduces force production, and hastens fatigue. $NaHCO_3$ is a buffer and, when ingested in high enough doses, can increase the bicarbonate $\left(HCO_3^-\right)$ concentration of the extracellular fluid from 25 to 30 mmol/L, which can slow acidosis-related fatigue (Jones 2014). Over two decades ago, Matson and Tran (1993) conducted a meta-analytic review of 29 investigations into the effects of $NaHCO_3$ supplementation on anaerobic exercise performance. They reported an effect size of 0.44, which is possibly a 0.8-sec improvement in a 1-min race. More recently, Peart et al. (2012) reported a slightly smaller effect size (0.36) in a meta-analysis of 40 studies, and Carr et al. (2011) demonstrated a 1.7% improvement in performance during a 1-min sprint in their meta-analysis. Thus, there is convincing evidence of a small benefit of $NaHCO_3$ supplementation on the performance of brief intense exercise. Although the benefits of $NaHCO_3$ ingestion are typically small, they can be very meaningful for an elite athlete. One unanswered question that remains is whether trained and untrained subjects experience similar benefits of supplementation, as both theories have been put forth (Carr et al. 2011; Peart et al. 2012).

$NaHCO_3$ ingestion of 0.3 to 0.5 g/kg body mass 1 to 2 h before exercise is a prudent recommendation, but athletes should practice supplementation strategies outside of competition. $NaHCO_3$ supplementation is well known to cause gastrointestinal disturbances in as much as 50% of research volunteers, which could be detrimental to performance. To maximize the benefit-to-risk ratio, it appears best to ingest $NaHCO_3$ in serial doses in combination with a carbohydrate meal or snack. In fact, it has been recommended that $NaHCO_3$ be ingested over 3 to 5 days at a dose of 100 to 150 mg/kg body mass. As Jones (2014) has noted, this might be best for athletes who have multiple events in the same day or over several days. Although acute $NaHCO_3$ supplementation has proven successful as an ergogenic aid in sprinting type activities lasting 1 to 7 min, there are few studies of $NaHCO_3$ supplementation with resistance training outcomes. Both Carr et al. (2013) and Duncan et al. (2014) reported improved resistance exercise performance (i.e., increased repetitions) following acute $NaHCO_3$ supplementation. This introduces the concept of more prolonged supplementation, which could improve resistance-training adaptations, and subsequently sports performance. However, this remains to be seen. Strength power athletes attempting to improve sports performance and athletes attempting to improve strength and power outcomes in the weight room should consider the benefit-to-risk ratio (improved performance vs. gastrointestinal distress) and whether their sport or training program supports a use for an enhanced buffer system based on exercise intensity (maximal vs. submaximal) and duration (1 to 7 min vs. less than 1 min).

Much like HCO_3^- is a strong extracellular buffer, the dipeptide carnosine (β-alanyl-L-histidine) is a robust intracellular buffer. Carnosine is more highly concentrated in type II vs. type I fibers, in sprinters vs. marathon runners, and in animals that rely heavily on anaerobic energy production for hunting or fleeing (e.g., canines, deer) or surviving under hypoxic conditions (e.g., whales) (reviewed in Harris et al. 2012). Additionally, muscle carnosine content may increase with sprint exercise training, but this has not been shown in every case. As plasma carnosine is quickly hydrolyzed by carnosinase in humans, carnosine supplementation as a means to increase muscle carnosine content is likely ineffective. However, the amino acid β-alanine, which is the limiting factor in endogenous carnosine synthesis, can be used to increase muscle carnosine content (Figure 5.3).

As with creatine monohydrate supplementation, the seminal research on β-alanine supplementation was conducted by Harris and colleagues (2006). Since 2006, research on β-alanine supplementation increased exponentially, and meta-analytic (Hobson et al. 2012), systematic (Quesnele et al. 2014), and narrative reviews have been published (Artioli et al. 2010; Harris and Sale 2012; Sale et al. 2010, 2013). Hobson et al. (2012) analyzed the results of 15 studies and reported a 2.85% improvement in performance following β-alanine supplementation. Thus, much like creatine monohydrate and NaHCO₃ supplementation, there appears to be a small absolute effect, but one that could be very meaningful to an elite athlete. In practical terms, time in a 1500-m run (about 4 min) could potentially be reduced by as much as 6 sec (Hobson et al. 2012), but an effect of this size is doubtful in an elite athlete. Interestingly, Hobson et al. (2012) separated performance outcomes into three distinct time periods, and found that exercise lasting >240 sec and from 60 to 240 sec was improved with supplementation, but there was no benefit in tasks lasting less than 60 sec. This makes sense, as the cause of fatigue in exercise lasting less than

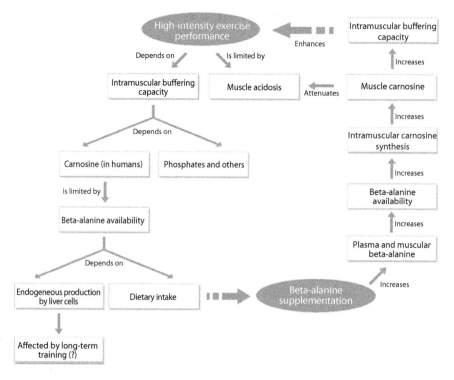

FIGURE 5.3   Overview of the role of β-alanine supplementation on high-intensity exercise performance. (From Artioli, G.G. et al. 2010. *Med Sci Sports Exerc* 42(6):1162–1173. With permission.)

60 sec is unlikely to be severe acidosis. Although β-alanine supplementation can increase power output in certain intense exercises, whether it can improve resistance exercise performance like creatine monohydrate is unclear (Kendrick et al. 2008). Any benefits on resistance training outcomes are likely dependent on the nature of the training program (repetitions, volume, rest periods, etc.).

In a systematic review of 19 studies, Quesnele et al. (2014) reported a range of supplement doses of 2.0 to 6.4 g per day for durations of 4 to 13 weeks. Although an exact recommended dose is currently unknown, a sensible supplementation regimen supported by research is 3 to 6 g per day for 4 to 8 weeks (Jones 2014). This appears adequate to increase muscle carnosine content by about 40% to 50%, and these levels remain elevated for about 10 to 15 weeks after supplementation is discontinued. There are few data on the safety of β-alanine supplementation; however, as it is an amino acid, serious adverse events would not be expected. The only known side effect to date is paresthesia (flushing), but this appears to have been resolved with timed-release supplements.

PROTEIN AND AMINO ACIDS

Dietary protein is made up of 20 different amino acids consisting of 9 essential amino acids (EAA), 3 of which are BCAAs, and 11 nonessential amino acids (NEAA). A complete review of the biochemistry of protein is beyond this chapter, which focuses on supplementation. A more detailed review of the effects of protein and amino acids is available in Chapter 4.

The recommended dietary allowance (RDA) of protein for adults is 0.8 g/kg body mass/d. It has been demonstrated, on many occasions, that this is not adequate to support the needs of intensely training athletes. The recommended intake of protein for strength power athletes is generally about 1.6 to 1.7 g/kg/d, or about twice the RDA. However, it appears that strength power athletes easily achieve at least this much in the diet (reviewed in Slater and Phillips 2011), with some ingesting as much as 3.2 g/kg/d (Chen et al. 1989). Fox and co-workers (2011) reported that collegiate male athletes are either completely unaware of the current protein intake recommendations (67%) or perceive them to be higher than they actually are (8.7 g/kg/d). The ingestion of dietary protein above 1.7 g/kg/d results in increased amino acid catabolism and protein oxidation and does not encourage greater muscle hypertrophy (Moore et al. 2009).

Muscle protein synthesis is increased following ingestion of an intact protein or a mixture of amino acids. Immediately following exercise, the consumption of about 20 g of protein (with about 8 to 10 g of EAA) is recommended to maximally stimulate protein synthesis, while increasing this amount to 40 g only serves to increase leucine oxidation (Moore et al. 2009). To promote protein synthesis throughout the day, consuming 0.25 to 0.30 g of protein/kg body mass/meal (about 20 to 25 g/meal) is recommended. In terms of protein type or quality, athletes should ingest proteins that have high levels of EEAs, in particular leucine, which are necessary for the best stimulation. In addition to EEA and leucine content, it appears that rate of digestion is an important factor in optimizing protein synthesis. For instance, Tang et al. (2009) reported that whey protein increased muscle mixed protein synthesis 93%

more than casein and 18% more than soy under resting conditions, and 122% and 31% more than casein and soy, respectively, after resistance exercise. Recently, van Loon and colleagues (Beelen et al. 2008; Res et al. 2012; van Loon 2013) reported that the consumption of protein following an evening training session was only enough to optimize protein synthesis acutely, and that overnight recovery was suboptimal. This group demonstrated a 22% higher rate of muscle protein synthesis during the overnight period with the consumption of 40 g of casein protein 30 min before sleep (Res et al. 2012). More research needs to be conducted, and long-term data are unavailable, but if a strength power athlete is training intensely, bedtime protein ingestion may help optimize overnight protein synthesis and help improve training adaptations.

A recent meta-analysis of 22 studies revealed that prolonged resistance training (>6 weeks) combined with protein supplementation resulted in larger increases in fat-free mass (38%), type I muscle fiber cross-sectional area (CSA) (45%), type II muscle fiber CSA (54%), and 1-RM leg press strength (20%) compared to training with placebo ingestion (Cermak et al. 2012). Thus, it appears that protein ingestion is a safe and effective way for strength power athletes to optimize recovery from, and adapt to, intense exercise training. Protein supplements appear beneficial, but whether they are necessary is unknown, especially given that most strength power athletes appear to ingest adequate protein. However, in terms of optimizing timing (consume immediately post-exercise, every 3 to 4 h, and before bedtime) and convenience, protein supplements provide an important nutritional option for strength power athletes. It is best if athletes viewed protein supplements as "supplements," and high protein foods as sources of EAAs as well as other important essential nutrients such as iron, zinc, and fatty acids.

β-HYDROXY β-METHYLBUTYRATE (HMB)

HMB is a metabolite of the EAA leucine. Much of the research on HMB supplementation focuses on the effects of HMB on body composition of farm animals (i.e., broiler chickens, cows, pigs, etc.). Since 1996, about 40 human supplementation studies have been published, and narrative (Zanchi et al. 2011) and systematic (Molfino et al. 2013) reviews are available. HMB, like leucine, is anti-catabolic, and can potentially decrease protein breakdown and muscle damage caused by stressful exercise. This would make HMB a valuable supplement for recovery from intense training or competition. The literature on HMB, however, is more difficult to interpret than for other strength power supplements.

Early studies and a meta-analysis (Nissen and Sharp 2003) of nine studies indicated that HMB supplementation reduced muscle damage and increased strength and lean mass. This analysis and early studies have been criticized because the nine studies were essentially completed by three groups. Additional criticisms were use of unreliable markers to assess muscle damage (e.g., creatine kinase instead of force production), overlooking the repeated bout effect (i.e., muscle damage decreases with training) in trained subjects, and failure to disclose conflicts of interest (financial relationships and patents). More recently, Molfino and colleagues (2013) analyzed 22 studies of HMB supplementation in healthy young adults, and reported that HMB supplementation increased fat-free mass in 4 of 10 studies and strength in 7 of 14 studies. Recommended daily dosage of HMB is about 3 g per day, and although it appears safe, there are few safety data available. HMB, like creatine monohydrate, may benefit older adults or individuals with certain atrophic diseases; however, unlike creatine monohydrate, the benefits of HMB for strength power athletes are unclear. In terms of sales, HMB has not experienced the same popularity as creatine monohydrate, protein, and β-alanine in strength power athletes. It is unclear if trained or untrained individuals benefit more from HMB ingestion, but it has been proposed that HMB supplementation would be more beneficial for beginning than for advanced trainers.

Recently, Wilson et al. (2014) reported greater increases in lean mass (7.4 vs. 2.1 kg), total strength (bench press + squat + deadlift) (77 vs. 25 kg), and power (991 vs. 630 watts) in HMB-Free Acid (HMB-FA) vs. placebo supplemented subjects following 12 weeks of resistance exercise. These results are promising, but gains such as these in trained subjects rival the improvements acquired from high dose testosterone administration (HMB-FA supplementation [3 g/d for 12 weeks] plus resistance training = 7.4 kg increase in lean mass; testosterone enanthate supplementation [600 mg/week for 10 weeks] plus resistance training = 6.1 kg increase in fat free mass [Bhasin et al. 1996]) in untrained subjects. Wilkinson and colleagues (2013) reported that consumption of about 3 g of HMB-FA stimulated muscle protein synthesis, increased anabolic signaling, and attenuated muscle protein breakdown, which highlights the mechanism through which HMB supplementation might alter lean mass during resistance exercise. Although promising, research on HMB-FA is in its infancy, and much more work needs to be done before it can be recommended.

CAFFEINE

As a potential ergogenic aid, caffeine (1, 3, 7-trimethylxanthine) has been studied for over a century, and today is a common ingredient of energy drinks and many pre-workout supplements. Most research has focused on the effects of caffeine supplementation on submaximal and endurance-based performance, with the majority of studies supporting a positive effect on such activities (Ganio et al. 2009; Spriet 2014). There is also evidence that caffeine supplementation enhances short duration, high intensity, anaerobic-based exercise, which would benefit the training or competition of many strength power athletes (Astorino and Roberson 2010; Davis and Green 2009; Spriet 2014; Warren et al. 2010).

In a review article on caffeine and anaerobic exercise performance, Davis and Green (2009) concluded that caffeine ingestion was most beneficial for speed endurance activities when the duration of the activity lasted between 60 and 180 sec. However, short duration activities (4 to 6 sec) can also be benefited when the activities are more sport specific. For instance, in a simulated rugby game, Stuart et al. (2005) demonstrated an improvement in sprint speed, agility performance, peak power, and throwing accuracy in male rugby players who ingested caffeine (6 mg/kg) compared to those who ingested placebo. Caffeine is likely also ergogenic to other team sports such as soccer, lacrosse, and football, with 65% of studies using team sports or power and sprint performance outcomes supporting significant improvements ranging from 1.0% to 20.0% (reviewed by Astorino and Roberson 2010).

There is some evidence that caffeine can benefit both muscular strength (1-RM, 3-RM, etc.) and resistance training performance (repetitions to failure at a given percentage of maximum or lifting volume), although these have not been unanimous outcomes (Astorino and Roberson 2010; Davis and Green 2009). A recent systematic review reported that 6 out of 11 studies supported a significant benefit to resistance training with a mean improvement of 9.4% (Astorino and Roberson 2010). It was also estimated that caffeine supplementation improved resistance training performance (measured by repetitions completed) more than muscular strength (measured by 1 or 3-RM). One study supported an increase in both 1-RM and repetitions to failure at 60% of 1-RM in collegiate male athletes following consumption of a moderate dose of caffeine (5 mg/kg) (Duncan and Oxford 2011). Therefore, there is some evidence to suggest that caffeine ingestion prior to resistance training may provide some advantages; however, more research is needed on the topic.

A full understanding of caffeine's mechanisms of action is currently unknown, although evidence suggests that multiple mechanisms are involved. It has been proposed that caffeine improved exercise performance by increasing the oxidation of fat and decreasing carbohydrate metabolism through a negative feedback loop, but this has been a controversial theory over the years and is no longer thought to be the primary mechanism of action (Spriet 2014). Further, even if caffeine supplementation resulted in glycogen sparing and increased fat oxidation during exercise, it would not explain performance enhancements that would occur during short-term high-intensity exercise. Caffeine is a powerful central nervous system stimulant, increases alertness, and may reduce perceived exertion and decrease pain perception (Astorino and Roberson 2010; Davis and Green 2009). In addition, caffeine can enhance Ca^{2+} release from the sarcoplasmic reticulum, excitation contraction coupling, force production, and motor unit recruitment (Warren et al. 2010).

Low to moderate doses of caffeine ranging from 2.5 to 7 mg/kg have been shown to be ergogenic for a variety of strength and power outcomes including resistance training, sprinting, agility, and sport-specific measures (Astorino and Roberson 2010; Sokmen et al. 2008; Spriet 2014). When caffeine is consumed from sources such as energy drinks, supplements, or gum, doses as low as 1.0 to 2.5 mg/kg are sufficient to improve performance; however, it appears that larger amounts are needed when only caffeine is consumed (Astorino and Roberson 2010). In addition, while low to moderate doses may provide optimal benefits, doses in excess of 6 to 9 mg/kg typically result in adverse effects such as jitters, tachycardia, anxiety, restlessness, insomnia, headaches, and performance decrements.

Plasma concentration levels peak between 30 and 60 min post-consumption, with benefits disappearing approximately 6 h after acute ingestion. Therefore, caffeine should be taken no sooner than 3 h before strength and power events to maximize benefits (Sokmen et al. 2008). Caffeine tolerance may blunt the effects of caffeine, and so habitual caffeine users may choose to withdraw from caffeine prior to an athletic event to maximize benefits. Caffeine withdrawal should begin a minimum of 1 week prior to competition with caffeine intake being slowly decreased over 3 or 4 days to reduce negative effects and training decrements, which can result from an abrupt cessation of caffeine use (Sokmen et al. 2008). Returning to normal levels of caffeine intake on the day of the athletic event will again provide an enhanced ergogenic effect.

CARBOHYDRATE

The ergogenic effects of carbohydrate ingestion for endurance athletes are well known. However, carbohydrate ingestion may be important for strength power athletes as well. High volume resistance training significantly decreases muscle glycogen content, which could increase fatigue and lead to deficits in performance (MacDougall et al. 1999; Robergs et al. 1991; Tesch et al. 1998). Muscle glycogen stores are reduced 20% to 40% during an acute bout of resistance exercise (MacDougall et al. 1999; Tesch et al. 1998), and carbohydrate restriction leads to a decrease in resistance exercise performance (Leveritt and Abernethy 1999). The hypertrophy or endurance phase of some athletes' resistance training programs is characterized by 3 to 20 repetitions, 3 to 5 sets, and 3 to 4 days per week, which relies heavily on carbohydrate for fuel. With that in mind, several research groups have examined the effects of carbohydrate ingestion on strength and power related outcomes (Haff et al. 1999, 2000, 2001; Lambert et al. 1991) (reviewed in Haff et al. 2003).

Carbohydrate (CHO) supplementation prior to (1.0 g CHO/kg body mass) and during (0.17 g CHO/kg body mass) resistance exercise enhanced resistance exercise performance by enabling more sets (+2.7) of leg extensions performed to volitional fatigue (80% of 10-RM) (Lambert et al. 1991). Also, carbohydrate ingestion prior to (1.0 g CHO/kg body mass) and in between sets (0.51 g CHO/kg body mass) increased work and torque during 16 sets of isokinetic leg extensions (10 reps at 120°/s) (Haff et al. 2001). Significant improvements in performance were also seen with consumption of 1.2 g CHO/kg body mass during and between multiple training sessions in one day, resulting in more sets, repetitions, and delayed muscular fatigue (Haff et al. 1999). Conversely, Haff et al. (2000) reported that carbohydrate supplementation prior to (1.0 CHO/kg body mass) and every 10 min during (0.51 g CHO/kg body mass) a 39-min resistance exercise bout did not improve isokinetic leg exercise performance (3 sets of 10 repetitions at 120°/s). Similarly, carbohydrate ingestion of 0.3 g/kg body mass before and after every set of five repetitions at 85% 1-RM did not improve performance or delay fatigue (Kulik et al. 2008).

The characteristics of a resistance exercise training program (intensity, duration, volume, etc.) influence the rate of glycogenolysis (Robergs et al. 1991) and may explain some of the discrepant findings in this small body of literature. For instance, the exercise completed in the studies where carbohydrate ingestion successfully improved resistance exercise performance tended to be longer in duration (56 to 77 min) than those where there was no ergogenic effect of the carbohydrate (28 to 39 min). Unfortunately, there are few studies of the effects of carbohydrate on strength power outcomes and resistance exercise performance, and they are difficult to compare due to differences in supplementation and exercise protocols. More research is warranted to establish the impact of carbohydrate supplementation prior to and during high intensity anaerobic activities such as resistance training.

CONCLUSION

Although the foundation for success in sports continues to be optimal diet and training, there are a small number of dietary supplements that appear to be worthwhile for strength power athletes. Supplements that appear to have a sensible benefit-to-risk ratio include creatine monohydrate, protein, and caffeine, and potentially beta-alanine, sodium bicarbonate, HMB, and carbohydrate. Collectively, these supplements may enhance strength and power performance in the weight room or on the playing field, or enhance recovery from stressful exercise. As with all dietary supplements, consumers must be conscious of quality control issues, legality, and the rules of their sporting organizations. Not enough data are available to conclude if the dietary supplements described in this chapter benefit elite athletes more than beginning or intermediate exercisers. In either scenario, the absolute benefit will be small. The supplements described in this review all work through different mechanisms and pathways, suggesting that their effects may be additive. While this is an alluring thought, and there is some evidence that the combination of some of these supplements may be more beneficial than ingestion of any one individual supplement, there are few data available. Overall, after taking into account the specifics of their sport, training, and diet, it appears that certain dietary supplements may be of benefit to strength power athletes. Athletes should be reminded that dietary supplements are just that, supplements to the diet, and that a poor diet or suboptimal training will place them at a far greater disadvantage than the absence of a particular sports supplement.

REFERENCES

Artioli, G.G., B. Gualano, A. Smith, J. Stout, and A.H. Lancha, Jr. 2010. Role of beta-alanine supplementation on muscle carnosine and exercise performance. *Med Sci Sports Exerc* 42(6):1162–1173.

Astorino, T.A., and D.W. Roberson. 2010. Efficacy of acute caffeine ingestion for short-term high-intensity exercise performance: A systematic review. *J Strength Cond Res* 24(1):257–265.

Beelen, M., M. Tieland, A.P. Gijsen et al. 2008. Coingestion of carbohydrate and protein hydrolysate stimulates muscle protein synthesis during exercise in young men, with no further increase during subsequent overnight recovery. *J Nutr* 138(11):2198–2204.

Bhasin, S., T.W. Storer, N. Berman et al. 1996. The effects of supraphysiologic doses of testosterone on muscle size and strength in normal men. *N Engl J Med* 335(1):1–7.

Branch, J.D. 2003. Effect of creatine supplementation on body composition and performance: A meta-analysis. *Int J Sport Nutr Exerc Metab* 13(2):198–226.

Carr, A.J., W.G. Hopkins, and C.J. Gore. 2011. Effects of acute alkalosis and acidosis on performance: A meta-analysis. *Sports Med* 41(10):801–814.

Carr, B.M., M.J. Webster, J.C. Boyd, G.M. Hudson, and T.P. Scheett. 2013. Sodium bicarbonate supplementation improves hypertrophy-type resistance exercise performance. *Eur J Appl Physiol* 113(3):743–752.

Cermak, N.M., P.T. Res, L.C. de Groot, W.H. Saris, and L.J. van Loon. 2012. Protein supplementation augments the adaptive response of skeletal muscle to resistance-type exercise training: A meta-analysis. *Am J Clin Nutr* 96(6):1454–1464.

Chen, J.D., J.F. Wang, K.J. Li et al. 1989. Nutritional problems and measures in elite and amateur athletes. *Am J Clin Nutr* 49(5 Suppl):1084–1089.

Davis, J.K., and J.M. Green. 2009. Caffeine and anaerobic performance: Ergogenic value and mechanisms of action. *Sports Med* 39(10):813–832.

Duncan, M.J., and S.W. Oxford. 2011. The effect of caffeine ingestion on mood state and bench press performance to failure. *J Strength Cond Res* 25(1):178–185.

Duncan, M.J., A. Weldon, and M.J. Price. 2014. The effect of sodium bicarbonate ingestion on back squat and bench press exercise to failure. *J Strength Cond Res* 28(5):1358–1366.

Fox, E.A., J.L. McDaniel, A.P. Breitbach, and E.P. Weiss. 2011. Perceived protein needs and measured protein intake in collegiate male athletes: An observational study. *J Int Soc Sports Nutr* 8:9.

Froiland, K., W. Koszewski, J. Hingst, and L. Kopecky. 2004. Nutritional supplement use among college athletes and their sources of information. *Int J Sport Nutr Exerc Metab* 14(1):104–120.

Ganio, M.S., J.F. Klau, D.J. Casa, L.E. Armstrong, and C.M. Maresh. 2009. Effect of caffeine on sport-specific endurance performance: A systematic review. *J Strength Cond Res* 23(1):315–324.

Giese, M.W., and C.S. Lecher. 2009. Non-enzymatic cyclization of creatine ethyl ester to creatinine. *Biochem Biophys Res Commun* 388(2):252–255.

Goston, J.L., and M.I. Correia. 2010. Intake of nutritional supplements among people exercising in gyms and influencing factors. *Nutrition* 26(6):604–611.

Gualano, B., H. Roschel, A.H. Lancha, Jr., C.E. Brightbill, and E.S. Rawson. 2012. In sickness and in health: The widespread application of creatine supplementation. *Amino Acids* 43(2):519–529.

Haff, G.G., M.H. Stone, B.J. Warren et al. 1999. The effect of carbohydrate supplementation on multiple sessions and bouts of resistance exercise. *J Strength Cond Res* 1(2):111–117.

Haff, G.G., A.J. Koch, J.A. Potteiger et al. 2000. Carbohydrate supplementation attenuates muscle glycogen loss during acute bouts of resistance exercise. *Int J Sport Nutr Exerc Metab* 10(3):326–339.

Haff, G.G., C.A. Schroeder, A.J. Koch, K.E. Kuphal, M.J. Comeau, and J.A. Potteiger. 2001. The effects of supplemental carbohydrate ingestion on intermittent isokinetic leg exercise. *J Sports Med Phys Fitness* 41(2):216–222.

Haff, G.G., M.J. Lehmkuhl, L.B. McCoy, and M.H. Stone. 2003. Carbohydrate supplementation and resistance training. *J Strength Cond Res* 17(1):187–196.

Harris, R.C., E. Hultman, and L.O. Nordesjö. 1974. Glycogen, glycolytic intermediates and high-energy phosphates determined in biopsy samples of musculus quadriceps femoris of man at rest. Methods and variance of values. *Scand J Clin Lab Invest* 33(2):109–120.

Harris, R.C., K. Söderlund, and E. Hultman. 1992. Elevation of creatine in resting and exercised muscle of normal subjects by creatine supplementation. *Clin Sci (Lond)* 83(3):367–374.

Harris, R.C., A.L. Almada, D.B. Harris, M. Dunnett, and P. Hespel. 2004. The creatine content of creatine serum and the change in the plasma concentration with ingestion of a single dose. *J Sports Sci* 22(9):851–857.

Harris, R.C., M.J. Tallon, M. Dunnett et al. 2006. The absorption of orally supplied beta-alanine and its effect on muscle carnosine synthesis in human vastus lateralis. *Amino Acids* 30(3):279–289.

Harris, R.C., and C. Sale. 2012. Beta-alanine supplementation in high-intensity exercise. *Med Sport Sci* 59:1–17.

Harris, R.C., J.A. Wise, K.A. Price, H.J. Kim, C.K. Kim, and C. Sale. 2012. Determinants of muscle carnosine content. *Amino Acids* 43(1):5–12.

Heikkinen, A., A. Alaranta, I. Helenius, and T. Vasankari. 2011. Use of dietary supplements in Olympic athletes is decreasing: A follow-up study between 2002 and 2009. *J Int Soc Sports Nutr* 8(1):1.

Hobson, R.M., B. Saunders, G. Ball, R.C. Harris, and C. Sale. 2012. Effects of beta-alanine supplementation on exercise performance: A meta-analysis. *Amino Acids* 43(1):25–37.

Huang, S.H., K. Johnson, and A.L. Pipe. 2006. The use of dietary supplements and medications by Canadian athletes at the Atlanta and Sydney Olympic Games. *Clin J Sport Med* 16(1):27–33.

Jäger, R., M. Purpura, A. Shao, T. Inoue, and R.B. Kreider. 2011. Analysis of the efficacy, safety, and regulatory status of novel forms of creatine. *Amino Acids* 40(5):1369–1383.

Jones, A.M. 2014. Buffers and their role in the nutritional preparation of athletes. *Gatorade Sports Science Exchange* 27(124):1–5.

Kendrick, I.P., R.C. Harris, H.J. Kim et al. 2008. The effects of 10 weeks of resistance training combined with beta-alanine supplementation on whole body strength, force production, muscular endurance and body composition. *Amino Acids* 34(4):547–554.

Kulik, J.R., C.D. Touchberry, N. Kawamori, P.A. Blumert, A.J. Crum, and G.G. Haff. 2008. Supplemental carbohydrate ingestion does not improve performance of high-intensity resistance exercise. *J Strength Cond Res* 22(4):1101–1107.

Lambert, C.P., M.G. Flynn, J.B. Boone, T.J. Michaud, and J. Rodriguez-Zayas. 1991. Effects of carbohydrate feeding on multiple-bout resistance exercise. *J Appl Sport Sci Res* 5(4):192–197.

Leveritt, M., and P.J. Abernethy. 1999. Effects of carbohydrate restriction on strength performance. *J Strength Cond Res* 13(1):52–57.

Lopez, R.M., D.J. Casa, B.P. McDermott, M.S. Ganio, L.E. Armstrong, and C.M. Maresh. 2009. Does creatine supplementation hinder exercise heat tolerance or hydration status? A systematic review with meta-analyses. *J Athl Train* 44(2):215–223.

Lun, V., K.A. Erdman, T.S. Fung, and R.A. Reimer. 2012. Dietary supplementation practices in Canadian high-performance athletes. *Int J Sport Nutr Exerc Metab* 22(1):31–37.

MacDougall, J.D., S. Ray, D.G. Sale, N. McCartney, P. Lee, and S. Garner. 1999. Muscle substrate utilization and lactate production. *Can J Appl Physiol* 24(3):209–215.

Matson, L.G., and Z.V. Tran. 1993. Effects of sodium bicarbonate ingestion on anaerobic performance: A meta-analytic review. *Int J Sport Nutr* 3(1):2–28.

Maughan, R.J., F. Depiesse, and H. Geyer. 2007. The use of dietary supplements by athletes. *J Sports Sci* 25(Suppl 1):S103–S113.

Molfino, A., G. Gioia, F. Rossi Fanelli, and M. Muscaritoli. 2013. Beta-hydroxy-beta-methylbutyrate supplementation in health and disease: A systematic review of randomized trials. *Amino Acids* 45(6):1273–1292.

Moore, D.R., M.J. Robinson, J.L. Fry et al. 2009. Ingested protein dose response of muscle and albumin protein synthesis after resistance exercise in young men. *Am J Clin Nutr* 89(1):161–168.

Newmaster, S.G., M. Grguric, D. Shanmughanandhan, S. Ramalingam, and S. Ragupathy. 2013. DNA barcoding detects contamination and substitution in North American herbal products. *BMC Med* 11:222.

Nissen, S.L., and R.L. Sharp. 2003. Effect of dietary supplements on lean mass and strength gains with resistance exercise: A meta-analysis. *J Appl Physiol (1985)* 94(2):651–659.

Peart, D.J., J.C. Siegler, and R.V. Vince. 2012. Practical recommendations for coaches and athletes: A meta-analysis of sodium bicarbonate use for athletic performance. *J Strength Cond Res* 26(7):1975–1983.

Persky, A.M., and E.S. Rawson. 2007. Safety of creatine supplementation. *Subcell Biochem* 46:275–289.

Quesnele, J.J., M.A. Laframboise, J.J. Wong, P. Kim, and G.D. Wells. 2014. The effects of beta-alanine supplementation on performance: A systematic review of the literature. *Int J Sport Nutr Exerc Metab* 24(1):14–27.

Rawson, E.S., and J.S. Volek. 2003. Effects of creatine supplementation and resistance training on muscle strength and weightlifting performance. *J Strength Cond Res* 17(4):822–831.

Rawson, E.S., and A.M. Persky. 2007. Mechanisms of muscular adaptations to creatine supplementation. *Int Sport Med J* 8(2):43–53.

Rawson, E.S., M.J. Stec, S.J. Frederickson, and M.P. Miles. 2011. Low-dose creatine supplementation enhances fatigue resistance in the absence of weight gain. *Nutrition* 27(4):451–455.

Res, P.T., B. Groen, B. Pennings et al. 2012. Protein ingestion before sleep improves post-exercise overnight recovery. *Med Sci Sports Exerc* 44(8):1560–1569.

Robergs, R.A., D.R. Pearson, D.L. Costill et al. 1991. Muscle glycogenolysis during differing intensities of weight-resistance exercise. *J Appl Physiol (1985)* 70(4):1700–1706.

Sale, C., B. Saunders, and R.C. Harris. 2010. Effect of beta-alanine supplementation on muscle carnosine concentrations and exercise performance. *Amino Acids* 39(2):321–333.

Sale, C., G.G. Artioli, B. Gualano, B. Saunders, R.M. Hobson, and R.C. Harris. 2013. Carnosine: From exercise performance to health. *Amino Acids* 44(6):1477–1491.

Slater, G., and S.M. Phillips. 2011. Nutrition guidelines for strength sports: Sprinting, weightlifting, throwing events, and bodybuilding. *J Sports Sci* 29(Suppl 1):S67–S77.

Sokmen, B., L.E. Armstrong, W.J. Kraemer et al. 2008. Caffeine use in sports: Considerations for the athlete. *J Strength Cond Res* 22(3):978–986.

Spriet, L.L. 2014. Exercise and sport performance with low doses of caffeine. *Sports Med* 44(Suppl 2):S175–S184.

Stuart, G.R., W.G. Hopkins, C. Cook, and S.P. Cairns. 2005. Multiple effects of caffeine on simulated high-intensity team-sport performance. *Med Sci Sports Exerc* 37(11): 1998–2005.

Tang, J.E., D.R. Moore, G.W. Kujbida, M.A. Tarnopolsky, and S.M. Phillips. 2009. Ingestion of whey hydrolysate, casein, or soy protein isolate: Effects on mixed muscle protein synthesis at rest and following resistance exercise in young men. *J Appl Physiol (1985)* 107(3):987–992.

Tesch, P., L. Ploutz Snyder, L. Ystrom, M. Castro, and G.A. Dudley. 1998. Skeletal muscle glycogen loss evoked by resistance exercise. *J Strength Cond Res* 12(2):67–73.

van Loon, L.J.C. 2013. Protein ingestion prior to sleep: Potential for optimizing post-exercise recovery. *Gatorade Sports Science Exchange* 26(117):1–5.

Volek, J.S., and E.S. Rawson. 2004. Scientific basis and practical aspects of creatine supplementation for athletes. *Nutrition* 20(7–8):609–614.

Warren, G.L., N.D. Park, R.D. Maresca, K.I. McKibans, and M.L. Millard-Stafford. 2010. Effect of caffeine ingestion on muscular strength and endurance: A meta-analysis. *Med Sci Sports Exerc* 42(7):1375–1387.

Wilkinson, D.J., T. Hossain, D.S. Hill et al. 2013. Effects of leucine and its metabolite beta-hydroxy-beta-methylbutyrate on human skeletal muscle protein metabolism. *J Physiol* 591(Pt 11):2911–2923.

Wilson, J.M., R.P. Lowery, J.M. Joy et al. 2014. The effects of 12 weeks of beta-hydroxy-beta-methylbutyrate free acid supplementation on muscle mass, strength, and power in resistance-trained individuals: A randomized, double-blind, placebo-controlled study. *Eur J Appl Physiol* 114(6):1217–1227.

Zanchi, N.E., F. Gerlinger-Romero, L. Guimaraes-Ferreira et al. 2011. HMB supplementation: Clinical and athletic performance-related effects and mechanisms of action. *Amino Acids* 40(4):1015–1025.

6 Nutrition and Dietary Supplements for Team Sport Athletes

Louise Burke, OAM, PhD, APD, FACSM
Australian Institute of Sport, Belconnen, ACT, Australia
MacKillop Institute for Health Research, Australian
Catholic University, Melbourne, Victoria, Australia

CONTENTS

Team sports essentially involve two groups of people competing for possession of a ball. At the elite level, they involve several other shared characteristics: huge popular appeal eliciting tribal or national fervor, and the elevation of the best players to the fame and fortune usually reserved for movie stars. The professionalism of the sport has created a range of new nutritional challenges for players, as well as promoted the development of the highly organized sports science/medicine support team dedicated to solving these challenges and developing optimal performance in players. This chapter will examine some of these challenges and solutions.

NUTRITION-DETERMINING CHARACTERISTICS OF TEAM SPORTS

The nutritional goals and requirements for team sport athletes are determined by a number of elements of training and covmpetition that vary between and within codes. Table 6.1 summarizes some of the important characteristics that will be discussed in brief below; for more in-depth analysis, readers are directed to other reviews (Burke

TABLE 6.1

Characteristics of Team Sports That Underpin Nutritional Goals and Practices

Game Characteristic	Effect on Nutrition	Examples of the Range Seen in Team Sports
Game environment	Environmental contribution (heat, humidity, altitude) to sweat losses and carbohydrate utilization	Basketball is played on a small court in a temperature-controlled stadium.
Season of play (winter, summer)		Football (soccer) is typically a winter sport but can be played in seasons or countries with hot climates. Rectangular field size varies but is typically 70–80 m wide and 110–120 m long.
Typical environment (outdoors, indoors, ice)	Physical limitations on distances covered in bursts or over whole game influencing energy and fuel demands	Oval field size for Australian football varies, but is typically 110–155 m wide and 135–155 m long. Code is also a winter sport but lengthy competition seasons and leagues include hot weather games.
Size of court or field		
Type of competition fixture	Periodization of preparation for competition goals over the year	Main Australian Rules seasonal fixture features a weekly match, with 25 games required to reach Grand Final playoff.
Seasonal fixture or tournament draw	Periodization of training between games in a weekly fixture or between tournaments	Teams in the National Basketball Association (U.S.) play 82 games in the regular season (~4 months) and 60–105 games in the playoffs (~6 weeks).
Number of games and period between matches	Opportunity for changes in physique (both positive during preseason and negative during off-season)	The winner of the World Cup (soccer), played every 4 years, will play 8 matches in 31 days.
Road trips		
Length of season or tournament	Opportunities for recovery (refueling, rehydration, repair) between matches	

(Continued)

TABLE 6.1 (Continued)
Characteristics of Team Sports That Underpin Nutritional Goals and Practices

Game Characteristic	Effect on Nutrition	Examples of the Range Seen in Team Sports
Game movement patterns	Heat production (sweat losses, fluid needs)	In soccer, midfielders and forwards complete greater distances during a game (~10.5–11 km) than the defenders (~9.5 km) and a greater distance at high intensity (2.2–2.5 km vs. 1.7 km). The goal keeper covers ~4 km.
Playing time and distance covered in a game	Fuel use: risk of muscle glycogen depletion, likely benefits of carbohydrate intake during game	Typical distance covered during a rugby union game is 5.8 km, with 2.2 km at walking pace, 1.6 km jogging, and 2.0 km sprinting. The typical sprint distance is ~20 m, with the backs covering greater distances, both over the total game and at sprinting speeds. Most high-intensity activities of the forwards involve body contact rather than running.
Number, duration, and frequency of high-intensity work bout during game	Opportunity for creatine loading to address limitation of resynthesis of phosphocreatine between high-intensity efforts	Basketball players make ~1000 different movements each game, changing their activities every 2 sec. About 100 high-intensity activities are undertaken by each player per game, occurring approximately every 20 s of actual playing time.
Work–recovery ratio between high-intensity work bouts and low-intensity activities	Opportunity for enhanced buffering capacity to address fatigue due to acid–base imbalances	
	Importance of low body fat content for speed, agility, and endurance	
Duration of playing periods within game time	Duration of time that players are exposed to playing environment	Australian Rules football is played in 4 quarters, each lasting 25–35 min. Soccer is played in 2 halves of 45 min.
	Duration of time that players may have limited access to nutritional support (e.g., opportunities for intake of fluid and carbohydrate)	Lacrosse consists of four 15-min quarters. Ice hockey is played in three 20-min periods with substantial added time.
Number of players on team/on field	Opportunities to periodically reduce workload (and rate of heat production and substrate utilization) in individual players	Field hockey has 11 players from each team on field at one time with a substitution bench of 5 players who have an unlimited number of substitutions.
Number of formal breaks during match (quarters, halves)	Opportunity for intake of fluid and carbohydrate between match play	Eleven soccer players from each team are on field at one time; substitution bench of three players allows replacements but benched player cannot return to field. The only break is at halftime.
Availability of rotational or unlimited player substitutions		

(Continued)

TABLE 6.1 *(Continued)*
Characteristics of Team Sports That Underpin Nutritional Goals and Practices

Game Characteristic	Effect on Nutrition	Examples of the Range Seen in Team Sports
Rules regarding carriage of fluids onto field Rules regarding access of trainers to field of play during playing time	Opportunity for intake of fluid and carbohydrate within match play	The rules of soccer prevent fluid from being carried on to the ground within the 45-min half. Australian Rules football permits trainers to be on the ground during breaks in play to provide players with a drink.
Diversity of positional or game style attributes between players in the same sport/team	Need to individualize nutritional practices and nutritional support for training and game	According to the style of team play, soccer features 11 players on the ground, with a goalkeeper and various numbers of defenders, midfielders, and forwards. American football features 11 players from each team on the field at one time with separate offensive and defensive teams alternating according to play. Basketball features 5 players on the court, playing positions designated into forwards, center, and defenders.
Body contact: tackling/scrums, pushing within game play	Importance of high body mass/lean body mass for strength and momentum Tolerance of higher body fat content Potential for direct muscle damage and contact injuries (interfering with muscle repair and refueling) Uniform characteristics: use of heavy protective gear (helmets, padding)	American football players and Rugby Union forwards spend a significant amount of game time and energy cost in pushing and tackling their opponents, and withstanding the same efforts. American football players wear thick padding and protective gear. In hot weather training, this adds to the thermoregulatory stress.

Source: Adapted from Burke, L. 2007. In *Practical Sports Nutrition*, L. Burke, Ed. Champaign IL: Human Kinetics Publishers. With permission.

2007a,b; Duthie et al. 2003; Reilly 1990; Reilly and Borrie 1992; Stølen et al. 2005; Ziv and Lidor 2009).

CHARACTERISTICS OF THE MATCH

Match play in all codes is characterized by high-intensity passages of play interspersed with low-intensity activities such as standing, walking, and jogging. Performance is determined by a complex and changing mixture of physical and skill-based talents. Players not only must be able to run to the ball or scene of play, but also must be able to execute skills involving cognitive function (e.g., reading the play, making tactical decisions) and fine motor control. In contact sports, players must possess the strength and speed to apply or withstand tackles, but even noncontact sport involves a considerable amount of jostling. Nutrition plays a key role in promoting optimal performance during competition by providing fuel for muscle and the central nervous system. It is likely that inadequate nutritional strategies during competition have a greater negative impact on performance than in continuous endurance sports such as running or cycling because these shortcomings will also affect the skill and cognitive function that overlay the player's performance.

Despite the importance of achieving optimal nutrition practices and the resources and rewards available at elite and professional levels of team sports, it is still complicated to pinpoint exact nutritional needs. This is ironic because at elite levels of play, match analysis is routinely undertaken by specialist coaches and performance analysts to produce reports of the movement patterns of each player (e.g., the total distance covered, time or distance spent at different running speeds) and their activities in each game. An important characteristic to note from these sophisticated data, however, is that the calculations of movement underestimate the true energy expenditure in a game ecause activities undertaken while moving (e.g., handling the ball, tackling, defending) add considerably to the energy cost. The energy cost of constantly accelerating, decelerating, and changing direction also needs to be taken into account.

One source of the challenge of working with team sports is that the actual requirements of a game are really only known retrospectively; each match is composed of some standard or anticipated elements, but many unpredictable and changing features. Teams sports include those that have a consistent playing time with formal breaks between set periods while others have the inconsistency of flexible playing periods due to the addition of considerable "extra time" while the ball is out of play or informal breaks such as substitutions and stoppages. These features are important in creating the energy, fuel, and fluid needs of the game, but also in creating the opportunities for intake of fluid and carbohydrate to address them. The game characteristics of different positions or playing styles within a team can also vary markedly. Therefore, even within a sport, players may have different physique characteristics and face different nutritional issues and challenges. However, even for the same player, the actual demands change from match to match because each is literally a new ball game. For these and other attributes summarized in Table 6.1, it can be difficult to make precise judgments of the nutritional challenges faced in a single match or in the larger competition scenarios that determine the winners of a league or championship.

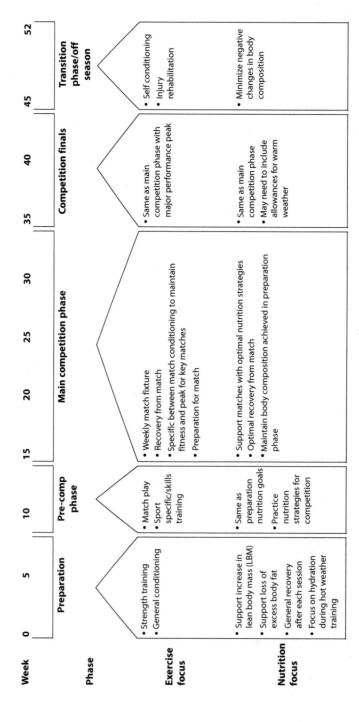

FIGURE 6.1 Overview of a simplistic periodization model for a team sport involved in a single seasonal fixture. (From Burke, L.M and N.A. Jeacocke. 2011. In *Nutrient Timing: Metabolic Optimisation for Health, Performance and Recovery*, CM. Kerksick, Ed. Boca Raton FL: CRC Press, 1–22. With permission.)

CHARACTERISTICS OF THE PERIODIZED YEAR

Typically, in team sports, competitions are undertaken under two different proto-cols: the seasonal fixture or the tournament. Both call for clever recovery tactics between matches because players may be required to play full-length games with a recovery period of 1 to 2 days up to a week. These shorter turnaround times occur during road trips and playoffs of seasonal fixtures (e.g., basketball), during a tournament, or in scenarios found in some professional codes where a team may be entered in several competitions at the same time (e.g., English soccer teams may play in the English Premier League, European Champions League, and FA cup in the same year). In the most extreme situation, the format of the international level Rugby Sevens World Series tournaments, added to the 2016 Olympic Games schedule, involves teams playing 3 matches a day over 2 to 3 days, with games of two 7- or 10-min halves. The various competition schedules not only provide a challenge to preparing and recovering from each game, but also to the organization of the annual schedule as in all elite sports, the systematic planning of the exercise stimulus known as periodization is crucial to the preparation of the team athlete.

The most simplistic model involves the macrocycles of an offseason, a preseason, and the season, culminating toward peak performance during finals or playoffs. Figure 6.1 provides an overview of this model comparing the different exercise and dietary focuses during each phase. While the majority of the conditioning work to gain the specific required characteristics of fitness and physique is undertaken during the preseason, the seasonal fixture needs to integrate continued training within the weekly microcycle of preparation and recovery for each game. This model of periodization becomes far more complex when the athlete is involved in several important competitions for the year, particularly the overlap or addition of a seasonal fixture and a tournament. This often occurs when athletes in professional team competitions are then called for national representation at an Olympic Games or World Championship.

PHYSIQUE CHARACTERISTICS

In most team sports, athlete physiques vary across playing positions or playing styles according to the characteristics of the game. Some sports favor a tall physique; while nutrition may not directly control the achievement of this characteristic, the growth needs of such athletes represent a significant factor in determining their nutritional needs. In sports in which team athletes play a fast and agile game, covering significant distances during a match, a lean physique is generally desirable. In recent years, there have been trends for a gradual reduction in body fat levels of professional team sport players (Duthie et al. 2003; Reilly 1990). Indeed, although team sport players generally do not reach the low levels of body fat associated with endurance athletes such as runners and cyclists, some professional team sport players in mobile positions (e.g., midfielders in soccer and Australian football) have set new standards of leanness for their codes. A common issue faced by many team sport athletes is the need to reverse the significant gain of body fat incurred during periods of inactivity, such as the off-season or an injury break. Even at elite levels of play, where team athletes are expected to retain a reasonable level of fitness and physique all year round and to fine-tune this during the preseason, there is a substantial change in body composition over the phases of the year. Reduced physical activity and poor lifestyle practices can quickly lead to excess body fat, and there are still (usually well-publicized) cases in which team sport players struggle to reduce their body fat levels to meet a team standard.

Finally, while team sports are not generally noted as "aesthetic" sports in which appearance plays a role in determining physique, the introduction of Lycra bodysuits as the game uniform in many female team sports has caused a noted increase in the desire of players to be lean. In some cases, this may lead to undue stress related to food intake and body image (personal communication, Jill McIntosh, former National Head Coach, Australian Netball team) for an issue not directly related to performance.

Strength, speed, and power are game characteristics favoring the development of lean body mass. These features are particularly important for sports or positions involving physical contact, with resistance training playing a core role in the preparation of most team sport players. In addition to desiring high levels of muscle mass, many players in contact sports strive simply to be big; for example, rugby union forwards and American football players often weigh in excess of 270 lbs. Higher levels of body fat are sometimes common in these players, and in some players and codes like American football, this appears to be tolerated. In certain games and playing positions, bulk is a desirable characteristic and the player must balance the advantages of increased momentum against a possible loss of speed and agility.

WHAT DO ELITE TEAM SPORT PLAYERS CURRENTLY EAT?

Anecdotal observations of elite level team sports include a range of models of nutrition practices. At one extreme are the professional teams, which offer high levels of nutrition support, including full time club dietitians/nutritionists and "performance kitchens" or "training tables" in which chefs provide players with several meals each day around the club schedule. Some teams even travel with their chefs to provide a consistent menu structure around their competition activities. In such scenarios, the club usually provides specialized sports foods and supplements to players with expert advice and systematic structures to ensure they are available and consumed with optimal protocols. Other nutrition services offered to players include practical education activities around shopping, meal planning, and cooking, which may be highly necessary in situations where young players have left home at an early age to pursue a career in an elite team sport. Of course, it should be recognized that at the highest levels of professional team sport, star players often reach a lifestyle in which the continuous travel, astronomical salaries, professional entourages (whether privately organized or club provided), sponsorships, and general fame mean that they have little opportunity to take much personal responsibility for their nutritional practices.

At the other end of the spectrum of elite team sport are the codes in which there is less public interest and financial support. This is more often the case for women's team sports, but can also apply to codes of men's sport in which national and international level competition is semiprofessional at best. In these situations, there may be few nutrition services or provisions available to players. Players may need to schedule their sporting commitments around work or study for an alternative career. In these situations, erratic or poorly chosen nutrition practices may arise from lack of knowledge, finances, time, or resources.

It should be noted that travel plays a large role in the lives of elite team sport athletes. They may be required to travel regionally or to other countries and continents to fulfill the requirements of the leagues or competitions in which they play. Depending on the distance, the draw, and the importance given to preparation for the upcoming match, the travel commitment may span one to several days and involve transport by plane, bus, train, or car. The mode of transport can create special nutritional needs (e.g., the need to increase fluid losses in pressurized or air-conditioned environments) as well as determine the opportunities for food intake. In the case of tournaments or specialized training camps, players may be required to leave their home base for substantial periods.

Few dietary surveys have been specifically designed to investigate the practices of elite team sport athletes in a sophisticated manner. Comprehensive reviews of the available literature (Burke 2007a,b) have found that it provides a simplistic picture of mean daily energy and nutrient intakes of groups of players without an appreciation of the specific nutritional goals of the individual or the phase of the periodized program. Typically, reported energy intakes are high in absolute terms in male players with large body mass (e.g., American football players, Rugby Union forwards), and high relative to body mass in players in mobile codes or positions (midfield soccer players). Highest energy intakes are typically expected during the preseason because of the two-a-day training schedules or aggressive hypertrophy programs to gain muscle size and strength.

Historical accounts of the daily carbohydrate intakes reported by groups of male team sport players include observations that meet or exceed the range of 5–7 g/kg body mass (BM) (Lundy et al. 2006; Rico-Sanz et al. 1998; Schena et al. 1995; Zuliani et al. 1996), as well as others that fail to meet this generic target (Bangsbo et al. 1992; Burke et al. 1991; Maughan et al. 1997; Schokman et al. 1999). Of course, these guidelines should be better fitted to the actual fuel cost of the phase of training or competition. Meanwhile, the universal assessment of reported protein intakes in all of these studies has been of adequacy based on a daily consumption exceeding 1.2 g/kg BM and in most cases >1.5 g/kg/d. A more modern assessment would judge optimal intake of protein in terms of the spread over the day and in relation to exercise. Most dietary surveys of elite male team sport players report mean intakes of micronutrients in excess of reference intakes (Burke et al. 1991; Lundy et al. 2006; Rico-Sanz et al. 1998). However, a recent study of Spanish professional basketball players found that more than half the team showed biochemical vitamin D deficiency as a result of poor sunlight exposure (indoor sport, winter time assessment) and low dietary intakes of vitamin D (Bescós-García and Rodríguez-Guisado 2011).

There is an almost complete absence of information on the dietary practices of female elite/professional team sport players. However, if surveys of sub-elite (e.g., collegiate) players are used as a guide, we would expect to see lower levels of reported energy intake (both absolute and relative to BM), as well as lower intakes of macronutrients and a high prevalence of reported intakes of micronutrient below reference standards (Burke 2007a,b). Whether the apparently low energy intakes of female team sport athletes reflects the inadequacy of dietary survey methodologies, a light training load attributable to the lower caliber of play, or a deliberate energy deficit to achieve loss of body fat is uncertain. Nevertheless, it is likely that female team athletes face greater challenges to meet nutritional goals than their male counterparts do, and it is of interest to undertake better studies of energy availability in these cohorts to see if problems exist as in other female athletes. A recent study conducted in collegiate volleyball players found that although mean energy availability was in the healthy range, 20% of players were assessed to have energy availability (EA) below the threshold of 30 kcal/kg fat-free mass (Woodruff and Meloche 2013).

One dietary practice that has been documented in sources ranging from formal studies to lay reports and newspaper headlines is the apparently high rates of excessive alcohol intake among team sport athletes. Alcohol has a strong relationship to sport through the sponsorship of events and teams by companies that produce beer and other alcoholic drinks and through the licensed clubs or fundraising strategies that often provide the financial underpinning of sports clubs. Some dietary surveys have shown that reported alcohol intakes are higher among team sports than other athletic groups, with the pattern of consumption involving binge drinking sessions after the game or during the off-season (Burke and Read 1988). Problems that may arise from these patterns include some level of direct impairment of the physiological processes underpinning recovery as well as the larger problem of indirect interference secondary to the failure to follow optimal nutritional and lifestyle practices while intoxicated (Burke and Maughan 2000). There is public documentation of the unfortunate outcomes of the poor judgment and high-risk behavior undertaken by athletes who are intoxicated, including loss of sponsorship value and public regard, injury, criminal and civil offences and, in extreme cases, death (Burke 2007a). Chronic episodes can lead to health problems and failure to achieve performance nutrition goals such as weight control. For these reasons, most professional clubs now run education programs related to alcohol and illicit drug use, which include information about the damaging effects on a sporting career via loss of performance and reputation.

The final word on our knowledge of dietary practices of team sport athletes should reiterate the earlier comments that most of the available dietary studies of elite team athletes are more than a decade old and reflect both older practices and assessment criteria. It is important that studies that are more contemporary be undertaken to investigate the effect of enhanced sports science/nutrition support on the nutrition practices and strategies of team sport players, and to provide an assessment against more modern concepts such as the periodized, individualized nutrition plan.

WHAT SHOULD ELITE TEAM SPORT ATHLETES EAT?

There is no such thing as a single set of dietary guidelines or ideal nutrition practices that can be offered to every athlete within a type of sport. The varying range of characteristics of each sport, each phase within the sporting calendar, and the specific needs of individuals means that a much more flexible approach is required. Nevertheless, some common themes of interest can be identified for various aspects of the preparation of the team sport athlete.

COMMENTS ON THE OFF-SEASON

At the highest levels of team sport, the off-season is short and may be mandated by the player unions or governing bodies of sport to occur at all. Clubs will differ in their expectations of players and the assistance provided to them to maintain fitness and conditioning during this time. In previous eras and in some current scenarios, the off-season can be a time of poor nutrition choices and sedentary behavior by team players, leading to significant loss of muscle mass and gain of body fat. Player education should target the philosophy and eating practices needed to combine some "down time" with maintenance of reasonable levels of physique and fitness. Of course, not all the physique change or sedentary behavior that occurs in the off-season is the result of poor lifestyle practices. Many players choose this time or, in the case where their team is out of contention for finals, the end of the competitive season to undergo elective surgery for injury repair. In this case, a different management approach is required.

The athlete who is injured or undergoing rehabilitation from injury must find a balanced approach to promoting a nutritional environment that promotes repair and regeneration, minimizes the wasting associated with a reduced training stimulus, and yet minimizes unnecessary gain of body fat. Certainly it is appropriate for the team athlete to alter their energy intake from one needed to support a high exercise load to a level that is more commensurate with their new energy needs. However, it is important that neither energy intake nor nutrient support be restricted too heavily during the early recovery phase. Adequate intake of energy and protein is important to support optimal rates of repair and regeneration (Tipton 2010). Although some athletes abandon any concern about energy balance, a more prudent approach may be to attempt to remain in energy balance during the immediate rehabilitation/post-operation phase or allow a small energy surplus to ensure adequate intakes of protein and other nutrients. Later phases of the rehabilitation may be more appropriate times to attempt correction of sub-optimal physique issues along with general and then more specific conditioning. For more information on nutrition for injury and rehabilitation, the reader is directed to Burke and Maughan (2012).

COMMENTS ON THE PRESEASON

The phase prior to competition provides the main opportunity for the team sport athlete to undertake major conditioning work (see Figure 6.1 periodization overview). Overall energy intakes during this phase need to take into account a potentially heavy training schedule, as well as the desire to gain muscle mass or lose fat mass. Nutrition and training plans are often individualized to each player, or groups with similar goals. Training for team sport involves a hybrid of the conditioning sessions undertaken by strength athletes and endurance athletes, and daily or sessional eating plans often need to switch between the strategies suited to each (see Chapters

2 and 4). As the preparation phase continues, there is usually an increase in the game-specific skill and tactical training, including "friendly" games or a preseason competition. During this phase, the player should focus on developing or fine-tuning the game day eating strategies that will be used during the main season.

Although nutritional strategies to achieve high carbohydrate availability are important for key training sessions and matches where it is important to perform optimally in both high-intensity and skill activities (Burke et al. 2011), there has been recent interest in the concept that training with low glycogen concentrations enhances the training response (Burke 2010). In some sports, athletes either deliberately or accidentally undertake some of their workouts with low glycogen concentrations, either by commencing a session with minimal refueling time after a prior workout, or by restricting dietary carbohydrate to prevent refueling for a specific period. Only one study has applied this "train low" theory to a team sport model. Morton and colleagues (2009) observed three groups of recreationally active men who undertook a set program of four high-intensity running sessions each week. One group undertook one session per day with high carbohydrate availability, another group trained twice a week with two sessions in succession (the second session was therefore done "low"), while the third group followed the "train low" protocol but consumed carbohydrate before and during the session. Although the group that trained with low glycogen and low blood glucose concentrations showed greater improvements in muscle content of oxidative enzymes, all groups recorded a similar improvement in VO_{2max} (~10%) and distance run during a Yo-Yo Intermittent Recovery Test 2 protocol (~18%). Further work is needed to see how this dietary periodization strategy could be integrated into the training program to enhance the performance outcome without impairing training capacity and comfort.

COMMENTS ON MATCH NUTRITION

During most team sports, there is evidence of the manifestation of fatigue or loss of performance (whether measured by distance run, speed of running, percentage of movement done at high speed, or ability to execute skills), including periods within play from which there is recovery as well as an irreversible decline over the course of the match. Theoretically, optimal performance is achieved by identifying the causes of the different types of fatigue, and taking steps to prevent or delay their onset. Of course, since the ultimate outcome of team sports is to score goals, a leap of faith is required to link the maintenance of speed, decision-making, or accuracy to a winning result. Table 6.2 summarizes some of the key causes of momentary or longer lasting fatigue, including the identification of the circumstances or athletes in which they are most likely to occur and strategies that can be used to reduce their occurrence or impact on performance. These strategies involve protocols that are chronically applied (i.e., enhancing the muscle stores of creatine fuel or carnosine buffer) as well as those that are undertaken acutely before, during, or in the recovery between matches.

Significant muscle glycogen depletion has been shown to occur over the course of some team sports, at least for the "running players." Indeed, low glycogen content has been found at the end of soccer matches, with reduced fuel stores being

TABLE 6.2
Factors Related to Nutrition That Could Produce Fatigue or Sub-Optimal Performance in Team Sports

Factor and Cause	Examples of High Risk/Common Occurrence in Team Sports	Strategies to Prevent/Delay Fatigue
Dehydration Failure to drink enough fluid to replace sweat losses during a game. May be exacerbated if player begins match in fluid deficit	Matches played in hot conditions, particularly in players with high activity patterns and/or heavy protective garments Repeated matches (e.g., tournaments) where there is a risk of compounding dehydration from one match to the next	The player should try to rehydrate from any previous deficits so that the game is commenced with a good hydration status. An individualized drinking plan should be developed that fits the logistics for fluid intake during the game and aims to keep the net deficit to an acceptable level.
Muscle glycogen depletion Depletion of important muscle fuel due to high utilization in a single match and/or poor recovery of stores from previous activity/match	"Running" players with large total distances covered at high intensities (e.g., midfield players in soccer, Australian Rules football) Repeated matches (e.g., tournament) may increase risk of poor refueling from one match to the next	The player should consume adequate carbohydrate during the 24–36 h prior to the game, and at the pre-match meal according to their anticipated muscle fuel needs. Additional carbohydrate consumed during the match can add to carbohydrate availability. In a tournament or situation of closely timed matches, the period immediately after the first match should be prioritized for proactive carbohydrate intake for optimal refueling.

(Continued)

TABLE 6.2 *(Continued)*

Factors Related to Nutrition That Could Produce Fatigue or Sub-Optimal Performance in Team Sports

Factor and Cause	Examples of High Risk/Common Occurrence in Team Sports	Strategies to Prevent/Delay Fatigue
Hypoglycemia and depletion of central nervous system fuels Reduction in blood glucose concentrations due to poor carbohydrate availability	May occur in players with high carbohydrate requirements (see above) who fail to consume carbohydrate during the match	Intake of carbohydrate should be factored into the athlete's tailored hydration plan, aiming for an intake of 30–60 g/h for matches of lengthy duration, high activity patterns, or risk of sup-optimal recovery from last game. Even in shorter duration matches which do not deplete glycogen or threaten blood glucose concentrations, there is evidence of better performance when small amounts of carbohydrate are consumed (or put into contact with the mouth) at frequent intervals.
Disturbance of muscle acid-base balance High rates of H+ production via anaerobic glycolytic power system	Prolonged or repeated intervals of high-intensity activities	Chronic supplementation with B-alanine can increase muscle carnosine content, presumably enhancing intracellular buffering capacity for matches as well as training sessions. Extra-cellular buffering can be enhanced by acute protocols of bicarbonate loading. This is generally not undertaken in team sports, but could theoretically enhance capacity for high intensity work if tolerated.
Depletion of phosphocreatine stores Inadequate recovery of phosphocreatine system of power production	Prolonged or repeated intervals of high-intensity sprints/activities	Chronic supplementation with creatine can increase muscle phosphocreatine content and enhance PCr resynthesis in the recovery between repeated sprints.

(Continued)

TABLE 6.2 (Continued)
Factors Related to Nutrition That Could Produce Fatigue or Sub-Optimal Performance in Team Sports

Factor and Cause	Examples of High Risk/Common Occurrence in Team Sports	Strategies to Prevent/Delay Fatigue
Gastrointestinal disturbances GI disturbances, including vomiting and diarrhea, may directly reduce performance as well as interfere with nutritional strategies aimed at managing fluid and fuel status	Poorly chosen intake of food and fluid before and/or during match Extreme tournament formats (e.g., Rugby Sevens) where there are hours between matches, and aggressive post-game recovery may interfere with gut comfort for next match	The player should experiment with the timing, amount, and type of intake pre- and during match to fine-tune a plan that does not cause gut problems. Practice with intake of fluid and carbohydrate during training sessions should help to build a tolerance for intake during exercise.
Salt depletion Inadequate replacement of sodium lost in sweat. There is anecdotal evidence that salt depletion may increase the risk of a specific type of whole body muscle cramp	Salty sweaters—individuals with high sweat rates and high sweat sodium concentrations who may acutely or chronically deplete exchangeable sodium pools Situations involving repeated sessions of high sweat loss (e.g., 2 a day training or tournament play)	In scenarios where all other risk factors for cramps have been ruled out, the player who loses large amounts of sweat sodium should experiment with higher sodium sports drinks during matches and well-judged intake of salt-rich foods in the recovery after matches. Note that this is an area of debate and discussion.
Water intoxication/hyponatremia (low blood sodium) Excessive intake of fluids can lead to hyponatremia ranging from mild (often asymptomatic) to severe (can be fatal)	Players with low sweat losses (e.g., low activity or game time) who overzealously consume fluid before and during a match	A player's hydration plan should not involve excessive intake of fluid (i.e., greater than rates of sweat loss); this situation is unlikely in elite team sports.

vassociated with a reduction in the distance covered or running speed during the second half of a match (see Ekblom 1986). This presumably occurs in other mobile team sport players, such as in the midfielders in Australian Rules. Several studies have confirmed the value of fueling up in preparation for team sport. In one investigation, professional soccer players completed an intermittent high-intensity protocol of field and treadmill running lasting ~90 min, after a 48-h intake of high carbohydrate (~8 g/kg/d) or moderate carbohydrate (~4.5 g/kg/d) diets (Bangsbo et al. 1992). The high-carbohydrate diet increased intermittent running to fatigue at the end of the protocol by ~1 km ($p < .05$), with the performance enhancement being more marked in some participants than in others. Two field-based studies have provided more real life evidence. In one, movement analysis of a 90-min four-a-side indoor soccer game showed that soccer players complete ~33% more high-intensity work during the game after 48 h of a high carbohydrate intake (~8 g/kg/d), which increased muscle glycogen content by 38%, compared with a control diet providing a moderate (~3 g/kg/d) carbohydrate supply (Balsom et al. 1999). In the other, players from two elite Swedish ice hockey teams were randomly allocated to either a carbohydrate-enriched (8.4 g/kg/d) or mixed (6.2 g/kg/d) diet in the recovery period between two games held 72 h apart (Akermark et al. 1996). Muscle glycogen concentrations were reduced after the first game for all players, but restoration levels were 45% higher in the carbohydrate-loaded players before the next game. Distance skated, number of shifts skated, amount of time skated within shifts, and skating speed were all increased in the carbohydrate-loaded players compared with the mixed diet group, with the differences being most marked in the third period.

Special consideration should be given to nutritional strategies that are undertaken during a match (i.e., warm up, play, and breaks in play) because these have the potential to address the nutritional factors in fatigue but are reliant on the rules and logistics of the sport to be implemented. Guidelines for fluid intake during sport have become topical and controversial in recent years due to assertions that recommendations to athletes to follow individualized hydration plans are unnecessary, underpinned more by commercial imperatives of sports drink companies than evidence of benefit, and are even deliberately harmful (Noakes 2012). This largely stems from the real observations that a small number of recreational athletes in endurance and ultra-endurance events consume excessive amounts of fluid during exercise leading to a potentially fatal condition of hyponatremia (Noakes 2003). We recently reviewed the published literature on observations of hydration practices across competitive sports, including the few studies on fluid balance in elite team sports of soccer, rugby league, rugby union, and basketball (Garth and Burke 2013). Studies of male team sports typically found mean sweat rates >500 mL/h across all weather conditions and levels of play, with sweat rates of ~2000 mL/h during matches played in hot conditions. Mean fluid intakes ranged from 300–800 mL/h across sports, although in games where the highest mean sweat rates were recorded, mean fluid intakes were ~1000 mL/h. Overall, mean BM changes over a match ranged from ~1 to 1.5% in cool to warm conditions, to >2% BM in cases of soccer and cricket played in hot conditions. Where studies reported ranges in BM changes over a match, there were instances where this exceeded 4% BM in individual players (Aragon-Vargas et al. 2009; Gore et al. 1993; Kurdak et al. 2010). Data sets on female team sports were fewer and tended to show lower rates of intake, sweat loss, and fluid mismatches.

Overall, among elite competitors in team sports, there is little evidence of excessive fluid intakes and it should be noted that there are some situations and individuals in which a smaller fluid deficit or a greater intake of carbohydrate-containing fluid to address fuel goals might arguably represent better practice. Indeed, interventional studies show benefits of fluid intake across intermittent exercise protocols and skill-based activities simulating team sport (Baker et al. 2007; Devlin et al. 2001; McGregor et al. 1999). Furthermore, observational studies of real matches have reported better performance capacity in players who maintained better hydration. For example, Mohr and colleagues (2010) found a net fluid loss of >2% BM during a football game in the heat, with a significant correlation between the fluid deficit and repeated sprint test fatigue index after the game. Therefore, team sport athletes should be encouraged to develop individualized hydration plans that address both their carbohydrate intake goals and likely sweat losses, using the unique and often unpredictable opportunities to consume fluids within their codes (Garth and Burke 2013). It should be noted that the rules in some team sports (e.g., soccer) limit access to fluid to the predictable warm-up and half-time breaks; this increases the risk of a significant fluid deficit during hot weather games and for players with the highest intensity playing styles. At the other end of the spectrum are indoor court sports such as basketball where the high sweat rates associated with high intensity exercise are countered by shorter game length, continual substitutions and drink breaks, and air-conditioned environments (Osterberg et al. 2009). Only in these sports does access to fluid intake reach a level that could support the opportunity for the athlete to rely on the so-called "ad libitum" or "drink to thirst" recommendation (Noakes 2003).

Carbohydrate intake is another nutritional characteristic that should be built into the hydration plans for match day. Carbohydrate supplementation can enhance the performance of sports lasting more than 60 min by a variety of mechanisms including fuel provision to the muscle, glycogen sparing, maintenance of blood glucose concentrations, and enhancement of central nervous system function (Karelis et al. 2010). Again, the opportunity to consume carbohydrate intake during a match is dependent on the rules and logistics of each code of sport, while the benefits of doing so will vary according to the fuel demands of the game (intensity and duration of game) and the players' initial carbohydrate stores.

Several studies have demonstrated the benefits of carbohydrate ingestion on movement patterns and skill maintenance during longer games or game simulations. Nicholas et al. (1995) reported that ingesting a 7% carbohydrate–electrolyte solution enhanced endurance capacity during a prolonged, intermittent, high-intensity shuttle running test. More recently, Ali and co-workers (2007) investigated the effect of ingesting a similar carbohydrate–electrolyte solution in subjects with reduced carbohydrate stores, during an intermittent shuttle running test, which combined football passing and shooting performance. The carbohydrate–electrolyte solution enabled subjects with compromised glycogen stores to better maintain skill and sprint performance than when ingesting fluid alone. An old field study that investigated the effect of carbohydrate intake during match play over two soccer games reported that during matches with carbohydrate, teams scored more goals in the second half and conceded fewer goals than in control matches. Further analysis showed that goal scoring fell by 20% to 50% in the last 30 min of control matches compared with CHO matches. Individual analysis showed enhanced number of ball contacts over the last 15 min of CHO matches compared with glucose control (Muckle 1973). Therefore, there is good evidence to promote carbohydrate intake from sports drinks and other products (gels, confectionery, etc.) for players in mobile positions in longer-duration games, or during tournaments in which there is insufficient opportunity for full refueling between matches. In such cases, carbohydrate consumed during the game addresses muscle substrate needs and the inability of glycogen stores to meet game demands.

Guidelines for carbohydrate intake during exercise have been expanded over recent years to note different recommendations for different types of events and the different mechanisms by which carbohydrate enhances performance. Typically, intakes of 30–60 g/h are considered adequate to supply additional muscle fuel substrate during events of ~90 to 120 min, which takes into account the majority of team sports (Burke et al. 2011). However, there is now clear evidence that carbohydrate intake enhances the performance of sports even where muscle glycogen stores are not limiting, with the benefit being mediated via the central nervous system. This effect can be achieved (and perhaps even magnified) by the frequent presence of carbohydrate in the oral cavity, whereby receptors communicate with reward centers in the brain to enhance the feeling of well-being and pacing (Jeukendrup and Chambers 2010). Therefore, athletes in sports involving 45 to 75 min of high intensity play—a common format for team sports—should experiment with the available opportunities to ingest (or "taste") carbohydrate to see if it leads to enhanced performance outcomes (Burke et al. 2011).

Recovery after each match needs to address the replacement of nutrients depleted during the game and the provision of building blocks to enable repair and adaptation to the exercise stress. When there is a brief time frame between matches, early intake of key nutrients such as fluid, electrolytes, protein, and carbohydrate can all enhance recovery processes.

SUPPLEMENTS AND SPORTS FOODS FOR TEAM SPORTS

Like most athletes, team players are often interested in the potential benefits that could be gained by means of special sports foods and supplements. The range of products that may be useful in assisting the athlete meet his or her everyday nutrition goals or address situations of potential or diagnosed nutrient deficiencies is summarized in Table 6.3. A much larger number of sports supplements claim to achieve direct ergogenic (performance enhancing) benefits, but only a few of these could be considered evidence based. The typical protocols of use, mechanisms of action, and examples of scientific support for these more credible ergogenic aids is summarized in Table 6.4. Note that judgments of the efficacy of these supplements are based on (1) the use of supplementation protocols that are sufficient to alter muscle substrate or biochemical characteristics or, in the case of caffeine, to alter the central nervous system response to exercise and (2) specific scenarios in team sports in which these muscle or central nervous system characteristics underpin fatigue and loss of performance. Therefore, it is critical that research scenarios are undertaken to properly mimic the specific game demands of various sports and their individual

TABLE 6.3
Sports Foods and Supplements That May Be of Use for Team Sport Athletes to Achieve Nutritional Goals

Product	Comment
Sport drinks	Convenient source of fluid and carbohydrate to refuel and rehydrate during prolonged training sessions and matches and to rehydrate after the session. Contains some electrolytes to help replace sweat losses and increase voluntary intake of fluid.
Sport gels	Convenient and compact carbohydrate source that can be used for additional refueling during matches and prolonged training sessions.
Sport bars	Convenient, portable, and easy-to-consume source of carbohydrate, protein, and micronutrients for pre-match meal or post-exercise recovery.
	Low-bulk and portable form of energy and nutrients that can contribute to high energy needs, especially to support resistance training program or growth.
	Convenient and compact source of energy and nutrients for the traveling athlete.
Liquid meal supplements	Convenient, portable, and easy-to-consume source of carbohydrate, protein, and micronutrients for post-exercise recovery, including "recovery" intake before resistance exercise.
	Low-bulk and practical form of energy and nutrients that can contribute to high energy needs, especially to support resistance training program or growth.
	Well-tolerated pre-match meal that can be consumed to provide a source of carbohydrate quite close to the start of a match or workout; seems to be better tolerated than solid food by some athletes with high risk of gastrointestinal problems.
	Convenient and compact source of energy and nutrients for the traveling athlete.
Protein supplements (especially whey powders)	Convenient, portable, and easy-to-consume source of high quality protein for post-exercise recovery, particularly for immediate intake after key sessions and matches, to provide a pre-sleep protein boost, and to add protein to meals/snacks where the available food choices cannot meet protein goals (20–30 g).
Multivitamin and mineral supplement	Supplemental source of micronutrients for traveling when food supply is not reliable.
	Supplemental source of micronutrients during prolonged periods of energy restriction (female athletes).
Electrolyte supplements, including high-sodium sports drinks	Convenient source of for during and post-exercise salt replacement for cramp-prone players with heavy sweat and electrolyte losses.
	Convenient way to consume fluid and electrolytes post-exercise to promote rapid rehydration and restoration of sweat losses.
Iron supplements	Source of iron to be used under medical supervision to treat or prevent iron deficiency.
Calcium supplements	Source of calcium to be used when sub-optimal intake cannot be met via dietary sources. If used in relation to poor bone status (especially female players), should be part of an interdisciplinary approach.
Vitamin D supplements	Source of vitamin D used under medical supervision in the treatment or prevention of vitamin D deficiency due to inadequate exposure to sunlight.

TABLE 6.4

Supplements That Have Good Evidence Base for Ergogenic Role When Used in Specific Situations in Team Sports

Product	Explanation	Examples of Studies Showing Performance Benefit
Creatine	Creatine loading increases muscle phosphocreatine stores and enhances capacity to repeat high-intensity workouts with short recovery intervals (<2 min recovery). May increase capacity for various training activities—resistance training undertaken to enhance muscle mass and strength, interval training undertaken to enhance anaerobic fitness, and specific match simulation activities. Some field studies have shown that supplementation acutely enhances the performance of match-simulation protocols, or movement patterns within actual field play, and may therefore be seen as a competition aid. Typical protocols for creatine use: loading dose of 20–30 g in multiple doses (e.g., 4 × 5 g) for 5 days followed by maintenance dose of 2–5 g/day. Uptake appears to be enhanced by consuming creatine with carbohydrate-rich meal or snack. Acute weight gain of about 1 kg occurs with creatine loading, presumably because of fluid retention.	Acute supplementation protocols have been shown to enhance performance of repeated sprint protocols in elite hockey players (Jones et al. 1999), elite female soccer players (Cox et al. 2002), elite rugby players (Ahmun et al. 2005), elite soccer players (Mujika et al. 2000), and young soccer players (Ostojic 2004). These studies include both weight bearing and non-weight bearing activities, and included some evidence of benefits to skill-related work and vertical jump height. These benefits were seen even when a gain in body mass was seen.
Caffeine	May enhance performance of prolonged exercise (e.g., matches) by reducing perception of fatigue; outcomes include an attenuation of the decline in high-intensity work and skills in the latter stages of the match. New studies show that intakes of small to moderate amounts of caffeine (2–3 mg/kg) may be as effective as the traditionally used larger doses (6 mg/kg), especially when taken during exercise, prior to the onset of fatigue. Caffeine may be consumed in cola and energy drinks or as an ingredient in some sport products (e.g., gels, gum, pre-workout supplements). It was removed from the World Anti-Doping Agency (WADA) list of Prohibited Substances in 2004, but use during competition continues to be monitored. The use of caffeine tablets, although they can provide a small measured dose, is not universally accepted in terms of public perception. Excessive use of caffeine in matches, especially those played in the evening, may contribute to post-match sleep difficulties and the further problem of reliance on sleeping tablets.	Caffeine ingestion by well-trained players has been shown to enhance aspects of team sport performance such as speed, power, intermittent sprint ability, jump performance, and passing accuracy in protocols designed to mimic rugby union (Roberts et al. 2010; Stuart et al. 2005) and soccer (Foskett et al. 2009; Gant et al. 2010). Although most studies have used larger caffeine doses taken before the game (6 mg/kg), studies that are more recent have found lower caffeine doses (3–4 mg/kg) to be beneficial. These include a field study in semi-professional soccer in which a pre-game dose of caffeine (3 mg/kg) from an energy drink was associated with greater total distance covered in a match, greater amounts of high intensity running and sprinting, and superior jump height in tests taken pre- and post-game (Del Coso et al. 2012). Similarly, GPS studies of movement patterns in female rugby players during a tournament found that a 3-mg/kg dose of caffeine enhanced total running and running at high-intensities during games (Del Coso et al. 2013).

(Continued)

TABLE 6.4 (Continued)

Supplements That Have Good Evidence Base for Ergogenic Role When Used in Specific Situations in Team Sports

Product	Explanation	Examples of Studies Showing Performance Benefit
Buffers: Bicarbonate (extra-cellular) B-alanine (intra-cellular)	The use of bicarbonate or citrate to increase blood-buffering capacity (e.g., 300 mg/kg body mass bicarbonate or 500 mg/kg body mass citrate 1–2 h pregame) might enhance the performance of team sports involving repeated sprints. Field studies are needed with high-level athletes to confirm benefits. Risk of gastrointestinal problems should be noted but appear to be reduced by taking dose with large volumes of fluid (1–2 L). There is also recent evidence that chronic bicarbonate loading—loading prior to each session of interval training—may enhance training adaptations. It may also allow the player to train harder. Note that intracellular buffering can be enhanced by chronic loading with b-alanine (300 g taken in split doses totaling 6–8 g/d for 6–10 weeks) to increase muscle carnosine stores. The commonly accepted mechanism of action is to increase muscle-buffering capacity, but carnosine may also directly enhance muscle contractility among other activities. May enhance training capacity or ability to tolerate repeated high-intensity activities during match play. Further research is needed to test this hypothesis adequately.	Although the theory and support from studies of these supplements in other sports is sound, a team sport will only benefit from intra- or extra-cellular protocols of enhanced buffering in scenarios in which high levels of muscle acidity limit performance. To date, the only study of b-alanine supplementation in team sports (non-elite players) failed to find an enhancement of repeated sprint performance during the Loughborough Intermittent Sprint Test following a 4-week supplementation protocol (Saunders et al. 2012). One study of acute bicarbonate supplementation in female players showed a trend to performance improvement in the second half of a cycling protocol mimicking the repeated sprint patterns of a team sport (Bishop and Claudius 2005). Further research is warranted. An interesting variant is the effect of chronic application of bicarbonate supplementation in a training program: one study that buffered all interval training sessions in an 8-week training program found an enhanced performance outcome, which was attributed to the protection of the muscle cell from disturbed homeostasis (Edge et al. 2006).
Beetroot juice	Source of nitrate which when taken acutely (8–10 mol, 2 h pre-exercise) or chronically (8–10 mol, daily) can increase production of nitric oxide, leading to increased exercise economy. Performance benefits seem to be more easily detected in sub-elite athletes, and it is unclear whether elite athletes respond differently or require a larger/different supplementation regimen. Further research is required to develop a better understanding of mechanisms, optimal protocols of use, and best scenarios of use. Commercial juices and concentrates are now marketed for sports performance, with optimal doses of nitrate being provided by 500–1000 mL of juice or 2 × 70 mL concentrates.	Recreational team sport players consumed 7 bottles of beetroot juice concentrate over the 24 h prior to a high-intensity test protocol (Yo-Yo recovery level 1 test). Performance was increased by 4% with nitrate-containing juice compared with a nitrate-depleted placebo juice ($p < 0.05$). The authors suggested that this effect was achieved via greater muscle glucose uptake or by better maintaining muscle excitability.

positions before decisions can be made about the potential value of such ergogenic aids. Furthermore, decisions made by team sport athletes regarding the use of such supplements should consider their individual game demands and experiences of use, as well as the general concerns about supplements such as expense and the risk of contamination with prohibited substances.

SUMMARY

Team sport covers a wide variety of games in which there is a range of nutrition-related characteristics that affect match performance across codes, players, and individual games. The unique and changing scenarios of these nutritional challenges requires a specific set of strategies for each individual player. The periodized annual calendar of training and competition also requires a flexible and individualized approach. Since professional team sport is among the most highly watched and rewarded activities in the world, there is clear value in having expert nutrition advice and systems in place to ensure that each athlete is able to follow an individualized nutrition plan. Nutritional strategies around each match may include individualized hydration and fueling plans, as well as the evidence-based use of a few supplements.

REFERENCES

Ahmun, R.P., R.J. Tong, and P.N. Grimshaw. 2005. The effects of acute creatine supplementation on multiple sprint cycling and running performance in rugby players. *J Strength Cond Res* 19:92–97.

Akermark, C., I. Jacobs, M. Rasmusson, and J. Karlsson. 1996. Diet and muscle glycogen concentration in relation to physical performance in Swedish elite ice hockey players. *Int J Sport Nutr* 6:272–284.

Ali, A., C. Williams, C.W. Nicholas, and A. Foskett. 2007. The influence of carbohydrate-electrolyte ingestion on soccer skill performance. *Med Sci Sports Exerc* 39:1969–1976.

Aragon-Vargas, L.F., J. Moncada-Jimenez, J. Hernandez-Elizondo, A. Barrenechea, and M. Monge-Alvarado. 2009. Evaluation of pre-game hydration status, heat stress, and fluid balance during professional soccer competition in the heat. *Eur J Sport Sci* 9:269–276.

Baker, L.B., K.A. Dougherty, M. Chow, and W.L. Kenney. 2007. Progressive dehydration causes a progressive decline in basketball skill performance. *Med Sci Sports Exerc* 39:1114–1123.

Balsom, P.D., K. Wood, P. Olsson, and B. Ekblom. 1999. Carbohydrate intake and multiple sprint sports: With special reference to football (soccer). *Int J Sports Med* 20:48–52.

Bangsbo, J., L. Norregaard, and F. Thorsoe. 1992. The effect of carbohydrate diet on intermittent exercise performance. *Int J Sports Med* 13:152–157.

Bescós-García, R., and F.A. Rodríguez-Guisado. 2011. Low levels of vitamin D in professional basketball players after wintertime: Relationship with dietary intake of vitamin D and calcium. *Nutr Hosp* 26(5):945–951.

Bishop, D., and B. Claudius. 2005. Effects of induced metabolic alkalosis on prolonged intermittent-sprint performance. *Med Sci Sports Exerc* 37:759–767.

Burke, L. 2007a. Field-based team sports. In *Practical Sports Nutrition*, L. Burke, Ed. Champaign, IL: Human Kinetics Publishers, 185–219.

Burke, L. 2007b. Court-based team sports. In *Practical Sports Nutrition*, L. Burke, Ed. Champaign, IL: Human Kinetics Publishers, 220–239.

Burke, L.M. 2010. Fuelling strategies to optimise performance—Training high or training low? *Scand J Med Sci Sports* 20(Suppl 2):48–58.

Burke, L.M., and R.S.D. Read. 1988. A study of dietary patterns of elite Australian football players. *Can J Sport Sci* 13(1):15–19.

Burke, L.M., R.A. Gollan, and R.S.D. Read. 1991. Dietary intakes and food use of groups of elite Australian male athletes. *Int J Sport Nutr* 1:378–394.

Burke, L.M., and R.J. Maughan. 2000. Alcohol in sport. In *Nutrition in Sport*, R.J. Maughan, Ed. Oxford, UK: Blackwell Science, 405–414.

Burke, L.M., J.A. Hawley, S.H. Wong, and A.E. Jeukendrup. 2011. Carbohydrates for training and competition. *J Sports Sci* 29(Suppl 1):S17–S27.

Burke, L.M., and N.A. Jeacocke. 2011. The basis of nutrient timing and its role in sport and metabolic regulation. In *Nutrient Timing: Metabolic Optimisation for Health, Performance and Recovery*, C.M. Kerksick, Ed. Boca Raton, FL: CRC Press, 1–22.

Burke, L., and R. Maughan. 2012. Sports nutrition and therapy. In *Sports Therapy Services*, J.E. Zachazewski, and D.J. Magee, Eds. London: John Wiley & Sons, 103–116.

Cox, G.R., I. Mujika, D. Tumilty, and L.M. Burke. 2002. Acute creatine supplementation and performance during a field test simulating match play in elite female soccer players. *Int J Sport Nutr Exerc Metab* 12:33–46.

Del Coso, J., V.E. Muñoz-Fernández, G. Muñoz et al. 2012. Effects of a caffeine-containing energy drink on simulated soccer performance. *PLoS One* 7(2):e31380.

Del Coso, J., J. Portillo, G. Muñoz, J. Abián-Vicén, C. Gonzalez-Millán, and J. Muñoz-Guerra. 2013. Caffeine-containing energy drink improves sprint performance during an international rugby sevens competition. *Amino Acids* 44:1511–1519.

Devlin, L.H., S.F. Fraser, N.S., Barras, and J.A. Hawley. 2001. Moderate levels of hypohydration impairs bowling accuracy but not bowling velocity in skilled cricket players. *J Sci Med Sport* 4:179–187.

Duthie, G., D.B. Pyne, and S. Hooper. 2003. Applied physiology and game analysis of rugby union. *Sports Med* 33:973–1001.

Edge, J., D. Bishop, and C. Goodman. 2006. Effects of chronic bicarbonate ingestion during interval training on changes to muscle buffering capacity and short-term endurance performance. *J Appl Physiol* 101:918–925.

Foskett, A., A. Ali, and N. Gant. 2009. Caffeine enhances cognitive function and skill performance during simulated soccer activity. *Int J Sport Nutr Exerc Metab* 19:410–423.

Gant, N., A. Ali, and A. Foskett. 2010. The influence of caffeine and carbohydrate coingestion on simulated soccer performance. *Int J Sport Nutr Exerc Metab* 20:191–197.

Garth, A.K., and L.M. Burke. 2013. What do athletes drink during competitive sporting activities? *Sports Med* 43:539–564.

Gore, C.J., P.C. Bourdon, S.M. Woolford, and D.G. Pederson. 1993. Involuntary dehydration during cricket. *Int J Sports Med* 14:387–395.

Jeukendrup, A.E., and E.S. Chambers. 2010. Oral carbohydrate sensing and exercise performance. *Curr Opin Clin Nutr Metab Care* 13:447–451.

Jones, A.M., T. Atter, and K.P. Georg. 1999. Oral creatine supplementation improves multiple sprint performance in elite ice-hockey players. *J Sports Med Phys Fitness* 39:189–196.

Karelis, A.D., J.W. Smith, D.H. Passe, and F. Péronnet. 2010. Carbohydrate administration and exercise performance: What are the potential mechanisms involved? *Sports Med* 40:747–763.

Kurdak, S.S., S.M. Shirreffs, R.J. Maughan et al. 2010. Hydration and sweating responses to hot-weather football competition. *Scand J Med Sci Sports* 20(Suppl 3):133–139.

Lundy, B., H. O'Connor, F. Pelly, and I. Caterson. 2006. Anthropometric characteristics and competition dietary intakes of professional rugby league players. *Int J Sport Nutr Exerc Metab* 16:199–213.

Maughan, R.J. 1997. Energy and macronutrient intake of professional football (soccer) players. *Br J Sports Med* 31:45–47.

McGregor, S.J., C.W. Nicholas, H.K.A. Lakomy, and C. Williams. 1999. The influence of intermittent high-intensity shuttle running and fluid ingestion on the performance of a soccer skill. *J Sports Sci* 17:895–903.

Mohr, M., I. Mujika, and J. Santisteban. 2010. Examination of fatigue development in elite soccer in a hot environment: A multi-experimental approach. *Scand J Med Sci Sports* 20(Suppl 3):125–132.

Morton, J.P., L. Croft, J.D. Bartlett et al. 2009. Reduced carbohydrate availability does not modulate training-induced heat shock protein adaptations but does upregulate oxidative enzyme activity in human skeletal muscle. *J Appl Physiol* 106:1513–1521.

Muckle, D.S. 1973. Glucose syrup ingestion and performance in soccer. *Brit J Sports Med.* 7:340–343.

Mujika, I., S. Padilla, J. Ibanez, M. Izquierdo, and E. Gorostiaga. 2000. Creatine supplementation and sprint performance in soccer players. *Med Sci Sports Exerc* 32:518–525.

Nicholas, C.W., C. Williams, H.K. Lakomy, G. Phillips, and A. Nowitz. 1995. Influence of ingesting a carbohydrate-electrolyte solution on endurance capacity during intermittent, high-intensity shuttle running. *J Sports Sci* 13:283–290.

Noakes, T.D. 2003. Overconsumption of fluid by athletes. *Br Med J* 327:113–114.

Noakes, T.D. 2012. *Waterlogged. The Serious Problem of Overhydration in Endurance Sports.* Champaign, IL: Human Kinetics.

Osterberg, K.L., C.A. Horswill, and L.B. Baker. 2009. Pregame urine specific gravity and fluid intake by National Basketball Association players during competition. *J Athl Train* 44:53–57.

Ostojic, S.M. 2004. Creatine supplementation in young soccer players. *Int J Sport Nutr Exerc Metab* 14:95–103.

Reilly, T. 1990. Football. In *Physiology of Sports*, T. Reilly, N. Secher, P. Snell, and C. Williams, Eds. London: E & FN Spon, 371–426.

Reilly, T., and A. Borrie. 1992. Physiology applied to field hockey. *Sports Med* 14:10–26.

Rico-Sanz, J., W.R. Frontera, P.A. Mole, M.A. Rivera, A. Rivera-Brown, and C.N. Meredith. 1998. Dietary and performance assessment of elite soccer players during a period of intense training. *Int J Sport Nutr* 8:230–240.

Roberts, S.P., K.A. Stokes, G. Trewartha, J. Doyle, P. Hogben, and D. Thompson. 2010. Effects of carbohydrate and caffeine ingestion on performance during a rugby union simulation protocol. *J Sports Sci* 28:833–842.

Saunders, B., C. Sale, R.C. Harris, and C. Sunderland. 2012. Effect of beta-alanine supplementation on repeated sprint performance during the Loughborough Intermittent Shuttle Test. *Amino Acids* 43:39–47.

Schena, F., A. Pattini, and S. Mantovanelli. 1995. Iron status in athletes involved in endurance and prevalently anaerobic sports. In *Sports Nutrition: Minerals and Electrolytes*, C.V. Kies, and J.A. Driskell, Eds. Boca Raton, FL: CRC Press, 65–79.

Schokman, C.P., I.H.E. Rutishauser, and R.J. Wallace. 1999. Pre- and postgame macronutrient intake of a group of elite Australian Rules football players. *Int J Sport Nutr* 9:60–69.

Stølen, T., K. Chamari, C. Castagna, and U. Wisløff. 2005. Physiology of soccer: An update. *Sports Med* 35:501–536.

Stuart, G.R., W.G. Hopkins, C. Cook, and S.P. Cairns. 2005. Multiple effects of caffeine on simulated high-intensity team-sport performance. *Med Sci Sports Exerc* 37:1998–2005.

Tipton, K.D. 2010. Nutrition for acute exercise-induced injuries. *Ann Nutr Metab* 57(Suppl 2):43–53.

Woodruff, S.J., and R.D. Meloche. 2013. Energy availability of female varsity volleyball players. *Int J Sport Nutr Exerc Metab* 23:24–30.

Wylie, L.J., M. Mohr, P. Krustrup et al. 2013. Dietary nitrate supplementation improves team sport-specific intense intermittent exercise performance. *Eur J Appl Physiol* 113:1673–1684.

Ziv, G., and R. Lidor. 2009. Physical attributes, physiological characteristics, on-court performances and nutritional strategies of female and male basketball players. *Sports Med* 39:547–568.

Zuliani, G., G. Baldo-Enzi, E. Palmieri et al. 1996. Lipoprotein profile, diet and body composition in athletes practicing mixed and anaerobic activities. *J Sports Med Phys Fitness* 36:211–216.

7 Nutrition and Dietary Supplements for Aesthetic and Weight-Class Sport Athletes

Jennifer Burris, MS, RD, CSG, CNSC, CSSD, CDE
Kathleen Woolf, PhD, RD, FACSM
Steinhardt School of Culture, Education and Human
Development, Department of Nutrition, Food Studies
and Public Health, New York University, New York

CONTENTS

INTRODUCTION

Elite athletes face tremendous pressures to perform and achieve success in sport. Although skill and talent are predictors of athletic achievement, body weight and body composition are also important contributors. Many elite athletes attempt to achieve an ideal body shape or weight in order to meet the demand of competition, conform to the standards or ideals of their sport, and improve performance. These pressures are especially high among athletes competing in aesthetic and weight-class sports (Bachner-Melman et al. 2006; Brownell et al. 1987; de Bruin et al. 2007; Pettersson et al. 2012; Sundgot-Borgen and Garthe 2011; Sundgot-Borgen and Torstveit 2010). These sports place an emphasis on leanness, aesthetic appeal, and/or achieving a specific body weight prior to competition. Due to these demands, the frequency of disordered eating and eating disorders is higher among athletes participating in sports that emphasize leanness and a thinner ideal body shape, compared to athletes participating in sports without such a focus (Bachner-Melman et al. 2006; de Bruin et al. 2007; Rosendahl et al. 2009; Smolak et al. 2000; Sundgot-Borgen and Torstveit 2004). Although the regulations and characteristics of aesthetic and weight-class sports differ, these sports report similar concerns regarding body shape and image.

Aesthetic sports, including gymnastics, figure skating, dance, synchronized swimming, and diving, require tremendous anaerobic and aerobic power to succeed. In addition to these skills, aesthetic sports emphasize physical appearance. In many aesthetic sports, leanness is a required component of technical skill. However, leanness may also contribute to artistic and visual appeal, encouraging athletes to conform to an ideal body shape and image. Moreover, athletes participating in aesthetic sports often compete in tight or revealing attire and are routinely evaluated by coaches and judges, augmenting the existing pressures to achieve this idealized shape (Sundgot-Borgen 1994). Due to the emphasis on physical attractiveness and the pressures to excel and conform to the standards or ideals of their sport, athletes participating in aesthetic sports are at an increased risk of weight concerns, body dissatisfaction, excessive dieting behaviors, and impaired health (Brooks-Gunn et al. 1988; Krentz and Warshburger 2011; Sundgot-Borgen and Garthe 2011; Sundgot-Borgen and Torstveit 2004, 2010; Zucker et al. 1999).

Weight-class sports, including rowing, wrestling, and mixed martial arts (judo, karate, and boxing), require athletes to achieve a specific body weight prior to competition. When used appropriately, weight classifications encourage fair competition among athletes, especially among sports in which body weight or size could be a considerable advantage. Unfortunately, athletes may attempt weight loss in order to participate in a lighter weight-class, thus gaining a competitive advantage over smaller components (Oppliger et al. 2003). To achieve a lower body weight, athletes may use dangerous or extreme weight loss techniques including fasting, restricting fluids, engaging in excessive exercise, exercising in the heat, vomiting, using diuretics or enemas, sauna-induced sweating, and wearing rubber/plastic suits, particularly in the days leading to competition (Artioli et al. 2010b; Oppliger et al. 2003; Pettersson et al. 2012). These techniques may lead to serious health consequences, including psychological effects or death. Researchers have observed negative physiological effects, such as mood changes, impairment of short-term memory, and increased confusion and tension, in both mixed martial arts and combat sport athletes after attempting rapid weight loss (Choma et al. 1998; Koral and Dosseville 2009). While preparing for the 1996 Olympic Games, a judo athlete died after undergoing a rapid weight loss program (Artioli et al. 2010a). In 1997, three collegiate wrestlers died from dehydration-induced hyperthermia when attempting excessive weight loss (Centers for Disease Control and Prevention 1998). In an effort to discourage dangerous weight loss practices, the National College Athletic Association

(NCAA) mandated a wrestling weight-certificate program in 1998. This program established minimum percentage body fat and weight classes, revised weight-loss guidelines, and initiated penalties for noncompliance (National Collegiate Athletic Association 2000). Despite these policies, the use of extreme dieting and rapid weight loss remains common among athletes competing in weight-class sports (Artioli et al. 2010b; Oppliger et al. 2003) and few athletes question the methods used to make weight (Hall and Lane 2001). Recently, Kazemi and colleagues (2005) examined the dietary practices of martial artists, observing over 50% of participants report dieting prior to competition in order to lose weight. Furthermore, many athletes continue to believe these weight loss techniques are a necessary component of the sport and are a determinant of success (Hall and Lane 2001).

ENERGY AND MACRONUTRIENT RECOMMENDATIONS

Only limited research provides sports-specific energy and macronutrient recommendations for aesthetic and weight-class athletes (Economos et al. 1993; Sundgot-Borgen and Garthe 2011). In addition, the existing research contains limitations including underreporting of dietary intakes (Burke 2001; Fogelholm et al. 1995; Hill and Davies 1999, 2001; Jonnalagadda et al. 2000; Magkos and Yannakoulia 2003; Thompson 1998) and small sample sizes (Artioli et al. 2009, 2010c; Chen et al. 1989; Dahlström et al. 1995; Degoutte et al. 2006; de Wijn et al. 1979; Ebine et al. 2000; Finaud et al. 2006; Fogelholm et al. 1993; Grandjean 1989; Gropper et al. 2003; Hassapidou and Manstrantoni 2001; Heinemann and Zerbes 1989; Hickson et al. 1986; Hill and Davies 2002; Howat et al. 1989; Leydon and Wall 2002; López-Varela et al. 2000; Morris and Payne 1996; Ohta et al. 2002; Roemmich and Sinning 1997; Slater et al. 2006; Smith et al. 2001; van Erp-Baart et al. 1989; Widerman and Hagan 1982; Wilson et al. 2012; Xia et al. 2001). In order to achieve a sports-specific ideal body shape or make a specific weight category, these athletes routinely practice rapid and dangerous weight loss techniques, report frequent fluctuations in body weight, and/or consume inadequate energy (Sundgot-Borgen and Garthe 2011). Further complicating matters, the dietary intake patterns of aesthetic and weight-class sport athletes fluctuate dramatically throughout the competitive season. This trend is likely due to the increased pressures to maintain or lose body weight and fat mass during peak competition. Consequently, these concerns make it difficult to use the existing literature to establish strong evidence-based dietary recommendations for aesthetic and weight-class sport athletes.

The energy requirements for aesthetic and weight-class sports vary depending on the sport, gender, time during the competitive season, and the intensity and duration of exercise. Collectively, athletes participating in aesthetic and weight-class sports are inclined to practice for long periods of time with multiple sessions per week or day. Thus, aesthetic and weight-class sport athletes should follow the general recommendation for athletes exercising >90 min per day, consuming approximately 45 to 50 kcal/kg body weight per day to meet the demands of intense exercise and provide fuel for physiological function (Sundgot-Borgen and Garthe 2011).

Although adequate energy intake is ideal for optimal performance, dieting is part of the culture of both aesthetic and weight-class sports. However, diets providing <30 kcal/kg fat free mass per day do not provide enough energy for elite athletes and are not recommended (Loucks et al. 2011). Low energy diets are associated with a decline in bone mineralization, decrease in insulin, insulin-like growth factor-1 and thyroid hormone concentrations, and may suppress immune function (Ihle and Loucks 2004; Loucks 2004; Loucks et al. 2011). Aesthetic and weight-class sport athletes attempting weight loss should follow a diet providing a minimum of 30 to 45 kcal/kg fat free mass per day to reduce body fat and maintain muscle mass (Loucks et al. 2011).

Athletes participating in aesthetic and weight-class sports predominantly utilize the anaerobic pathway for fuel during competition. Because these athletes typically exercise or compete in multiple, short-duration, high-intensity exercise bouts over a condensed period of time, carbohydrate is the primary fuel (Burke et al. 2011). In general, aesthetic and weight-class athletes should follow the same carbohydrate recommendations of non-endurance athletes, consuming approximately 5 to 7 g carbohydrate/kg body weight per day (American College of Sports Medicine et al. 2009; Burke et al. 2011; Sundgot-Borgen and Garthe 2011). Athletes competing in power sports lasting >1 to 10 min, including lightweight rowing, may require up to 6 to 12 g/kg/d body weight of carbohydrate, especially during periods of intense training (exercise time of 1 to 5 h/day) (Stellingwerff et al. 2011).

Pre-exercise carbohydrate recommendations for aesthetic and weight-class sport athletes are similar to the recommendations for active individuals. To increase carbohydrate availability during exercise, athletes should strive to consume 1 to 4 g/kg body weight of carbohydrate 1 to 4 h before exercise to maintain high carbohydrate availability and fuel working muscles and the central nervous system (Burke et al. 2011; Karelis et al. 2010). Each athlete's individual preferences and experiences, as well as the practical needs of the sport, should be taken into account when determining the timing, quality, and quantity of pre-exercise carbohydrate foods or drinks (Burke et al. 2011).

Because aesthetic and weight-class sport athletes primarily utilize the anaerobic fuel system and competition is <45 min, carbohydrate consumption during exercise may not be necessary (Burke et al. 2011). However, aesthetic and weight-class sport athletes may train for long periods or multiple times per day when preparing for competition. In these situations, carbohydrates consumed during exercise will provide an exogenous fuel source to working muscles and the central nervous system, ultimately sparing glycogen and enhancing performance (Burke et al. 2011; Karelis et al. 2010). During exercise lasting 60 to 150 min, aesthetic and weight-class sport athletes should follow the general recommendations for active individuals, consuming 30 to 60 g carbohydrate per hour (Burke et al. 2011). Aesthetic and weight-class sport athletes may want to use both carbohydrate foods and drinks to meet carbohydrate needs during exercise.

Recently, experimental evidence demonstrates benefits to consuming small amounts of carbohydrate or a mouth rinse of carbohydrate during intense practice sessions lasting 45 to 75 min (Burke et al. 2011; Carter et al. 2004). Rinsing the mouth with carbohydrate may stimulate the central nervous system, enhancing performance by approximately 2% to 3% (Jeukendrup and Chambers 2010). To date, the effect of carbohydrate consumption or a carbohydrate mouth rinse on high-intensity, repeated events, including aesthetic or weight-class sports, is not well known.

Carbohydrate consumption after exercise maximizes glycogen resynthesis and is important when recovery time (between events or practices) is <8 h (Burke et al.

2011). Because aesthetic and weight-class sport athletes may participate or compete in multiple events per day, recovery nutrition, especially carbohydrate consumption, is critical. Aesthetic and weight-class athletes should aim to consume 1.0 to 1.2 g/kg body weight/hour of carbohydrate during the first 4 h after activity to replenish muscle glycogen stores and prepare for the next exercise session (Burke et al. 2011). Power sports lasting >1 to 10 min, including rowing, may require up to 1.2 to 1.5 g/kg body weight/hour of carbohydrate in the first 2 h after activity for optimal recovery (Burke et al. 2011). When the time between exercise and competition is >24 h, the timing and quantity of carbohydrate consumption are not as critical (Burke et al. 2011).

Most athletes, including aesthetic and weight-class sport athletes, require more protein than the Recommended Daily Allowance (RDA) designed for a healthy, sedentary population (Friedman and Lemon 1989; Lemon et al. 1992; Phillips and Van Loon 2011; Stellingwerff et al. 2011). Aesthetic and weight-class sport athletes should consume 1.2 to 1.7 g protein/kg body weight per day, spread throughout the day, to maximize muscle protein synthesis and repair muscle damage associated with weight resistive activities (American College of Sports Medicine et al. 2009; Phillips and Van Loon 2011).

Athletes following a diet for weight loss may require a higher protein intake, especially if carbohydrate intake is low (Krieger et al. 2006; Sundgot-Borgen and Garthe 2011). In order to maintain lean body mass and promote glycogen resynthesis, athletes following a low energy diet require a minimum protein and carbohydrate intake of 1.4 to 1.8 g/kg body weight and 4 g/kg body weight per day, respectively (Sundgot-Borgen and Garthe 2011). Some research suggests an even greater protein consumption (1.8 to 2.7 g/kg body weight per day) by athletes following a low energy diet in order to maintain muscle mass (Mettler et al. 2010).

Dietary fat is not the primary fuel for athletes competing in aesthetic or weight-class sports, due to the nature of these sports. However, dietary fat provides essential fatty acids, insulates/protects internal organs, maintains cell membrane integrity, facilitates absorption and transportation of fat-soluble vitamins, and synthesizes steroid hormones (Hargreaves et al. 2004). In addition, dietary fat increases satiety and flavor, making eating more enjoyable for athletes. These functions are important roles, particularly for aesthetic and weight-class athletes who are at a higher risk of disordered eating habits or eating disorders. Total dietary fat intake should be sufficient to provide the essential fatty acids and fat-soluble vitamins as well as contributing energy for weight maintenance (American College of Sports Medicine et al. 2009). Thus, aesthetic and weight-class sport athletes should follow the Acceptable Macronutrient Distribution Range of the Dietary Reference Intakes, consuming 20% to 35% of total energy as dietary fat (Burke et al. 2004; Food and Nutrition Board 2002).

DIETARY INTAKE PATTERNS

Tables 7.1 to 7.9 summarize the research literature on the reported dietary intakes of aesthetic and weight-class sports. Reported dietary intakes of athletes have been well documented in some, but not all, aesthetic and weight-class sports, and include studies investigating dancers, figure skaters, gymnasts, synchronized swimmers, jockeys, mixed martial artists, rowers, ski jumpers, and wrestlers. These studies use a variety of dietary assessment methodology, including food frequency questionnaires, 24-h dietary recalls, dietary histories, and food records (weighed and non-weighed, ranging from 1 to 14 days). Unfortunately, many athletes, especially those participating in aesthetic sports, may underreport dietary intakes (Burke 2001; Fogelhom et al. 1995; Hill and Davies 1999; Jonnalagadda et al. 2000; Magkos and Yannakoulia 2003; Thompson 1998). In addition, the research investigating reported dietary intake patterns of aesthetic and weight-class sport athletes cover a large period of time, with some research published during the 1970s. The variety in the study designs, the scarcity of research in some sports, the potential of underreporting of dietary intakes, and the limited recent research generates challenges when interpreting this literature.

AESTHETIC SPORTS

DANCERS

Success in dance is determined aesthetically through movement and shape. In order to achieve an ideal body shape, many dancers, especially ballet dancers, restrict energy intake and engage in disordered eating patterns (Benson et al. 1985; Hincapié and Cassidy 2010; Koutedakis and Jamurtas 2004). As a result, elite and professional dancers often consume energy intakes less than dietary recommendations (Bonbright 1989; Dahlström et al. 1990) and weigh 10% to 12% below ideal body weight (Kaufman et al. 2002). These methods of weight control may lead to long-term consequences. Recent research observed a significantly lower mean absolute and relative (kcal/kg body weight) resting metabolic rate among elite female dancers compared to sedentary controls matched by age, BMI, and fat-free mass (Doyle-Lucas and Davy 2011). The reduction in resting metabolic rate may be the result of chronic energy restriction.

Over the last 20 years, research evaluating the dietary patterns of elite dancers consistently reports a relatively low energy intake, ranging from 26.6 to 37.9 kcal/kg body weight (Bonbright 1989; Dahlström et al. 1990, 1995; Doyle-Lucas et al. 2010; Frusztajer et al. 1990; Hassapidou and Manstrantoni 2001; Quintas et al. 2003; Short and Short 1983; Soric et al. 2008; Van Marken Lichtenbelt et al. 1995; Warren et al. 2002; Yannakoulia et al. 2004) (Table 7.1). Reported mean carbohydrate intakes ranged from 3.1 to 4.5 g/kg body weight, representing 33% to 67% of total energy intake. Dancers typically reported mean protein intakes of 1.0 to 1.3 g/kg body weight, representing 11% to 25% of total energy intake and dietary fat intakes of 19% to 48% total energy intake. Most studies focused on adult ballet dancers; thus, the results may not be applicable to dancers of all ages or types of dance.

To date, only limited research examines the dietary patterns of young dancers, and the results are mixed (Bonbright 1989; Quintas et al. 2003; Soric et al. 2008). Soric et al. (2008) examined dietary intakes of 16 female ballet dancers, 9 to 13 years of age. Using a food frequency questionnaire, the young ballet dancers reported a mean energy intake of 1731 ± 432 kcal/day (51.4 ± 16.6 kcal/kg body weight). The mean reported carbohydrate intake was 6.6 ± 2.5 g/kg body weight (51 ± 4% of total energy

TABLE 7.1
Studies Investigating Reported Dietary Intakes of Dancers

Ref.	Participants	Dietary Assessment Method	Energy	Carbohydrate	Protein	Fat
Bonbright 1989	32 female ballet dancers, 16.4 years, 48.6 kg	5-day food record	1584 kcal/d (range 642–2611 kcal/d), 32.6 kcal/kg BW	210 g/d, 4.3 g/kg BW, 33–67% total energy	64.8 g/d, 1.3 g/kg BW, 11–25% total energy	58.4 g/d, 19–48% total energy
Dahlström et al. 1990	14 female dancers, 23.7 ± 2.1 years, BW = 57.9 ± 5.3 kg, BMI = 20.7 ± 1.7 kg/m²	Diet history interview	1989 ± 455 kcal/d BW, 34.4 kcal/kg BW	236 ± 52 g/d, 4.1 g/kg/d BW, 48 ± 3% total energy	73 ± 16 g/d, 1.3 g/kg/d BW, 15 ± 2% total energy	78 ± 22 g/d, 36 ± 3% total energy
Dahlström et al. 1995	8 female dancers, 24 ± 2 years, BW = 58.5 ± 9 kg, BMI = 21.0 ± 19.4 kg/m²	7-day food record	2142 ± 514 kcal/d, 36.6 kcal/kg BW	264 ± 67 g/d, 4.5 g/kg BW, 49 ± 6% total energy	65 ± 22 g/d, 1.1 g/kg BW, 13 ± 2% total energy	84 ± 24 g/d, 36 ± 5% total energy
Doyle-Lucas et al. 2010	15 female ballet dancers, 24.3 ± 5.0 years, BW = 51.9 ± 2.7 kg, BMI = 18.9 ± 0.8 kg/m²	4-day food record	1557 ± 345 kcal/d, 30.0 kcal/kg BW	56 ± 12% total energy	17 ± 4% total energy	26 ± 8% total energy

(Continued)

TABLE 7.1 (Continued)
Studies Investigating Reported Dietary Intakes of Dancers

Ref.	Participants	Dietary Assessment Method	Energy	Carbohydrate	Protein	Fat
Frusztajer et al. 1990	Group 1: 10 female ballet dancers with a stress fracture history, 20.5 ± 3.9 years, BW = 49.2 ± 4.9 kg, BMI = 18.0 ± 1.7 kg/m² Group 2: 10 female ballet dancers without stress fracture history, 20.5 ± 4.0 years, BW = 50.9 ± 3.4 kg, BMI = 19.0 ± 1.3 kg/m²	Two 24-h dietary recalls; FFQ	Group 1: 24-h dietary recall = 1482 ± 524 kcal/d, 30.1 kcal/kg BW; FFQ = 1139 ± 265 kcal/d, 23.1 kcal/kg BW Group 2: 24-h dietary recall = 1692 ± 505 kcal/d, 33.2 kcal/kg BW; FFQ = 1432 ± 500 kcal/d, 28.1 kcal/kg BW			Group 1: 31 ± 12 g/d Group 2: 53 ± 26 g/d
Hassapidou and Manstrantoni 2001	7 female ballet dancers, 22.5 ± 2.3 years Time 1 (in training): BW = 54.5 ± 3.9 kg, BMI = 20.1 ± 1.3 kg/m² Time 2 (during competition): BW = 51.5 ± 4.8 kg, BMI = 19.7 ± 1.3 kg/m²	Two 7-day weighed food records	Time 1: 1701 ± 580 kcal/d, 31.2 kcal/kg BW Time 2: 1506 ± 468 kcal/d, 29.2 kcal/kg BW	Time 1: 168 ± 65 g/d, 3.1 g/kg BW, 44 ± 8% total energy Time 2: 199 ± 77 g/d, 3.9 g/kg BW, 53 ± 12% total energy	Time 1: 68 ± 16 g/d, 1.2 g/kg BW, 17 ± 3% total energy Time 2: 51 ± 13 g/d, 1.0 g/kg BW, 14 ± 2% total energy	Time 1: 78 ± 35 g/d, 41 ± 7% total energy Time 2: 62 ± 30 g/d, 37 ± 11% total energy

(Continued)

TABLE 7.1 (*Continued*)
Studies Investigating Reported Dietary Intakes of Dancers

Ref.	Participants	Dietary Assessment Method	Energy	Carbohydrate	Protein	Fat
Quintas et al. 2003	33 female ballet dancers, 16.2 ± 2.0 years, BW = 49.5 ± 3.9 kg, BMI = 18.7 ± 1.1 kg/m²	5-day food record	1891 ± 422 kcal/d, 38.2 kcal/kg BW		1.7 ± 0.4 g/kg BW	
Short and Short 1983	9 female dancers	1- to 14-day food record	1909 kcal/d (range 898–2909 kcal/d)	256 g/d (range 67–415 g/d), 52% total energy (range 29–72% total energy)	82 g/d (range 39–122 g/d), 17% total energy (range 13–20% total energy)	65 g/d (range 21–113 g/d), 31% total energy (range 16–52% total energy)
Soric et al. 2008	16 female ballet dancers, 11 years (range 9–13 years), BW = 34.6 ± 4.7 kg	FFQ	1731 ± 432 kcal/d, 51.4 ± 16.6 kcal/kg BW	6.6 ± 2.5 g/kg BW, 51 ± 4% total energy	2.1 ± 0.6 g/kg BW, 2% total energy	1.9 ± 0.6 g/kg, 34 ± 4% total energy
Van Marken Lichtenbelt et al. 1995	24 female ballet dancers, 22.6 ± 4.5 years, BW = 52.4 ± 4.6 kg, BMI = 18.9 ± 1.0 kg/m²	7-day food record	1552 kcal/d, 29.6 kcal/kg BW			
Warren et al. 2002	54 female ballet dancers Group 1: 32 with eumenorrhea, 22.0 ± 4.7 years, BW = 53.4 ± 6.8 kg Group 2: 22 with amenorrhea, 19.2 ± 3.4 years, BW = 46.6 ± 5.5 kg	2-day diet history; FFQ	Group 1: 1620 ± 598 kcal/d, 30.3 kcal/kg BW Group 2: 1765 ± 643 kcal/d, 37.9 kcal/kg BW			Group 1: 55 ± 31 g/d Group 2: 57 ± 50 g/d

(*Continued*)

TABLE 7.1 (Continued)
Studies Investigating Reported Dietary Intakes of Dancers

Ref.	Participants	Dietary Assessment Method	Energy	Carbohydrate	Protein	Fat
Yannakoulia et al. 2004	31 female dancers, 20.7 ± 1.8 years, BMI = 20.0 ± 1.1 kg/m² Group 1: 21 with eumenorrhea, 19.8 ± 1.2 years, BW = 53.2 ± 3.6 kg, BMI = 20.0 ± 1.2 kg/m² 10 with oligoamenorrhea/amenorrhea, 21.3 ± 2.0 years, BW = 53.7 ± 4.5 kg, BMI = 20.1 ± 1.1 kg/m²	3-day food record	Group 1: 1409 ± 482 kcal/d, 26.6 ± 9.2 kcal/kg BW Group 2: 1593 ± 401 kcal/d, 30.0 ± 8.0 kcal/kg BW	Group 1: 50 ± 10% total energy Group 2: 52 ± 8% total energy	Group 1: 1.0 ± 0.4 g/kg BW, 15 ± 6% total energy Group 2: 1.0 ± 0.3 g/kg BW, 13 ± 2% total energy	Group 1: 35 ± 6% total energy Group 2: 34 ± 7% total energy

Note: All values are means or mean ± SD. BMI = body mass index, BW = body weight, FFQ = food frequency questionnaire.

intake) and the mean reported protein intake was 2.1 ± 0.6 g/kg body weight (16 ± 2% of total energy intake). Quintas et al. (2003) also examined the reported dietary intakes of young female ballet dancers (n = 33; age: 16.2 ± 2.0 years), using 5-day food records. This group of adolescent ballet dancers reported mean energy and protein intakes of 1891 ± 422 kcal/day (38.2 kcal/kg body weight) and 1.7 ± 0.4 g/kg body weight, respectively. Bonbright (1989) observed similar results in a group of young ballet dancers (n = 32; age: 16.4 years). After completing a 5-day food record, this group of dancers reported consuming only 1584 kcal/day (32.6 kcal/kg body weight), 4.3 g/kg body weight carbohydrate (range 33% to 67% total energy), and 1.3 g/kg body weight protein (range 11% to 25% total energy). Total dietary fat ranged from 19% to 48% total energy. The reported energy intakes varied widely with the lowest reported energy intake of just 642 kcal/day. Collectively, these studies suggest young dancers tend to consume a higher relative energy (kcal/kg body weight) compared to adult dancers. However, few studies have investigated the dietary patterns of young dancers and these studies utilized different dietary assessment methodologies, making it difficult to summarize the dietary practices of young dancers.

Aesthetic sports that emphasize a low body weight are associated with an increased risk of the female athlete triad. This condition includes low energy availability with or without disordered eating, menstrual dysfunction, and low bone mineral density (Nattiv et al. 2007). The low energy availability may lead to exercise-induced amenorrhea (Nattiv et al. 2007; Torstveit and Sundgot-Borgen 2005), possibly due to the body adapting an energy-conserving technique to protect other physiological functions. Studies examining the dietary patterns of dancers have also assessed the female athlete triad, due to the low energy intakes typically seen in dancers. For example, two studies examined differences in reported dietary intake among adult ballet dancers grouped by menstrual status (Warren et al. 2002; Yannakoulia et al. 2004). Warren and colleagues (2002) studied female ballet dancers with eumenorrhea (EU) (n = 32; age: 22.0 ± 4.7 years; body weight: 53.4 ± 6.8 kg) and amenorrhea (AM) (n = 22; age: 19.2 ± 3.4 years; body weight: 46.6 ± 5.5 kg). In this study, no significant differences were observed in reported mean energy intakes between the two groups of dancers (EU: 1620 ± 598 kcal/day, 30.3 kcal/kg body weight; AM: 1765 ± 643 kcal/day, 37.9 kcal/kg). Yannakoulia et al. (2004) also examined usual dietary intakes of female dancers by menstrual status and observed similar results. Thirty-one female dancers were categorized as being EU (n = 21; age: 19.8 ± 1.2 years; BMI: 20.0 ± 1.2 kg/m^2) or oligoamenorrheic/amenorrheic (OA) (n = 10; age = 21.3 ± 2.0 years; BMI: 20.1 ± 1.2 kg/m^2). The researchers did not observe any differences in mean total energy intake between the two groups of dancers (EU: 1409 ± 482 kcal/day, 26.6 ± 9.2 kcal/kg body weight; OA: 1593 ± 401 kcal/day, 30.0 ± 8.0 kcal/kg body weight). Although these two studies found no differences in energy intake by menstrual status, the adult female ballet dancers consistently reported low energy availability.

FIGURE SKATING

The sport of figure skating emphasizes technique, artistic expression, and aesthetic appeal, placing an importance on leanness, low body weight, and an ideal body shape. For instance, 72% of female and 39% of male young figure skaters reported a desire to lose weight (Ziegler et al. 1998c). This aspiration is particularly problematic given many elite figure skaters are competing and training during their peak growing years. Restricted dietary intakes are potentially detrimental to long-term growth, development, and maturation and are not encouraged.

Researchers have assessed dietary intakes of both adolescent and adult male figure skaters (Jonnalagadda et al. 2004; Rucinski 1989; Ziegler et al. 1998b,c, 1999, 2001, 2002a, 2003, 2005b) (Table 7.2). Compared to female figure skaters, the body of literature examining male figure skaters is less robust. Adult male figure skaters report energy intakes ranging from 30.8 to 36.0 kcal/kg body weight (Jonnalagadda et al. 2004; Rucinski 1989; Ziegler et al. 2001, 2005b). Carbohydrate consumption ranged from 4.2 to 5.1 g/kg body weight, representing 47% to 57% of total energy intake. Protein consumption ranged from 1.2 to 1.3 g/kg body weight, contributing 15% to 17% of total energy. Reported dietary fat contributed 30% to 33% of total energy intake.

Although the total number of studies is small, adolescent male figure skaters appear to meet nutrient needs more consistently than adult male figure skaters do (Ziegler et al. 1998b,c, 1999, 2002a, 2003). The reported energy intakes of male adolescent figure skaters ranged from 37.0 to 40.4 kcal/kg body weight. Carbohydrate consumption typically ranged from 4.8 to 5.7 g/kg body weight, representing 47% to 67% of total energy. Reported protein consumption of adolescent male figure skaters ranged from 1.4 to 1.7 g/kg body weight, contributing 15% to 18% of total energy whereas reported dietary fat contributed 27% to 33% of total energy intake.

Reported dietary intakes for adolescent female figure skaters have been examined extensively in the research literature (Delistraty et al. 1992; Fogelholm et al. 1995; Jonnalagadda et al. 2004; Reading et al. 2002; Rucinski 1989; Ziegler et al. 1998a,b,c, 1999, 2001, 2002a,b, 2003, 2005b). Although there is some variance, reported dietary intakes of adolescent female figure skaters generally reflect a pattern of energy restriction and low dietary fat consumption. The reported energy intakes of female adolescent figure skaters ranged from 26.0 to 41.9 kcal/kg body weight. Reported carbohydrate intakes ranged from 4.1 to 5.5 g/kg body weight (51% to 64% of total energy intake), protein consumption ranged from 0.9 to 1.6 g/kg body weight (12% to 19% of total energy), and reported dietary fat intakes ranged from 23% to 36% of total daily energy intake.

The current research suggests dietary intakes of female figure skaters decline throughout adolescence. For example, Delistraty et al. (1992) observed the dietary intakes of 13 young female figure skaters using a 3-day food record (age: 12.9 ± 2.1 years; body weight: 47.8 ± 11.4 kg). The athletes reported an energy intake of 2003 ± 493 kcal/day (41.9 kcal/kg body weight). Likewise, Ziegler and colleagues (1998b) found that young female figure skaters (n = 19; age: 14.0 ± 1.6; body weight: 44.0 ± 7.0 kg) reported consuming 1674 ± 684 calories/day (38.0 kcal/kg body weight). In contrast, female figure skaters in their late teens tend to report a lower energy intake. Ziegler and colleagues (2005a) observed the dietary intakes of a relatively large sample of female figure skaters (n = 123; age: 17.4 ± 2.1 years; body weight: 59.0 ± 6.4 kg). The athletes reported consuming 1552 ± 45 kcal/day, just 26.0 kcal/kg body weight. In a similar study, Ziegler et al. (2005b) surveyed the dietary intakes of 80 female

TABLE 7.2
Studies Investigating Reported Dietary Intakes of Figure Skaters

Ref.	Participants	Dietary Assessment Method	Energy	Carbohydrate	Protein	Fat
Delistraty et al. 1992	13 female figure skaters, 12.9 ± 2.1 years, BW = 47.8 ± 11.4 kg	3-day food record	2003 ± 493 kcal/d, 41.9 kcal/kg BW	260 ± 67 g/d, 5.4 g/kg BW, 52 ± 8% total energy	70 ± 19 g/d, 1.6 ± 0.5 g/kg BW, 14 ± 2% total energy intake	75.4 ± 30.0 g/d, 34 ± 8% total energy
Fogelholm et al. 1995	12 female figure skaters, 17.1 ± 1.2 years, BW = 51.7 ± 5.9 kg, BMI = 19.6 ± 1.6 kg/m²	7-day food record	1682 ± 533 kcal/d, 32.5 kcal/kg BW			
Grandjean 1989	29 female figure skaters, 15 male figure skaters (individual demographics not provided)	3-day food record	Females: 1809 ± 489 kcal/d; Males: 2660 ± 845 kcal/d	Females: 52 ± 7% total energy; Males: 47 ± 9% total energy	Females: 15 ± 3% total energy; Males: 17 ± 6% total energy	Females: 33 ± 8% total energy; Males: 33 ± 6% total energy
Jonnalagadda et al. 2004	23 male figure skaters, 19 ± 4.0 years, BW = 68.6 ± 10.5 kg, BMI = 22.9 ± 3.3 kg/m²; 26 female figure skaters, 15.5 ± 2.6 years, BW = 46.4 ± 7.6 kg, BMI = 18.6 ± 2.0 kg/m²	3-day food record	Males: 2112 ± 802 kcal/d, 30.8 kcal/kg BW; Females: 1490 ± 461 kcal/d, 32.1 kcal/kg BW	Males: 291 ± 129 g/d, 4.2 g/kg BW, 53 ± 11% total energy; Females: 238 ± 72 g/d, 5.1 g/kg BW, 64 ± 9% total energy	Males: 82 ± 29 g/d, 1.2 g/kg BW, 16 ± 3% total energy; Females: 54 ± 19 g/d, 1.2 g/kg BW, 15 ± 3% total energy	Males: 73 ± 32 g/d, 32 ± 9% total energy; Females: 39 ± 21 g/d, 23 ± 7% total energy

(Continued)

TABLE 7.2 (Continued)
Studies Investigating Reported Dietary Intakes of Figure Skaters

Ref.	Participants	Dietary Assessment Method	Energy	Carbohydrate	Protein	Fat
Reading et al. 2002	22 female figure skaters Group 1: 10 with oligo/ amenorrhea (5 figure skaters), 15.7 ± 0.7 years, BW = 52.8 ± 11.7 kg Group 2: 12 with eumenorrhea (5 figure skaters), 16.4 ± 1.0 years, BW = 53.1 ± 4.9 kg	3-day food record	Group 1: 1191 ± 665 kcal/d, 37.8 ± 14.2 kcal/kg BW Group 2: 2076 ± 401 kcal/d, 38.6 ± 8.0 kcal/kg	Group 1: 63 ± 7% total energy EA: 63 ± 9% total energy	Group 1: 12 ± 2% total energy Group 2: 14 ± 2% total energy	Group 1: 25 ± 6% total energy Group 2: 25 ± 6% total energy
Rucinski 1989	17 male figure skaters, 21.1 years (range 16–26 years) 23 female figure skaters, 17.6 years (range 13–22 years)	3-day food record	Males: 2897 ± 1065 kcal/d Females: 1174 ± 454 kcal/d	Males: 56% total energy Females: 60% total energy	Males: 15% total energy Females: 15% total energy	Males: 30% total energy Females: 25% total energy
Ziegler et al. 1998a	21 female figure skaters, 13.7 ± 1.4 years, BW = 50.3 ± 8.4 kg, BMI = 19.9 ± 2.4 kg/m²	3-day food record	1781 ± 417 kcal/d, 35.4 kcal/kg BW	229 ± 50 g/d, 4.6 g/kg BW, 51% total energy	70 ± 19 g/d, 1.4 g/kg BW, 15% total energy	68 ± 9 g/d, 33% total energy

(Continued)

TABLE 7.2 (Continued)
Studies Investigating Reported Dietary Intakes of Figure Skaters

Ref.	Participants	Dietary Assessment Method	Energy	Carbohydrate	Protein	Fat
Ziegler et al. 1998b	15 male figure skaters, 16 ± 1 years, BW = 60 ± 6 kg; 19 female figure skaters 14 ± 2 years, BW = 44 ± 7 kg	4-day food record	Males: 2325 ± 907 kcal/d, 38.8 kcal/kg BW; Females: 1674 ± 684 kcal/d, 38.0 kcal/kg BW	Males: 308 ± 126 g/d, 5.1 g/kg BW, 53% total energy; Females: 241 ± 88 g/d, 5.4 g/kg BW, 58% total energy	Males: 94 ± 35 g/d, 1.6 g/kg BW, 16% total energy; Females: 66 ± 27 g/d, 1.5 g/kg BW, 16% total energy	Males: 82 ± 43 g/d, 32% total energy; Females: 53 ± 34 g/d, 28% total energy
Ziegler et al. 1998c	19 male figure skaters, 17.8 ± 2.6 years, BW = 66.7 ± 10.5 kg, BMI = 22.4 ± 2.2 kg/m²; 20 female figure skaters, 15.9 ± 2.7 years, BW = 45.9 ± 5.8 kg, BMI = 18.4 ± 2.2 kg/m²	4-day food record	Males: 2477 ± 876 kcal/d, 37.1 g/kg BW; Females: 1422 ± 487 kcal/d, 31.0 kcal/kg BW	Males: 355 ± 124 g/d, 5.3 g/kg BW, 58 ± 6% total energy; Females: 221 ± 76 g/d, 4.8 g/kg BW, 63 ± 8% total energy	Males: 96 ± 48 g/d, 1.4 g/kg BW, 15 ± 3% total energy; Females: 56 ± 18 g/d, 1.2 g/kg BW, 16 ± 3% total energy	Males: 78 ± 34 g/d, 28 ± 6% total energy; Females: 38 ± 21 g/d, 23 ± 8% total energy
Ziegler et al. 1999	21 male figure skaters, 16.5 ± 1.6 years, BW = 63.6 ± 8.9 kg; 20 female figure skaters, 14.1 ± 1.7 years, BW = 46.5 ± 7.1 kg	4-day food record	Males: 2365 ± 869 kcal/d, 37.0 kcal/kg BW; Females: 1536 ± 620 kcal/d, 33.0 kcal/kg BW	Males: 307 ± 110 g/d, 4.8 g/kg BW, 52% total energy; Females: 216 ± 77 g/d, 4.6 g/kg BW, 56% total energy	Males: 106 ± 50 g/d, 1.7 g/kg BW, 18% total energy; Females: 61 ± 33 g/d, 1.0 g/kg BW, 16% total energy	Males: 82 ± 45 g/d, 31% total energy; Females: 49 ± 32 g/d, 29% total energy

(Continued)

TABLE 7.2 (Continued)
Studies Investigating Reported Dietary Intakes of Figure Skaters

Ref.	Participants	Dietary Assessment Method	Energy	Carbohydrate	Protein	Fat
Ziegler et al. 2001	80 male figure skaters, 18.4 ± 3.6 years, BW = 65.2 ± 8.9 kg, BMI = 22.0 ± 16.1 kg/m² 81 female figure skaters, 15.9 ± 3.6 years, BW = 47.8 ± 6.3 kg, BMI = 19.3 ± 13.5 kg/m²	3-day food record	Males: 2329 kcal/d (range 748–4438 kcal/d), 36.0 ± 12.0 kcal/kg BW Females: 1545 kcal/d (range 465–3303 kcal/d), 33.0 ± 11.0 kcal/kg BW	Males: 5.1 ± 1.7 g/kg BW, 57 ± 7% total energy Females: 5.0 ± 1.8 g/kg BW, 60 ± 10% total energy	Males: 1.3 ± 0.5 g/kg BW, 15 ± 3% total energy Females: 1.3 ± 0.4 g/kg BW, 16 ± 4% total energy	Males: 30 ± 7% total energy Females: 25 ± 9% total energy
Ziegler et al. 2002a	46 male figure skaters, 17.2 ± 3.0 years, BW = 65.5 ± 8.9 kg, BMI = 21.2 ± 2.0 kg/m² 48 female figure skaters, 15.0 ± 2.4 years, BW = 45.0 ± 8.1 kg, BMI = 18.5 ± 2.0 kg/m²	3-day food record	Males: 2649 ± 861 kcal/d, 40.4 kcal/kg BW Females: 1632 ± 734 kcal/d, 36.3 kcal/kg BW	Males: 374 ± 122 g/d, 5.7 k/kg BW, 67 ± 10% total energy Females: 243 ± 111 g/d, 5.5 g/kg BW, 58 ± 14% total energy	Males: 104 ± 41 g/d, 1.6 g/kg BW, 16 ± 7% total energy Females: 70 ± 35 g/d, 1.6 g/kg BW, 17 ± 7% total energy	Males: 86 ± 34 g/d, 29 ± 7% total energy Females: 45 ± 28 g/d, 24 ± 7% total energy

(Continued)

TABLE 7.2 (Continued)
Studies Investigating Reported Dietary Intakes of Figure Skaters

Ref.	Participants	Dietary Assessment Method	Energy	Carbohydrate	Protein	Fat
Ziegler et al. 2002b	18 female figure skaters, 14–16 years Time 1 (preseason): 15 ± 1 years, BW = 50.1 ± 5.2 kg Time 2 (competition): 16 ± 1 years, BW = 51.9 ± 5.8 kg Time 3 (off season): 16 ± 1 years, BW = 52.6 ± 5.3 kg	3-day food record	Time 1: 1678 kcal/d, 33.5 kcal/kg BW Time 2: 1630 kcal/d, 31.4 kcal/kg BW Time 3: 1673 kcal/d, 31.8 kcal/kg BW	Time 1: 214 g/d, 4.3 g/kg BW, 51% total energy Time 2: 212 g/d, 4.1 g/kg BW, 52% total energy Time 3: 218 g/d, 4.1 g/kg BW, 52% total energy	Time 1: 64 g/d, 1.3 g/kg BW, 15% total energy Time 2: 64 g/d, 1.2 g/kg BW, 16% total energy Time 3: 59 g/d, 1.1 g/kg BW, 14% total energy	Time 1: 65 g/d, 35% total energy Time 2: 62 g/d, 34% total energy Time 3: 66 g/d, 36% total energy
Ziegler et al. 2003	30 male figure skaters and dietary supplement users (DSU), 17 ± 2 years, BMI = 21.8 ± 2.2 kg/m² 16 male figure skaters and non-dietary supplement users (NSU), 16 ± 2 years, BMI = 20.9 ± 2.4 kg/m² 45 female figure skaters and DSU, 15 ± 1 year, BMI = 18.4 ± 1.3 kg/m² 14 female figure skaters and NSU, 16 ± 3 years, BMI = 19.2 ± 1.5 kg/m²	3-day food record	Male DSU: 2535 ± 811 kcal/d Male NSU: 2164 ± 1092 kcal/d Female DSU: 1493 ± 389 kcal/d Female NSU: 1673 ± 501 kcal/d	Male DSU: 311 ± 110 g/d, 50 ± 11% total energy Male NSU: 315 ± 184 g/d, 57 ± 8% total energy Female DSU: 216 ± 67 g/d, 56 ± 13% total energy Female NSU: 233 ± 60 g/d, 57 ± 7% total energy	Male DSU: 107 ± 27 g/d, 17 ± 5% total energy Male NSU: 87 ± 32 g/d, 17 ± 4% total energy Female DSU: 63 ± 20 g/d, 19 ± 11% total energy Female NSU: 70 ± 22 g/d, 17 ± 4% total energy	Male DSU: 98 ± 44 g/d, 33 ± 5% total energy Male NSU: 65 ± 28 g/d, 27 ± 4% total energy Female DSU: 44 ± 20 g/d, 27 ± 7% total energy Female NSU: 54 ± 15 g/d, 27 ± 7% total energy

(Continued)

TABLE 7.2 (Continued)
Studies Investigating Reported Dietary Intakes of Figure Skaters

Ref.	Participants	Dietary Assessment Method	Energy	Carbohydrate	Protein	Fat
Ziegler et al. 2005a	123 female figure skaters, 17.4 ± 2.1 years, BW = 59.0 ± 6.4 kg, BMI = 21.3 ± 2.0 kg/m²	3-day food record	1552 ± 45.0 kcal/d, 26.0 kcal/kg BW	241 ± 9 g/d, 4.1 g/kg BW, 62 ± 1% total energy	56 ± 2 g/d, 0.9 g/kg BW, 14 ± 0.3% total energy	41 ± 2 g/d, 24 ± 1% total energy
Ziegler et al. 2005b	79 male figure skaters, 18.4 years, BMI = 22.3 kg/m² (range 15.6–26.7 kg/m²) 80 female figure skaters, 15.9 years, BMI = 19.2 kg/m² (range 14.9–24.3 kg/m²)	3-day food record	Males: 2326 kcal/d (range 748–4438 kcal/d) Females: 1545 kcal/d (range 465–3303 kcal/d)	Males: 56% total energy Females: 60% total energy	Males: 15% total energy Females: 15% total energy	Males: 30% total energy Females: 25% total energy

Note: All values are means or mean ± SD. BMI = body mass index, BW = body weight, FFQ = food frequency questionnaire.

figure skaters (age: 15.9 years) using a 3-day food record. Four of the female figure skaters reported an average energy intake of less than 1000 kcal/day, well below the recommendations for active females. Energy intakes ranged from 465 to 3303 kcal/day (mean energy intake: 1545 kcal day), demonstrating the severe energy restriction practiced by some female figure skaters, especially among elite athletes.

Gymnastics

In competitive gymnastics, success is influenced by technical skill and body aesthetics. Thus, gymnasts experience considerable pressures to achieve and maintain an ideal body shape. These demands increase by level of competition, with elite gymnasts facing the most pressure (de Bruin et al. 2007). The ideal body of elite female gymnasts represents a prepubertal shape and has influenced the decline in age of competitive gymnasts. In 1997, the Federation Internationale de Gymnastique raised the minimum age limit for international competition from 15 to 16 years of age due to a concern to protect the musculoskeletal development of elite young gymnasts (Anderson 1997). Despite this change, gymnasts continue to face tremendous pressure to achieve an ideal body shape. The drive to diet and achieve the lean and ideal body shape is so intense, approximately 65% of collegiate gymnasts display asymptomatic eating disorders (Anderson and Petrie 2012). Even more unsettling, 28.9% and 6.1% of gymnasts surveyed were classified with subclinical and clinical eating disorders, respectively. Because gymnasts compete in a sport where body size and appearance are a large determinant of success, the preoccupation and concern with achieving an ideal body shape often continues for years, even after retirement (O'Connor et al. 1996).

Dietary intakes of female gymnasts have been well examined in the research literature (Benardot et al. 1989; Benson et al. 1990; Chen et al. 1989; Cupisti et al. 2000; D'Alessandro et al. 2007; Ersoy 1991; Filaire and Lac 2002; Fogelholm et al. 1995; Grandjean 1989; Gropper et al. 2003; Hickson et al. 1986; Howat et al. 1989; Jonnalagadda et al. 1998, 2000; Kirchner et al. 1995; Lindholm et al. 1995; Loosli and Benson 1990; López-Varela et al. 2000; Michopoulou et al. 2011; Moffatt 1984; Reading et al. 2002; Reggiani et al. 1989; Short and Short 1983; Soric et al. 2008; Sundgot-Borgen 1996; van Erp-Baart et al. 1989; Weimann et al. 2000) (Table 7.3). However, the existing literature is challenging to interpret, with research suggesting that gymnasts underreport energy intake (Jonnalagadda et al. 2000; Thompson 1998). In one study, over 60% of the female gymnasts underreported energy intake (Jonnalagadda et al. 2000). This misrepresentation of dietary intake may be due to the preoccupation with body image and a prepubertal body shape. Additionally, most research evaluating self-reported dietary intakes in gymnasts is at least a decade old. Thus, these results may not be generalizable to contemporary gymnasts and must be interpreted with caution. Despite these limitations, the existing literature consistently portrays a low or moderate energy intake among female gymnasts, suggesting these athletes do not meet estimated energy and macronutrient recommendations. Benardot (2000) summarized studies examining dietary intake in gymnasts, varying in age and level of competition. Gymnasts involved in the highest level of competition had the greatest disparity between energy intake and energy requirement. This trend is likely due to the increasing pressures that occur with higher levels of

TABLE 7.3
Studies Investigating Reported Dietary Intakes of Gymnasts

Ref.	Participants	Dietary Assessment Method	Energy	Carbohydrate	Protein	Fat
Benardot et al. 1989	22 female gymnasts, 11–14 years	2-day food record	1706 ± 421 kcal/d	227 ± 64 g/d, 7.3 g/kg, 53 ± 6% total energy	67 ± 20 g/d, 2.0 g/kg, 15 ± 2% total energy	62 ± 18 g/d, 32 ± 5% total energy
Benson et al. 1990	12 females gymnasts, 12.5 ± 1.1 years, BW = 34.9 ± 6.0 kg	7-day food record	1544 ± 398 kcal/d, 39.4 ± 13.3 kcal/kg BW	205 g/d, 5.9 g/kg BW, 53 ± 6% total energy	69 g/d, 2.0 g/kg BW, 17 ± 3% total energy	55 g/d, 31 ± 6% total energy
Chen et al. 1989	5 female gymnasts, 18 ± 1 year, 45 ± 2 kg, 4 male gymnasts, 21 ± 3 years, 59 ± 6 kg	3- to 5-day weighed food record	Females: 2298 ± 326 kcal/d, 51 ± 7 kcal/kg BW, Males: 3310 ± 56 kcal/d, 56 ± 9 kcal/kg BW	Females: 242 ± 49 g/d, 5.4 ± 1.1 g/kg BW, 42 ± 9% total energy, Males: 357 ± 77 g/d, 6.1 ± 1.3 g/kg BW, 43 ± 9% total energy	Females: 94 ± 25 g/d, 2.1 ± 0.6 g/kg BW, 16 ± 4% total energy, Males: 151 ± 28 g/d, 2.6 ± 0.5 g/kg BW, 18 ± 3% total energy	Females: 106 ± 14 g/d, 42 ± 6% total energy, Males: 141 ± 18 g/d, 38 ± 5% total energy
Cupisti et al. 2000	20 female rhythmic gymnasts, 15.7 ± 1.3 years, BW = 46.7 ± 5.1 kg, BMI = 17.5 ± 1.3 kg/m²	3-day food record	1315 ± 97 kcal/d, 28.5 ± 5.6 kcal/kg BW	53 ± 6% total energy	~1.1 g/kg BW, 15 ± 1% total energy	31 ± 6% total energy
D'Alessandro et al. 2007	55 female rhythmic gymnasts, 15.2 ± 2.2 years, BW = 49.0 ± 6.1 kg, BMI = 18.9 ± 1.8 kg/m²	3-day food record	28.8 ± 10.8 kcal/kg BW	55 ± 6% total energy	1.2 ± 0.4 g/kg BW	28 ± 6% total energy

(Continued)

TABLE 7.3 (Continued)
Studies Investigating Reported Dietary Intakes of Gymnasts

Ref.	Participants	Dietary Assessment Method	Energy	Carbohydrate	Protein	Fat
Ersoy 1991	20 female gymnasts, 11.5 ± 0.5 years, BW = 31.6 ± 1.5 kg	3-day food record	1568 kcal/d, 49.6 kcal/kg BW	224 g/d, 7.1 g/kg BW, 57% total energy	60 g/d, 1.9 g/kg BW, 15% total energy	48 g/d, 27% total energy
Filaire and Lac 2002	12 female gymnasts, 10.1 ± 0.3 years, BW = 25.3 ± 1.2 kg	7-day food record	2006 ± 143 kcal/d, 74 kcal/kg BW	241 ± 14 g/d, 9.4 ± 0.2 g/kg BW, 48 ± 4% total energy	69 ± 3 g/d, 2.7 ± 0.4 g/kg BW, 14 ± 1% total energy	81 ± 6 g/d, 38 ± 3% total energy
Fogelholm et al. 1995	12 female gymnasts, 17.1 ± 1.2 years, BW = 51.7 ± 5.9 kg, BMI = 19.6 ± 1.6 kg/m²	7-day food record	1682 ± 533 kcal/d, 32.5 kcal/kg BW			
Grandjean 1989	10 female gymnasts (individual demographics not presented)	3-day food record	1935 ± 398 kcal/d	49 ± 5% total energy	15 ± 2% total energy	36 ± 4% total energy
Gropper et al. 2003	10 female gymnasts, 19.4 ± 1.1 years, BW = 56.6 ± 5.5 kg, BMI = 22.0 ± 2.1 kg/m²	3-day food record	1711 ± 498 kcal/d, 30.2 kcal/kg BW		61 ± 12 g/d, 1.1 g/kg BW, 14% total energy	
Hickson et al. 1986	9 female gymnasts, 19.1 ± 0.6 years, BW = 58.0 ± 3.0 kg	Three 24-hour dietary recalls	1827 ± 182 kcal/d, 32.0 ± 12.0 kcal/kg BW			

(Continued)

TABLE 7.3 (Continued)
Studies Investigating Reported Dietary Intakes of Gymnasts

Ref.	Participants	Dietary Assessment Method	Energy	Carbohydrate	Protein	Fat
Howat et al. 1989	10 females (9 gymnasts, 1 body builder) Group 1: 5 with eumenorrhea, 19.2 ± 0.5 years, BW = 55.4 ± 2.4 kg Group 2: 5 with oligomenorrhea/amenorrhea, 19.6 ± 1.4 years, BW = 52.3 ± 1.8 kg	7-day food record	Group 1: 1933 kcal/d, 34.9 kcal/kg BW; Group 2: 1551 kcal/d, 29.7 kcal/kg BW			
Jonnalagadda et al. 1998	29 female gymnasts, 15.1 ± 1.3 years, BW = 48.8 ± 8.3 kg	3-day food record	1678 ± 543 kcal/d, 34.4 kcal/kg BW	283 ± 96 g/d, 5.8 g/kg BW, 66% total energy	72 ± 23 g/d, 1.5 g/kg BW, 17% total energy	32 ± 17 g/d, 18% total energy
Jonnalagadda et al. 2000	Group 1 (low energy reporters): 17 female artistic gymnasts, 15.1 ± 1.5 years, BW = 48.7 ± 8.6 kg, BMI = 20.8 ± 2.3 kg/m² Group 2 (adequate energy reporters): 11 female artistic gymnasts, 15.0 ± 0.8 years, BW = 42.9 ± 7.2 kg, BMI = 19.0 ± 1.9 kg/m²	3-day food record	Group 1: 1306 ± 270 kcal/d, 26.8 kcal/kg BW; Group 2: 2209 ± 373 kcal/d, 51.5 kcal/kg BW	Group 1: 67 ± 3% total energy; Group 2: 64 ± 7% total energy	Group 1: 18 ± 3% total energy; Group 2: 16 ± 2% total energy	Group 1: 16 ± 4% total energy; Group 2: 19 ± 7% total energy

(Continued)

TABLE 7.3 (Continued)
Studies Investigating Reported Dietary Intakes of Gymnasts

Ref.	Participants	Dietary Assessment Method	Energy	Carbohydrate	Protein	Fat
Kirchner et al. 1995	26 female gymnasts, 19.7 ± 1.0 years, BW = 54.1 ± 6.1 kg	FFQ	1381 ± 556 kcal/d, 25.5 kcal/kg BW	180 ± 61 g/d, 3.3 g/kg BW, 52% total energy	53 ± 20 g/d, 1.0 g/kg BW, 15% total energy	48 ± 29 g/d, 31% total energy
Lindholm et al. 1995	22 female gymnasts, 14.8 years (median) (range 13.5–16.6 years), BW = 46.8 kg (median) (range 37.3–60.0 kg), BMI = 18.8 kg/m^2 (median) (range 16.0–22.3 kg/m^2)	Two 7-day weighed food records	1930 ± 455 kcal/d, 41.2 kcal/kg BW	259 ± 50 g/d, 5.5 g/kg BW	72 ± 17 g/d, 1.5 g/kg BW	72 ± 25 g/d
Loosli and Benson 1990	97 female gymnasts, 13.1 years, 43 kg	3-day food record	1838 kcal/d, 42.7 g/kg BW	220 g/d, 5.1 g/kg BW, 49% total energy	71 g/d, 1.6 g/kg BW, 15% total energy	74 g/d, 36% total energy
López-Varela et al. 2000	10 female gymnasts, 15.8 ± 0.5 years, BW = 42.4 ± 3.8 kg, BMI = 16.3 ± 0.9 kg/m^2	7-day food record	1267 ± 136 kcal/d, 29.9 kcal/kg BW	156 ± 22 g/d, 3.7 ± 0.5 g/kg BW, 47 ± 6% total energy	81 ± 15 g/d, 1.9 ± 0.3 g/kg BW, 26 ± 5% total energy intake	39 ± 12 g/d, 28 ± 6% total energy
Michopoulou et al. 2011	40 female rhythmic gymnasts, 11.0 ± 0.6 years, BW = 32.7 ± 3.1 kg, BMI = 16.4 ± 1.9 kg/m^2	7-day food record	1642 ± 420 kcal/d, 50.0 ± 13.0 kcal/kg BW	235 g/d, 7.2 g/kg BW, 57 ± 7% total energy	57 ± 20 g/d, 1.7 g/kg BW, 14 ± 3% total energy	40 ± 12 g/d, 28 ± 5% total energy
Moffatt 1984	13 female gymnasts, 15.2 ± 4.1 years, BW = 50.4 ± 6.5 kg	Two 3-day food records	1923 ± 674 kcal/d, 38.2 kcal/kg BW	222 ± 77 g/d, 4.4 g/kg BW, 46 ± 4% total energy	74 ± 23 g/d, 1.4 g/kg BW, 15 ± 2% total energy	82 ± 17 g/d, 38 ± 5% total energy

(Continued)

TABLE 7.3 (Continued)
Studies Investigating Reported Dietary Intakes of Gymnasts

Ref.	Participants	Dietary Assessment Method	Energy	Carbohydrate	Protein	Fat
Reading et al. 2002	22 female gymnasts Group 1: 12 with eumenorrhea (5 gymnasts), BW = 16.4 ± 1.0 years, 53.1 ± 4.9 kg Group 2: 10 with oligo/amenorrhea (5 gymnasts), 15.7 ± 0.7 years, BW = 52.8 ± 11.7 kg	3-day food record	Group 1: 2076 ± 401 kcal/d, 38.6 ± 8.0 kcal/kg Group 2: 1191 ± 665 kcal/d, 37.8 ± 14.2 kcal/kg	Group 1: 63 ± 9% total energy Group 2: 63 ± 7% total energy	Group 1: 14 ± 2% total energy Group 2: 12 ± 2% total energy	Group 1: 25 ± 6% total energy Group 2: 25 ± 6% total energy
Reggiani et al. 1989	26 female gymnasts, 12.3 ± 1.7 years, BW = 37.9 ± 6.9 kg, BMI 17.7 ± 1.5 kg/m²	6-day food record	1552 ± 502 kcal/k, 42.8 ± 17.6 kcal/kg	194 g/d, 5.1 g/kg, 48 ± 7% total energy	61.8 ± 25.4 g/d, 1.5 g/kg, 15 ± 3% total energy	62 g/d, 36 ± 7% total energy
Short and Short 1983	10 male gymnasts	1- to 14-day food record	2080 kcal/d (range 586–4249 kcal/d)	231 g/d (range 94–557 g/d), 44% total energy (range 24–60% total energy)	77 g/d (range 11–145 g/d), 15% total energy (range 8–26% total energy)	92 g/d (range 20–211 g/d), 39% total energy (range 34–49% total energy)
Soric et al. 2008	23 female gymnasts, 11 years (range 9–13 years) Group 1: 9 artistic, BW = 32.2 ± 7.5 kg Group 2: 14 rhythmic, BW = 39.3 ± 10.3 kg	FFQ	Group 1: 1941 ± 680 kcal/d, 63.4 ± 28.7 kcal/kg BW Group 2: 1647 ± 677 kcal/d, 44.9 ± 22.1 kcal/kg BW	Group 1: 9.1 ± 4.2 g/kg BW, 57 ± 6% total energy Group 2: 5.6 ± 3.1 g/kg BW, 48 ± 6% total energy	Group 1: 2.3 ± 1.2 g/kg BW, 14 ± 2% total energy Group 2: 1.8 ± 0.8 g/kg BW, 16 ± 2% total energy	Group 1: 29 ± 5% total energy Group 2: 36 ± 5% total energy

(Continued)

TABLE 7.3 (Continued)
Studies Investigating Reported Dietary Intakes of Gymnasts

Ref.	Participants	Dietary Assessment Method	Energy	Carbohydrate	Protein	Fat
Sundgot-Borgen 1996	12 female rhythmic gymnasts, 15.3 years (range 13–20 years), BW = 42 kg (range 33–58 kg)	4-day weighed food record	1703 kcal/d (range 1200–2374 kcal/d), 40.5 kcal/kg BW			
van Erp-Baart et al. 1989	52 female gymnasts Group 1: 11 females, 15 ± 1 years, BW = 46.9 ± 6.3 kg Group 2: 41 females, 13 ± 1 years, BW = 39.8 ± 11.1 kg	4- or 7-day food record	Group 1: 37.8 kcal/kg BW (range 21.7–51.6 kcal/kg BW) Group 2: 49.2 kcal/kg BW (range 27.0–79.8 kcal/kg BW)	Group 1: ~53% total energy Group 2: ~51% total energy	Group 1: ~14% total energy Group 2: ~15% total energy	Group 1: ~32% total energy Group 2: ~36% total energy
Weimann et al. 2000	22 female gymnasts, 13.6 ± 1.0 years 18 male gymnasts, 12.4 ± 1.6 years	3-day food record	Females: 1390 ± 515 kcal/d Males: 2116 ± 41 kcal/d	Females: 194 ± 81 g/d, 55% total energy Males: 158 ± 63 g/d, 47% total energy	Females: 47 ± 18 g/d, 13% total energy Males: 74 ± 12 g/d, 13% total energy	Females: 49 ± 20 g/d, 31% total energy Males: 91 ± 17 g/d, 36% total energy

Note: All values are means or mean ± SD. BMI = body mass index, BW = body weight, FFQ = food frequency questionnaire.

competition. Because elite females often reach the highest competitive level before adulthood, the present discussion will categorize the research literature examining usual dietary intakes of female gymnasts by age (≤14 years, 15 to 17 years, and ≥18 years). Male gymnasts do not appear to follow this trend. Consequently, the literature investigating usual dietary intakes among male gymnasts is categorized into two groups: young and adult male gymnasts.

The dietary intakes of female gymnasts ≤14 years are inconsistent, with some gymnasts reporting extremely low energy and macronutrient intakes (Benson et al. 1990; Ersoy 1991; Filaire and Lac 2002; Loosli and Benson 1990; Michopoulou et al. 2011; Reggiani et al. 1989; Soric et al. 2008; van Erp-Baart et al. 1989; Weimann et al. 2000). The reported energy intakes of female gymnasts ≤14 years ranged from 39.4 to 74.0 kcal/kg body weight. The highest relative energy intake was reported by young female gymnasts with a low body mass (age: 10.1 ± 0.3 years; body weight: 25.3 ± 1.2 kg) (Filaire and Lac 2002). Gymnasts in this age category typically reported carbohydrate intakes of 5.1 to 9.4 g/kg body weight or 48% to 57% of total energy. Reported protein intakes ranged from 1.5 to 2.7 g/kg body weight, contributing 13% to 17% of total energy intake. Total dietary fat intakes ranged from 27% to 28% of total energy.

Most research investigating the dietary intake patterns of female gymnasts does not identify if the gymnasts participate in artistic or rhythmic gymnastics. Therefore, the differences in dietary intake patterns of artistic or rhythmic gymnasts are not well established. Soric and colleagues (2008) investigated reported energy intakes among 23 artistic and rhythmic young gymnasts (artistic n = 9; rhythmic n = 14; age: 11 years) using a food frequency questionnaire. Artistic gymnasts reported consuming 1941 ± 680 kcal/day (63.4 ± 28.7 kcal/kg body weight), whereas rhythmic gymnasts reported consuming 1647 ± 677 kcal/day (44.9 ± 22.1 kcal/kg body weight). Carbohydrate intakes were statistically different between the gymnasts (artistic gymnasts: 9.1 ± 4.2 g/kg body weight, 57 ± 6% of total energy; rhythmic gymnasts: 5.6 ± 3.1 g/kg body weight, 48 ± 6% of total energy). Although this represents just one study, these results suggest the macronutrient distribution may differ between these groups of gymnasts. Additional research is necessary to determine the dietary intake patterns of both artistic and rhythmic gymnasts.

Other research has focused on the dietary intakes of female gymnasts between the ages of 15 and 17 years (Cupisti et al. 2000; D'Alessandro et al. 2007; Jonnalagadda et al. 1998, 2000; López-Varela et al. 2000; Moffatt 1984; Reading et al. 2002; Sundgot-Borgen 1996; van Erp-Baart et al. 1989). Using a variety of dietary assessment methods, these athletes reported energy intakes of 26.8 to 51.5 kcal/kg body weight, suggesting gymnasts ages 15 to 17 years do not consume adequate energy to cover the cost of training. For instance, Jonnalagadda et al. (1998) examined dietary intakes in female elite gymnasts (n = 29; age: 15.1 ± 1.3 years) and determined that the athletes reported an energy intake 20% below their estimated energy requirements. Unfortunately, athletes with the lowest self-reported energy intakes are at a greater risk of poor nutrient status. The research literature reports daily carbohydrate intakes of female gymnasts 15 to 17 years of age ranged from 3.7 to 5.8 g/kg body weight, contributing 46% to 67% of total energy intake (Cupisti et al. 2000; D'Alessandro et al. 2007; Jonnalagadda et al. 1998, 2000; López-Varela et al. 2000; Moffatt 1984; Reading et al. 2002; Sundgot-Borgen 1996; van Erp-Baart et al. 1989). Protein consumption ranged from 1.1 to 1.9 g/kg body weight, representing 14% to 26% of total dietary intake. Reported dietary fat intake contributed 16% to 38% of total energy, with several studies observing intakes ≤25% of total energy (Jonnalagadda et al. 1998, 2000; Reading et al. 2002). Moreover, dietary fat intakes remained below recommendations even when these gymnasts are grouped into categories based on energy intakes (low energy reporters n = 17: 26.8 kcal/kg body weight, dietary fat: 16 ± 4% of total energy intake; adequate energy reporters n = 11: 51.5 kcal/kg body weight, dietary fat: 19 ± 7% of total energy intake) (Jonnalagadda et al. 2000).

Other researchers have examined the dietary intakes of older female gymnasts (≥18 years of age), typically those participating in collegiate gymnastics (Chen et al. 1989; Gropper et al. 2003; Hickson et al. 1986; Howat et al. 1989; Kirchner et al. 1995). At this level of competition, reported energy intakes ranged from 25.5 to 51.0 kcal/kg body weight. Adult female gymnasts reported carbohydrate intakes of approximately 3.3 to 5.4 g/kg body weight (42% to 52% of total energy intake) and protein intakes of 1.0 to 2.1 g/kg body weight (14% to 16% of total energy). Reported dietary fat ranged from 31% to 42% of total energy. Gropper and colleagues (2003) conducted one of the most recent and well-designed studies examining the macro-nutrient and micronutrient intakes of 10 female collegiate gymnasts, using a 3-day food record. These adult gymnasts reported consuming just 1711 ± 498 kcal/day (30.2 kcal/kg body weight). Reported protein intakes were 1.1 g/kg body weight, contributing 14% of total daily energy. Unfortunately, reported carbohydrate and fat intakes were not included in the results of this study. Similar to younger gymnasts, collegiate gymnasts reported inadequate energy and macronutrient intakes.

Few studies have examined the dietary intakes of male gymnasts (Chen et al. 1989; Short and Short 1983; Weimann et al. 2000). Unfortunately, the existing research investigating reported dietary intakes of male gymnasts contains consider-able limitations, making it challenging to interpret the existing literature. For exam-ple, the authors utilized a variety of dietary assessment methods and the majority of the research was completed during the 1980s. Despite these concerns, male gym-nasts reported carbohydrate, protein, and fat intakes ranging from 43 to 47%, 13% to 18%, and 36% to 39% of total energy intake, respectively. The most extensive dietary study of male gymnasts was completed with only four athletes (age: 21 ± 3 years), using weighed food records for three to five days (Chen et al. 1989). The male gym-nasts reported a mean energy intake of 3310 ± 56 kcal/day (56 ± 9 kcal/kg body weight). The reported dietary intakes for carbohydrate and protein were 6.1 ± 1.3 g/kg body weight (43 ± 9% of total energy) and 2.6 ± 0.5 g/kg body weight (18 ± 3% of total energy), respectively. The athletes reported dietary fat intakes of 38 ± 5% of total energy. Although these results represent just one study, they are strikingly dif-ferent from the dietary intakes observed among female gymnasts, suggesting male gymnasts are more likely to meet nutrient recommendations.

SYNCHRONIZED SWIMMING

Synchronized swimmers require a high level of aerobic and anaerobic fitness, flex-ibility, strength, power, and acrobatic skills in order to succeed (Mountjoy 2009). In addition to these physiological needs, synchronized swimming emphasizes a

TABLE 7.4
Studies Investigating Reported Dietary Intakes of Synchronized Swimmers

Ref.	Participants	Dietary Assessment Method	Energy	Carbohydrate	Protein	Fat
Ebine et al. 2000	9 female synchronized swimmers, 16–21 years, BW = 52.5 ± 2.7 kg, BMI = 20.7 ± 0.7 kg/m^2	7-day food record	2128 ± 395 kcal/d, 40.5 kcal/kg BW			
Reading et al. 2002	22 females (3 synchronized swimmers) Group 1: 12 with eumenorrheic (1 synchronized swimmer), 16.4 ± 1.0 years, BW = 53.1 ± 4.9 kg Group 2: 10 with oligomenorrheic/amenorrheic (2 synchronized swimmers), 15.7 ± 0.7 years, BW = 52.8 ± 11.7 kg	3-day food record	Group 1: 2076 ± 401 kcal/d, 38.6 ± 8.0 kcal/kg BW Group 2: 1191 ± 665 kcal/d, 37.8 ± 14.2 kcal/kg BW	Group 1: 63 ± 9% total energy Group 2: 63 ± 7% total energy	Group 1: 14 ± 2% total energy Group 2: 12 ± 2% total energy	Group 1: 25 ± 6% total energy Group 2: 25 ± 6% total energy

Note: All values are means or mean ± SD. BMI = body mass index, BW = body weight, FFQ = food frequency questionnaire.

lean and athletic appearance, low body weight, and a uniformity of physique within the team (Lundy 2011). Synchronized swimmers have a higher prevalence of disordered eating and eating disorders, menstrual dysfunction, and low bone mineral density compared to other aquatic sport athletes and non-athletes (Douka et al. 2008; Ferrand et al. 2005, 2007; Lundy 2011). Unfortunately, the dietary practices of synchronized swimmers remain relatively unknown due to the scarcity of research.

To date, only two studies have investigated dietary intakes among female synchronized swimmers (Table 7.4) (Ebine et al. 2000; Reading et al. 2002). Ebine and colleagues (2000) conducted the largest study observing reported dietary patterns and energy expenditure among female synchronized swimmers. The researchers examined the reported dietary intakes in just nine female synchronized swimmers (age: 16 to 21 years; body weight: 52.5 ± 2.7 kg; BMI: 20.7 ± 0.7 kg/m^2) using a 7-day food record and energy expenditure using doubly labeled water. The average reported energy intake of the nine synchronized swimmers was 2128 ± 395 kcal/day (40.5 kcal/kg body weight) and the mean energy expenditure was 2738 ± 673 kcal/day (52.2 kcal/kg body weight). Because the synchronized swimmers were weight stable throughout the study, the athletes appear to have underreported dietary intake, a problem well documented in other aesthetic and weight-class sports (Burke 2001; Fogelhom et al. 1995; Hill and Davies 1999; Jonnalagadda et al. 2000; Magkos and Yannakoulia 2003; Thompson 1998). Reading et al. (2002) also observed self-reported dietary intakes among a larger group of athletes, including synchronized swimmers, which were further categorized according to menstrual status. Among the 22 female athletes, only three were synchronized swimmers and the dietary intakes were not separated by sport. Future research examining dietary intakes of athletes should include synchronized swimmers.

WEIGHT-CLASS SPORTS

JOCKEYS

Horse racing jockeys participate in a sport that requires them to weigh-in 30 min prior to competition. Jockeys must be weighed fully clothed with riding boots, back protector, and saddle. Jockeys may be reweighed after the race to validate body weights, decreasing the time to rehydrate or refuel before events. Thus, excessive dehydration and low energy availability resulting from extreme weight loss practices certainly impact performance. Although minimum weight guidelines for competition have been established and vary depending on the event, the weight targets of jockeys are still considerably low, often much less than the jockey's ideal body weight.

The weigh-in procedures of jockeys are arguably the most severe of all weight-class sports. The pressures to achieve a specific weight are so intense that many jockeys report making weight for competition takes precedence over all other concerns in their life (Cotugna et al. 2011; King and Mezey 1987). Not surprisingly, the act of rapidly and repeatedly making weight places horse racing jockeys at a high risk to develop disordered eating behaviors (King and Mezey 1987). In fact, the mean weight of horse racing jockeys is 13% below the population average for weight for height, with the lightest jockey weighing 21% below the population average (King

TABLE 7.5
Studies Investigating Reported Dietary Intakes of Jockeys

Ref.	Participants	Dietary Assessment Method	Energy	Carbohydrate	Protein	Fat
Dolan et al. 2011	27 male jockeys (n = 18 completed food records), 27.3 ± 6.8 years, BW = 58.0 ± 7.4 kg, BMI = 20.7 ± 1.5 kg/m²	7-day food record	1803 ± 564 kcal/d, 31.1 kcal/kg BW	75 ± 29 g/d, 3.7 ± 1.3 g/kg BW, 44% total energy	211 ± 72 g/d, 1.3 ± 0.5 g/kg BW, 17% total energy	68 ± 24 g/d, 33% total energy
Labadarios et al. 1993	93 male jockeys, 27.8 years (range 19–55 years)	7-day food record	1936 kcal/d	43% total energy	15% total energy	34% total energy
Leydon and Wall 2002	6 male jockeys, 23.5 ± 4.3 years, BW = 52.8 ± 2.4 kg, BMI = 20.1 ± 1.5 kg/m²; 14 female jockeys, 24.5 ± 6.7 years, BW = 49.3 ± 3.4 kg, BMI = 20.2 ± 1.5 kg/m²	7-day weighed food record	Males: 1618 ± 320 kcal/d, 30.6 kcal/kg; Females: 1485 ± 429 kcal/d, 30.1 kcal/kg	Males: 179 ± 56 g/d, 3.4 g/kg BW, 43 ± 12% total energy; Females: 174 ± 50 g/d, 3.5 g/kg BW, 46 ± 6% total energy	Males: 58 ± 12 g/d, 1.1 g/kg BW, 15 ± 4% total energy; Females: 47 ± 16 g/d, 1.0 g/kg BW, 13 ± 3% total energy	Males: 54 ± 23 g/d, 31 ± 11% total energy; Females: 59 ± 20 g/d, 36 ± 5% total energy
Wilson et al. 2012	1 male jockey, 22 years, 70.3 kg	7-day food record	1951 kcal/d, 27.8 kcal/kg	169 g/d, 2.4 g/kg BW, 42% total energy	49 g/d, 0.7 g/kg BW, 22% total energy	91 g/d, 36% total energy

Note: All values are means or mean ± SD. BMI = body mass index, BW = body weight, FFQ = food frequency questionnaire.

and Mezey 1987). In addition to the negative health consequences associated with disordered eating behaviors, rapid weight loss may affect the psychological well being of jockeys. Caufield and Karageorghis (2008) observed that jockeys who excessively restrict their weight through rapid weight loss techniques report more negative moods compared to those maintaining weight.

The existing research literature consistently documents poor dietary intakes for both male and female jockeys (Table 7.5) (Dolan et al. 2011; Labadarios et al. 1993; Leydon and Wall 2002; Wilson et al. 2012). Reported energy intakes among male jockeys ranged from 27.8 to 31.1 kcal/kg body weight (Dolan et al. 2011; Labadarios et al. 1993; Leydon and Wall 2002; Wilson et al. 2012). The reported carbohydrate intake for male jockeys ranged from 2.4 to 3.7 g/kg body weight (42% to 44% of total energy) whereas protein intake ranged from 0.7 to 1.3 g/kg body weight (15% to 22% of total energy). The reported dietary fat intake for male jockeys usually ranged from 31% to 36% of total energy. Interestingly, the proportion of reported dietary fat, relative to carbohydrate and protein consumption, was high among male jockeys.

To date, only one study has observed the dietary intakes of female jockeys (Leydon and Wall 2002). The findings for female jockeys are similar to the reported dietary intake patterns among male jockeys, suggesting female jockeys also practice energy restriction. For example, 14 female jockeys (age: 24.5 ± 6.7 years; BMI: 20.2 ± 1.5 kg/m^2) completed a 7-day weighed food record. The female jockeys reported total energy intakes of 1485 ± 429 kcal/day (30.1 kcal/kg body weight). The reported carbohydrate and protein intake was just 3.5 g/kg body weight ($46 \pm 6\%$ of total daily energy) and 1.0 g/kg body weight ($13 \pm 3\%$ total daily intake), respectively. Due to the low reported carbohydrate and protein consumption, participants reported a higher total dietary fat, $36 \pm 5\%$ of total energy intake. Although the research examining usual dietary intake patterns of female jockeys is limited, the existing literature highlights the extreme pressures among female horse racing jockeys to maintain dangerously low body weights.

MIXED MARTIAL ARTS

Mixed martial arts encompass many different activities, including judo, karate, tae kwon do, and boxing. Since lean body mass is considered an indicator of power, body weight may be an advantage in combat sports. Therefore, requiring these sports to establish weight classifications promotes fair competition and helps eliminate the iniquitous advantages of larger athletes. The number of weight classifications in mixed martial arts varies, depending on the sport and level of competition. Due to the enticement to compete in lower weight classes, athletes competing in mixed martial arts may engage in a variety of unhealthy or dangerous weight-loss strategies. For example, recent research reported that judo athletes attempt rapid weight loss using hypohydration techniques, increased physical activity, and decreased food intake (Artioli et al. 2010b; Brito et al. 2012). Boxers also engage in drastic weight loss behaviors to make weight, using dangerous strategies, such as abstaining from all fluid for greater than 24 h (Hall and Lane 2001). Other mixed martial arts athletes (judo, jujitsu, karate, and tae kwon do) use similar drastic rapid weight loss techniques, including unapproved or prohibited methods, such as diuretics, saunas, and plastic clothing (Brito et al. 2012). Even more alarming, these weight loss strategies are accepted as an essential component of the sport (Hall and Lane 2001) and many athletes begin losing weight at a young age, typically during adolescence (Brito et al. 2012). Moreover, some athletes competing in mixed martial arts consider weight loss prior to competition an important component of the precompetition preparation, providing the athlete with a feeling of increased focus and commitment to the sport (Pettersson et al. 2013). Because these techniques are engrained as culture within these sports, it is difficult to convince athletes of the dangers of participating in weight making practices.

The effect of rapid weight loss and dehydration on performance differs according to the sport and is influenced by a variety of environmental factors and weigh-in regulations. For example, the weigh-in time before competition varies by sport (i.e., first day of competition, day before competition, post season). These regulations certainly influence refueling and recovery strategies and impact performance. However, success in mixed martial arts is based on performance relative to the competitor, who may also be engaging in dangerous weight loss techniques. Thus, it is difficult to convince athletes to avoid rapid and dangerous weight loss techniques.

The literature examining dietary intakes of mixed martial arts reports a wide variability of energy, carbohydrate, protein, and fat consumption as summarized in Table 7.6 (Artioli et al. 2009, 2010c; Degoutte et al. 2003, 2006; Finaud et al. 2006; Fogelholm et al. 1993; Grandjean 1989; Ohta et al. 2002; Smith et al. 2001; Teshima et al. 2002; Umeda et al. 2004; van Erp-Baart et al. 1989). The large discrepancy is likely due to the time period during the season when the athletes were surveyed. The reported energy intakes for males participating in mixed martial arts ranged from 13.3 to 45.2 kcal/kg body weight. These athletes typically reported carbohydrate intakes of 2.2 to 7.2 g/kg body weight, representing approximately 43% to 61% of total energy intake. Protein intakes ranged from 0.3 to 1.9 g/kg body weight, representing approximately 14% to 22% of total energy intake. The reported range of dietary fat was more consistent, compared to other macronutrients, and ranged from 26% to 38% of total energy intake. Ohta and colleagues (2002) reported the lowest dietary intakes among male mixed martial artists. This group of researchers examined dietary intakes among 10 male athletes participating in judo at various times before and after competition. The mean energy intake, three weeks prior to competition, was 2747 ± 1212 kcal/day (37.2 kcal/kg body weight). Reported dietary energy intake decreased dramatically to just 930 ± 708 kcal/day (13.3 kcal/kg body weight) one day before competition. Umeda et al. (2004) observed similar results among male judo athletes attempting to make weight for competition (n = 11; body weight: 78.5 ± 13.6 kg). These judo athletes were separated into groups based on weight loss practices and the weight loss goals prior to competition. Each athlete completed two 3-day food records (20 days and 1 day before competition). Among the athletes attempting excessive weight reduction, total reported energy intakes decreased from 43.0 to 23.4 kcal/kg body weight, 20 days and 1 day before competition, respectively.

Few studies have examined the dietary patterns of females participating in mixed martial arts (Artioli et al. 2009; Teshima et al. 2002). The largest study evaluating the dietary intake of female mixed martial artists included 16 females (age: 19.7 ± 10.0 years) using 3-day food records (Teshima et al. 2002). The reported average energy intake was 1947 ± 398 kcal/day, 34.9 ± 8.1 kcal/kg body weight. Participants reported intakes of 4.8 ± 1.1 and 1.2 ± 0.4 g/kg body weight of carbohydrate and

TABLE 7.6
Studies Investigating Reported Dietary Intakes of Mixed Martial Artists

Ref.	Participants	Dietary Assessment Method	Energy	Carbohydrate	Protein	Fat
Artioli et al. 2009	10 male kung-fu athletes, 26 ± 4 years, BW = 76.9 ± 11.3 kg; 4 female kung-fu athletes, 25 ± 4 years, BW = 60.1 ± 5.0 kg	Semi-quantitative FFQ	Males: 2230 ± 1406 kcal/d, 41.5 ± 21.2 kcal/kg BW; Females: 2817 ± 893 kcal/d, 47.2 ± 15.3 kcal/kg BW	Males: 4.5 ± 1.9 g/kg BW, 48 ± 10% total energy; Females: 7.2 ± 2.0 g/kg BW, 61 ± 7% total energy	Males: 1.9 ± 1.1 g/kg BW, 16 ± 3% total energy; Females: 1.6 ± 0.6 g/kg BW, 18 ± 3% total energy	Males: 35 ± 7% total energy; Females: 25 ± 7% total energy
Artioli et al. 2010c	7 male judo athletes, 22 ± 4 years, BW = 67.3 ± 5.8 kg	3-day food record	38.7 ± 5.5 kcal/kg BW (range 32.6–45.3 kcal/kg BW)	5.6 ± 0.9 g/kg BW (range 4.8–7.1 g/kg BW)	1.7 ± 0.4 g/kg BW (range 1.2–2.3 g/kg BW)	
Degoutte et al. 2003	16 male judo athletes, 18.4 ± 6.4 years, BW = 74.9 ± 18.8 kg	7-day food record	3203 ± 764 kcal/d, 42.8 kcal/kg BW	333 ± 368 g/d, 4.4 g/kg BW, 51 ± 18% total energy	103 ± 104 g/d, 1.4 g/kg BW, 15 ± 8% total energy	100 ± 125 g/d, 33 ± 17% total energy
Degoutte et al. 2006	10 male judo athletes, BW = 74.7 ± 6.7, BMI = 23.6 ± 1.5 kg/m²	7-day food record		334 g ± 76 g/d, 4.5 g/kg BW		
Finaud et al. 2006	10 male judo athletes, BW = 75.9 ± 3.1 kg, BMI = 24.9 ± 0.8 kg/m²	7-day food record	2639 kcal/day, 34.8 kcal/kg BW	63% total energy	22% total energy	26% total energy
Fogelholm et al. 1993	10 males (3 judo athletes) 21.6 years (range 17–31 years), 73.4 kg (range 55.1–93.0 kg)	4-day food record		302 ± 48 g/d, 4.1 g/kg BW, 48% total energy	107 ± 17g, 1.5 g/kg BW, 17% total energy	35% total energy
Grandjean 1989	275 athletes, 13–35 years (13 male judo athletes)	3-day food record	3357 ± 769 kcal/d	46 ± 5% total energy	16 ± 2% total energy	38 ± 5% total energy

(Continued)

TABLE 7.6 (Continued)

Studies Investigating Reported Dietary Intakes of Mixed Martial Artists

Ref.	Participants	Dietary Assessment Method	Energy	Carbohydrate	Protein	Fat
Ohta et al. 2002	10 male judo athletes, 20 years Time 1 (<3 weeks before competition): BW = 73.9 ± 11.1 kg Time 2 (<1 week before competition): BW = 72.3 ± 10.3 kg Time 3 (1 day before competition): BW = 69.7 ± 10.8 kg Time 4 (5 days after competition): BW = 72.6 ± 10.0 kg	Weighed food records (number of days not recorded)	Time 1: 2747 ± 1212 kcal/d, 37.2 kcal/kg BW Time 2: 2249 ± 890 kcal/d, 31.1 kcal/kg BW Time 3: 930 ± 708 kcal/d, 13.3 kcal/kg BW Time 4: 3278 ± 226 kcal/d, 45.2 kcal/kg BW	Time 1: 446 ± 210 g/d, 6.0 g/kg BW Time 2: 340 ± 142 g/d, 4.7 g/kg BW Time 3: 153 ± 16 g/d, 2.2 g/kg BW Time 4: 503 ± 366 g/d, 6.9 g/kg BW	Time 1: 80 ± 41 g/d, 1.1 g/kg BW Time 2: 71 ± 31 g/d, 1.0 g/kg BW Time 3: 21 ± 17 g/d, 0.3 g/kg BW Time 4: 95 ± 70 g/d, 1.3 g/kg BW	Time 1: 69 ± 40 g/d Time 2: 61 ± 51 g/d Time 3: 25 ± 28 g/d Time 4: 92 ± 60 g/d
Smith et al. 2001	8 male (amateur) boxers, 23.5 ± 3.2 years Time 1: BW = 73.3 ± 8.3 kg Time 2: No body weight reported	Three 5-day food records	Time 1: 2294 ± 759 kcal/d, 31.3 kcal/kg BW Time 2: 2241 ± 361 kcal/d	Time 1: 307 ± 103 g/d, 4.2 ± 1.4 g/kg BW, 54% total energy Time 2: 294 ± 51 g/d, 4.0 ± 0.7 g/kg BW, 52% total energy	Time 1: 91 ± 28 g/d, 1.2 ± 0.4 g/kg BW, 16% total energy Time 2: 88 ± 16 g/d, 1.2 ± 0.2 g/kg BW, 16% total energy	Time 1: 78 ± 29 g/d, 31% total energy Time 2: 79 ± 15 g/d, 32% total energy
Teshima et al. 2002	29 male karate athletes, 20.1 ± 1.3 years, BW = 66.2 ± 7.5 kg, BMI = 22.0 ± 2.0 kg/m² 16 female karate athletes, 19.7 ± 1.0 years, BW = 56.3 ± 6.8 kg, BMI = 22.3 ± 2.6 kg/m²	3-day food record	Males: 2763 ± 741 kcal/d, 42.3 ± 12.7 kcal/kg BW Females: 1947 ± 398 kcal/d, 34.9 ± 8.1 kcal/kg BW	Males: 375 ± 109 g/d, 5.7 ± 1.8 g/kg BW Females: 267 ± 61 g/d, 4.8 ± 1.1 g/kg BW	Males: 90 ± 24 g/d, 1.4 ± 0.5 g/kg BW Females: 65 ± 16, 1.2 ± 0.4 g/kg BW	Males: 83 ± 29 g/d Females: 65 ± 19 g/d

(Continued)

TABLE 7.6 (Continued)
Studies Investigating Reported Dietary Intakes of Mixed Martial Artists

Ref.	Participants	Dietary Assessment Method	Energy	Carbohydrate	Protein	Fat
Umeda et al. 2004	27 male judo athletes, 19.3 ± 0.6 years	3-day food record	Group 1, Time 1: 3376 ± 920 kcal/d, 43.0 kcal/kg BW	Group 1, Time 1: 562 ± 160 g/d, 7.2 g/kg BW	Group 1, Time 1: 117 ± 33 g/d, 1.5 g/kg BW	Group 1, Time 1: 71 ± 23 g/d
	Group 1 (n = 11) (participants attempting excess weight reduction)		Time 2: 1761 ± 703 kcal/d, 23.4 kcal/kg BW	Time 2: 296 ± 124 g/d, 3.9 g/kg BW	Time 2: 63 ± 21 g/d, 0.8 g/kg BW	Time 2: 38 ± 17 g/d
	Time 1 (20 days before competition): BW = 78.5 ± 13.6 kg		Group 2, Time 1: 3099 ± 454 kcal/d, 38.4 g/kg BW	Group 2, Time 1: 545 ± 98 g/d, 6.7 g/kg BW	Group 2, Time 1: 101 ± 14 g/d, 1.3 g/kg BW	Group 2, Time 1: 59 ± 15 g/d
	Time 2 (1 day before competition): BW = 75.3 ± 12.4 kg		Time 2: 292 ± 86 g/d, 3.7 g/kg BW			Time 2: 42 ± 12 g/d
	Group 2 (n = 11) (participants attempting minimal weight reduction)		Group 3, Time 1: 2615 ± 360 kcal/d, 33.2 kcal/kg BW	Group 3, Time 1: 460 ± 84 g/d, 5.8 g/kg BW	Group 3, Time 1: 96 ± 21 g/d, 1.2 g/kg BW	Group 3, Time 1: 49 ± 11 g/d
	Time 1 (20 days before competition): BW = 80.7 ± 13.1 kg		Time 2: 3140 ± 986 kcal/d, 39.7 kcal/kg BW	Time 2: 527 ± 153 g/d, 6.7 g/kg BW	Time 2: 100 ± 31 g/d, 1.3 g/kg BW	Time 2: 73 ± 30 g/d
	Time 2 (1 day before competition): BW = 78.3 ± 12.8 kg					
	Group 3 (n = 5) (participants maintaining weight)					
	Time 1 (20 days before competition): BW = 78.7 ± 8.8 kg					
	Time 2 (1 day before competition): BW = 79.0 ± 8.9 kg					

(Continued)

TABLE 7.6 (Continued)
Studies Investigating Reported Dietary Intakes of Mixed Martial Artists

Ref.	Participants	Dietary Assessment Method	Energy	Carbohydrate	Protein	Fat
van Erp-Baart et al. 1989	32 male judo athletes Group 1 (n = 4): 23 ± 1 year, BW = 82.5 ± 11.6 kg Group 2 (n = 28): 18 ± 1 year, BW = 68.7 ± 10.0 kg	4- or 7-day food record	Group 1: 37.5 kcal/kg BW (range 11–50 kcal/kg BW) Group 2: 42.3 kcal/kg BW (range 14–78 kcal/kg BW)	Group 1: ~43% total energy Group 2: ~48% total energy	Group 1: ~16% total energy Group 2: ~14% total energy	Group 1: ~36.5% total energy Group 2: ~37% total energy

Note: All values are means or mean ± SD. BMI = body mass index, BW = body weight, FFQ = food frequency questionnaire.

protein, respectively. Future research examining the usual dietary intakes and patterns of athletes should include female athletes competing in mixed martial arts.

ROWING

Rowers compete in open weight (heavyweight) or lightweight categories. Athletes participating in open weight competitions do not have weight restrictions. However, lightweight rowers have weight restrictions for the individual athletes and team. Men competing in lightweight rowing cannot weigh more than 160 lb (72.5 kg). The average weight for the entire team or crew cannot exceed 155 lb (70 kg). Women competing in lightweight rowing cannot weigh more than 130 lb (59 kg) and the average weight of the entire team or crew cannot exceed 125 lb (57 kg). Coxswains (the member of the rowing team who steers the boat and generates rowing commands) must weigh at least 121 lb (55 kg) and 110 lb (50 kg) for men and women, respectively. Coxswains that do not meet the minimum weight may be required to carry up to 10 kg of dead weight. In an attempt to discourage rapid weight loss, all weigh-ins are held 1 to 2 h before each race. However, this procedure does not always prevent athletes from practicing extreme weight loss techniques.

The weight-making practices of rowing athletes are similar to other aesthetic and weight-class sports athletes. Morris et al. (1999) observed a loss of nearly 10% body weight in female lightweight rowers over the competitive season. This same group of researchers also observed female and male lightweight rowers losing approximately 6% and 8% body weight, respectively, during a single competitive season in an attempt to make weight (Morris and Payne 1996). This weight loss was achieved using a variety of techniques including exercise (73.3%), food restriction (71.4%), and fluid restriction (62.9%). The observed weight loss was primarily due to a decrease in body fat, not lean muscle mass. The authors concluded the excessive weight loss limited the athlete's potential to increase fat-free mass during the competitive season, possibly hindering overall rowing performance. Although extreme, the weight making practices of these rowers are not uncommon. Slater and colleagues (2005) examined the weight loss strategies of 100 lightweight rowers. Over 75% of males and nearly 85% of females reported routinely losing weight prior to competition, suggesting male and female rowers regularly restrict energy intake.

A reasonable number of studies have examined the dietary surveys of rowers (Desgorces et al. 2008, de Wijn et al. 1979; Heinemann and Zerbes 1989; Hill and Davies 2002; McCargar et al. 1993; Morris and Payne 1996; Short and Short 1983; Slater et al. 2006; Steen et al. 1995; Talbott and Shapses 1998; van Erp-Baart et al. 1989; Xia et al. 2001) (Table 7.7). Most authors identified participants as either lightweight or open weight/heavyweight athletes (Desgorces et al. 2008; Hill and Davies 2002; Morris and Payne 1996; Slater et al. 2006; Steen et al. 1995; Talbott and Shapses 1998; Xia et al. 2001). When the weight category of the rowers was not identified, mean body weights were used to categorize the athletes (de Wijn et al. 1979; Heinemann and Zerbes 1989; McCargar et al. 1993; Short and Short 1983; van Erp-Baart et al. 1989). The distinction between these two weight categories must be considered because the pressures to make weight, particularly among lightweight rowers, will likely have an effect on dietary intakes and patterns.

TABLE 7.7

Studies Investigating Reported Dietary Intakes of Rowers

Ref.	Participants	Dietary Assessment Method	Energy	Carbohydrate	Protein	Fat
Desgorces et al. 2008	13 male heavyweight rowers, 21.5 ± 0.8 years; Time 1 (beginning of season): BW = 82.2 ± 9 kg; Time 2 (end of season): BW = 81.8 ± 8.2 kg	3-day food record	Time 1: 2890 ± 430 kcal/d, 35.3 kcal/kg BW; Time 2: 3343 ± 334 kcal/d, 40.9 kcal/kg BW	Time 1: 375 ± 37 g/d, 4.7 ± 0.4 g/kg BW, 55 ± 5% total energy; Time 2: 458 ± 38g/d, 5.6 ± 0.4 g/kg BW, 57 ± 3% total energy	Time 1: 86 ± 12 g/d, 1.1 ± 0.1 g/kg BW, 17 ± 1% total energy; Time 2: 97 ± 13 g/d, 1.2 ± 0.1 g/kg BW, 16 ± 1% total energy	Time 1: 88 ±25 g/d, 28 ± 5% total energy; Time 2: 94 ± 18 g/d, 26 ± 3% total energy
de Wijn et al. 1979	8 male rowers (age not reported); Time 1 (peak season): 87.3 ± 5.4 kg; Time 2 (post season): 86.1 ± 5.9 kg	7-day food record	Time 1: 4140 ± 504 kcal/d, 46 kcal/kg BW; Time 2: 3190 ± 507 kcal/d, 37 kcal/kg BW	Time 1: 467 g/d, 5.4 g/kg BW, 43.2% total energy (range 37–50% total energy); Time 2: 4.0 g/kg, 43.5% total energy (range 40–52% total energy)	Time 1: 139 g/d, 1.6 g/kg (range 0.8–2.2 g/kg) 13% total energy (range 9–17% total energy); Time 2: 1.0 g/kg (range 0.8–1.4 g/kg) 11% total energy (range 9–13% total energy)	Time 1: 192 g/d, 43% total energy (38–48% total energy); Time 2: 38% total energy (range 34–42% total energy)
Heinemann and Zerbes 1989	3 male rowers, 18–23 years, BW = 88 kg (range 85–93 kg)	3-day food record	~72 kcal/kg BW	~52% total energy	~14% total energy	~35% total energy
Hill and Davies 2002	7 female lightweight rowers, 20.1 ± 1.1 years, BW = 60.9 ± 2.3 kg	4-day weighed food record	2214 ± 313 kcal/d, 36.4 kcal/kg BW			

(Continued)

TABLE 7.7 (Continued)
Studies Investigating Reported Dietary Intakes of Rowers

Ref.	Participants	Dietary Assessment Method	Energy	Carbohydrate	Protein	Fat
McCargar et al. 1993	14 female lightweight rowers Group 1 (n = 7) (weight cyclers), 22 ± 1 years, BW = 61.8 ± 2.1 kg Group 2 (n = 7) (non-weight cyclers), 21 ± 2 years, BW = 60.9 ± 4.4 kg	3-day food record	Group 1: Time 1: ~2030 kcal/d Time 2: ~1750 kcal/d Time 3: ~2200 kcal/d Group 2: Time 1: ~1500 kcal/d Time 2: ~1575 kcal/d Time 3: ~1625 kcal/d	Group 1: Time 1: 61 ± 3% total energy Time 2: 65 ± 8% total energy Time 3: 57 ± 6% total energy Group 2: Time 1: ~62% total energy Time 2: ~59% total energy Time 3: ~57% total energy	Group 1: Time 1: ~12% total energy Time 2: ~14% total energy Time 3: ~12% total energy Group 2: Time 1: ~12% total energy Time 2: ~14% total energy Time 3: ~13% total energy	Group 1: Time 1: 64 ± 19 g/d, 28 ± 3% total energy Time 2: 41 ± 42 g/d, 22 ± 8% total energy Time 3: 75 ± 32 g/d, 32 ± 5% total energy Group 2: Time 1: 48 ± 11 g/d, ~29% total energy Time 2: 52 ± 16 g/d, ~27% total energy Time 3: 73 ± 40 g/d, ~32% total energy

(Continued)

TABLE 7.7 (Continued)
Studies Investigating Reported Dietary Intakes of Rowers

Ref.	Participants	Dietary Assessment Method	Energy	Carbohydrate	Protein	Fat
Morris and Payne 1996	6 female lightweight rowers, 23.1 ± 4.5 years, Time 1 (preseason): BW = 61.3 ± 2.9 kg Time 2 (competition): BW = 57.0 ± 1.1 kg 12 male lightweight rowers, 23.5 ± 3.5 years Time 1 (preseason): BW = 75.6 ± 3.1 kg Time 2 (competition): BW = 69.8 ±1.6 kg	4-day food record	Females: Time 1: 1641 ± 1281 kcal/d, 26.8 kcal/kg BW Time 2: 1188 ± 1249 kcal/d, 20.8 kcal/kg BW Males: Time 1: 2628 ± 1853 kcal/d, 34.8 kcal/kg BW Time 2: 2341 ± 4056 kcal/d, 33.5 kcal/kg BW	Females: Time 1: 260 g/d, 4.2 g/kg BW, 58% total energy Time 2: 214 g/d, 3.8 g/kg BW, 68% total energy Males: Time 1: 354 g/d, 4.7 g/kg BW, 52% total energy Time 2: 415 g/d, 5.9 g/kg BW, 67% total energy	Females: Time 1: 73 g/d, 1.2 g/kg BW, 17% total energy Time 2: 37 g/d, 0.6 g/kg BW, 15% total energy Males: Time 1: 98 g/d, 1.3 g/kg BW, 15% total energy Time 2: 100 g/d, 1.4 g/kg BW, 18% total energy	Females: Time 1: 48 g/d, 21% total energy Time 2: 32 g/d, 15% total energy Males: Time 1: 86 g/d, 28% total energy Time 2: 33 g/d, 14% total energy

(Continued)

TABLE 7.7 (Continued)
Studies Investigating Reported Dietary Intakes of Rowers

Ref.	Participants	Dietary Assessment Method	Energy	Carbohydrate	Protein	Fat
Short and Short 1983	27 male collegiate rowers, BW = 81.8 kg Group 1 (n = 19) Group 2 (n = 8) Group 3 (n = 7) 24 female collegiate rowers, BW = 67.7 kg (range 45–77.2 kg)	1- to 14-day food record	Males: Group 1: 4104 kcal/d (range 1421–7337 kcal/d) Group 2: 3905 kcal/d (range 2388–5381 kcal/d) Group 3: 5267 kcal/d (range 2771–7162 kcal/d) Females: 2339 kcal/d (range 1262–3577 kcal/d), 34.5 kcal/kg BW	Males: Group 1: 474 g/d (range 143–1029 g/d) Group 2: 413 g/d (range 229–612g/d), 44% total energy (range 22–58% total energy) Group 3: 667 g/d (range 324–1029 g/d), 50% total energy (range 42–58% total energy) Females: 272 g/d (range 146–476 g/d), 4.0 g/kg BW, 46% total energy (range 29–62% total energy)	Males: Group 1: 183 g/d (range 65–465 g/d) Group 2: 185 g/d (range 110–241 g/d), 26% total energy (range 16–36% total energy) Group 3: 186 g/d (106–288 g/d), 14% total energy (12–16%) Females: 96 g/d (range 49–160 g/d), 1.4 g/kg BW, 16% total energy (9–23% total energy)	Males: Group 1: 170 g/d, (range 12–320 g/d) Group 2: 165 g/d (range 112–265 g/d), 38% total energy (range 19–43% total energy) Group 3: 212 g/d (range 115–322 g/d), 36% total energy (range 29–45% total energy) Females: 96 g/d (range 45–171 g/d), 36% total energy (range 21–51% total energy)

(Continued)

TABLE 7.7 (Continued)
Studies Investigating Reported Dietary Intakes of Rowers

Ref.	Participants	Dietary Assessment Method	Energy	Carbohydrate	Protein	Fat
Slater et al. 2006	3 male lightweight rowers, 20.3 ± 2.2 years, BW = 78.3 ± 1.7 kg	Food record (number of days not reported)	34.7 ± 11.7 kcal/kg BW		1.9 ± 0.6 g/kg BW	
Steen et al. 1995	16 female heavyweight rowers, 21.0 ± 1.1 years, BW = 68.6 ± 4.2 kg	5-day food record	2633 ± 449 kcal/d, 38.4 kcal/kg BW	337 ± 68 g/d, 4.9 g/kg BW, 51% total energy	88 ± 15 g/d, 0.8 g/kg BW, 13% total energy	104 ± 25 g/d, 36% total energy
Talbott and Shapses 1998	13 male lightweight rowers, 19.6 ± 1.4 years, BW = 70.8 ± 1.1 kg	1-day food record	2771 ± 1429 kcal/d, 39.1 kcal/kg BW	71 ± 10% total energy	74 ± 37 g/d, 1.0 g/kg BW, 11 ± 4% total energy	18 ± 8% total energy
van Erp-Baart et al. 1989	18 males rowers, 22 ± 2 years, BW = 77.2 ± 6.7 kg 8 female rowers, 23 ± 2 years, BW = 69.8 ± 5.8 kg	4- or 7-day food record	Males: 3487 kcal/d, 45.2 kcal/kg BW (range 40–54 kcal/kg BW) Females: 3102 kcal/d, 44.5 kcal/kg BW (range 26–48 kcal/kg BW)	Males: ~52% total energy Females: ~46% total energy	Males: ~14% total energy Females: ~15% total energy	Males: ~31% total energy Females: ~35% total energy
Xia et al. 2001	1 male lightweight rower, BW = 75.5 kg	3-day weighed food record	4088 kcal/d, 54.1 kcal/ kg BW	613 g/d, 8.1 g/kg BW, 51% total energy intake	3 g/kg BW, 19% total energy intake	30% total energy intake

Note: All values are means or mean ± SD. BMI = body mass index, BW = body weight, FFQ = food frequency questionnaire.

To date, few researchers have examined reported dietary intakes of female lightweight rowers (Hill and Davies 2002; McCargar et al. 1993; Morris and Payne 1996). The reported average energy intakes for these athletes ranged from 20.8 to 36.4 kcal/kg body weight. The typical mean carbohydrate intake ranged from 3.8 to 4.2 g/kg body weight, contributing 57% to 68% of total energy. The reported protein intakes ranged from 0.6 to 1.2 kcal/kg body weight, representing 12% to 17% of total energy intake. There was a large variability in reported dietary fat intakes (approximately 15% to 32% of total energy), with the lowest intakes reported during the competitive season (Morris and Payne 1996). Collectively, these results suggest female lightweight rowers regularly restrict energy and macronutrient intake.

The usual dietary intake patterns of female rowers competing in the open or heavyweight category have also been examined (Short and Short 1983; Steen et al. 1995; van Erp-Baart et al. 1989). Although the researchers did not categorize these athletes by weight-class, the reported average body weights of these female rowers ranged from 67.7 to 69.8 kg, suggesting these female athletes competed primarily in the open or heavyweight category. The female rowers reported an average energy intake of 34.5 to 44.5 kcal/kg body weight. Unfortunately, these studies did not always include extensive dietary intake information or body weights, making it difficult to make conclusions on dietary patterns. In two studies, the weight classifications of the athletes were not specified and the reported range of body weights suggested the sample included both lightweight and open or heavyweight athletes (Short and Short 1983; van Erp-Baart et al. 1989). Because lightweight and open or heavyweight athletes experience distinct weight pressures, their dietary intake patterns may differ. In 1995, Steen et al. (1995) published the most complete dietary assessment of female collegiate heavyweight rowers (n = 16; age: 21.0 ± 1.1 years; body weight: 68.6 ± 4.2 kg) using a 5-day food record. The female rowers reported an average energy intake of 2633 ± 449 kcal/day (38.4 kcal/kg body weight). The athletes reported a mean carbohydrate intake of 4.9 g/kg body weight (51% of total energy) and protein intake of 0.8 g/kg body weight (13% of total energy). The reported mean dietary fat intake was 36% of total energy. The high percentage of dietary fat was primarily due to a large consumption of fatty foods including mayonnaise, salad dressing, cream sauces, cakes, cookies, and chips. Although these results represent just one study, the reported dietary intakes of female open or heavyweight rowers are noticeably different when compared to female lightweight rowers, especially when considering macronutrient distributions.

Few studies have evaluated the dietary intakes and patterns of male lightweight rowers and the results are inconsistent (Morris and Payne 1996; Slater et al. 2006; Talbott and Shapses 1998; Xia et al. 2001). In addition, these studies have limitations in research design and the sample sizes are small, making it difficult to summarize the dietary patterns among this group of athletes. For instance, Xia et al. (2001) completed a case study of one world-class lightweight rower. Although this athlete met dietary recommendations based on body weight and activity level, the 3-day food record was measured during the off-season. Thus, the reported dietary intake may not reflect the dietary patterns that occur during the competitive season, especially among athletes attempting to make weight. In addition, because this was a case study of a single athlete, the results may not be generalizable to all lightweight rowers. In another study, Slater and colleagues (2006) followed three heavyweight rowers over

16 weeks as they attempted to transition from the heavyweight to the lightweight rowing category. These athletes reported an average energy intake of 34.7 kcal/kg body weight and protein intake of 1.9 g/kg body weight. During the study, all the athletes successfully decreased body weight in order to compete in the lightweight rowing category (weight loss range 2.0 to 8.0 kg). The authors observed the greatest decrease in performance among the athletes with the largest weight losses, suggesting the most severe weight-making practices had a greater impact on performance.

A larger number of studies have evaluated dietary intakes of male open or heavyweight rowers (Desgorces et al. 2008; de Wijn et al. 1979; Heinemann and Zerbes 1989; Short and Short 1983; van Erp-Baart et al. 1989). Unfortunately, the majority of these studies were conducted prior to 1990. Thus, the reported dietary intakes of these athletes may not reflect present-day heavyweight rowing athletes. The typical reported energy intakes of male heavyweight rowers were approximately 35.3 to 72.0 kcal/kg. These athletes reported dietary carbohydrates of 4.7 to 5.6 g/kg body weight (43% to 57% of total energy intake). Reported daily protein intakes ranged from 1.0 to 1.6 g/kg body weight (11% to 26% of total energy intake) and dietary fat intakes ranged from 26% to 43% total energy intake.

Unfortunately, the existing literature investigating the reported dietary intakes of male heavyweight rowers varied widely, further complicating the interpretation of the usual dietary patterns of these athletes. For example, Heinemann and Zerbes (1989) examined the dietary intakes of a large sample of athletes and non-athletes, which included three heavyweight rowers (age: 18 to 23 years; body weight: 88 kg), using a 3-day food record (Heinemann and Zerbes 1989). This group of researchers observed male heavyweight collegiate rowers to consume approximately 72 kcal/kg body weight. The macronutrient distribution was approximately 54% carbohydrate, 14% protein, and 35% fat. This reported energy intake is substantially higher compared to other research examining dietary intakes of rowers. However, these results represent just one study, conducted on a small sample prior to 1990. Therefore, the results of this study may not be generalizable and additional research is warranted.

Ski Jumping

During the 1980s, changes in the technique of ski jumping resulted in a greater emphasis on body mass. Around this time, the V-technique of ski jumping replaced the classic ski jump style of holding the skis parallel, increasing the athletes' dependence on the flight dynamics of lift and drag. Athletes with a lower body mass may have an advantage, producing an incredible incentive for these athletes to be extremely lean. Consequently, sporting organizations have established weight regulations, linking ski length to body mass.

Few studies have examined usual dietary intakes or weight-making practices of elite ski jumpers (Rankinen et al. 1998) (Table 7.8). Thus, the usual dietary intake patterns of these athletes are not well known. Rankinen and colleagues (1998) used a 4-day food record to examine reported dietary intakes of 21 male ski jumpers (age: 19.7 ± 3.9 years). The participants reported an average energy intake of 1815 ± 788 kcal/day or 29.3 kcal/kg body weight. The average reported dietary protein intake was 1.3 ± 0.5 g/kg body weight, representing 18% of total energy. The average

TABLE 7.8
Studies Investigating Reported Dietary Intakes of Ski Jumpers

Ref.	Participants	Dietary Assessment Method	Energy	Carbohydrate	Protein	Fat
Rankinen et al. 1998	21 male ski jumpers, 19.7 ± 3.9 years, BW = 61.9 ± 4.8 kg	4-day food record	1815 ± 788 kcal/d, 29.3 kcal/kg BW	51 ± 6% total energy	1.3 ± 0.5 g/kg BW, 18 ± 4% total energy	28 ± 5% total energy

Note: All values are means or mean ± SD. BMI = body mass index, BW = body weight, FFQ = food frequency questionnaire.

reported carbohydrate and fat intakes were 51 ± 6% and 28 ± 5% of total energy, respectively. Although this study suggests male ski jumpers consume a relatively low energy intake, further research is necessary to determine the regular dietary patterns of male and female ski jumpers.

WRESTLERS

The anxieties and controversies regarding the weight-making practices of wrestlers have a well-documented history. As early as 1943, researchers expressed concern over excessive weight loss due to dehydration and food restriction on wrestling performance (Steen and Brownell 1990; Tuttle 1943). In the late 1960s, Tipton and Tcheng (1970) evaluated the weight loss practices of 747 high school wrestlers, and observed an average weight loss of 6.8 lb (3.1 kg), nearly 5% of body weight, over a 17-day period prior to competition. The most common methods for weight loss included food restriction (83%), fluid restriction (77%), and increased exercise (83%). Other studies of high school and college wrestlers have demonstrated similar and often dangerous or inappropriate weight-making practices, including the use of fasting, saunas, rubber suits, laxatives, and vomiting (Alderman et al. 2004; Oppliger et al. 2003; Steen and Brownell 1990). Weight-loss practices are more extreme among collegiate wrestlers, compared to high school wrestlers, possibly due to the increased pressures that occur at higher levels of competition. Unfortunately, even very young wrestlers are not exempt from the pressures to lose weight in order to compete at a lower weight class. A study published as recently as 2005 reported a 5-year-old boy was pressured by his father, a former wrestler, to lose weight in order to compete at a lower weight class (Sansone and Sawyer 2005).

Many wrestlers attempt to lose weight multiple times throughout the season in order to compete in a lower weight category. Steen and Brownell (1990) investigated the weight-making practices of 368 high school and 63 college wrestlers. College wrestlers reported losing weight for competition an average of 15 times per competitive season, whereas high school wrestlers reported undergoing weight loss practices an average of nine times per competitive season. Over 40% of the college wrestlers reported weekly weight fluctuations of 5 to 9 kg and nearly 45% of high school wrestlers reported weekly weight fluctuations of 2.7 to 4.5 kg. Even more stunning, 35% of the collegiate wrestlers reported losing at least 4.5 kg greater than 100 times. The magnitude of repeated weight loss among high school and collegiate wrestlers is especially concerning. These findings were reported in 1990, before the NCAA implemented new weight loss rules and regulations. Since these policies were initiated, college wrestlers report a lower prevalence of fasting, vomiting, and use of diuretics, laxatives, and sweat suits (Oppliger et al. 2003). Although these changes are certainly an improvement, wrestlers continue to participate in extreme weight loss practices, including fluid and food restriction.

Numerous dietary surveys have examined the weight-making strategies and usual dietary intakes of wrestlers (Enns et al. 1987; Fogelholm et al. 1993; Grandjean 1989; Heinemann and Zerbes 1989; Horswill et al. 1990; McCargar and Crawford 1992; McMurray et al. 1991; Rankin et al. 1996; Roemmich and Sinning 1997; Rokitzki et al. 1994a,b; Short and Short 1983; Widerman and Hagan 1982) (Table 7.9). The

TABLE 7.9

Studies Investigating Reported Dietary Intakes of Wrestlers

Ref.	Participants	Dietary Assessment Method	Energy	Carbohydrate	Protein	Fat
Daneshvar et al. 2013	28 male wrestlers, 17–25 years	FFQ	3162 ± 946 kcal/d	473 ± 169 g/d	121 ± 35 g/d	103 ± 25 g/d
Enns et al. 1987	26 male wrestlers, 18–21 years Time 1 (n = 26): BW = 81.9 ± 14.3 kg, BMI = 26.1 ± 2.9 kg/m² Time 2 (n = 19): BW = 77.9 ± 10.5 kg	Two 3-day food records	Time 1: 3074 ± 959 kcal/d, 37.5 kcal/kg BW Time 2: 2125 ± 1035 kcal/d, 27.3 kcal/kg BW			
Fogelholm et al. 1993	10 males (7 wrestlers), 21.6 years (range 17–31 years), 73.4 kg (range 55.1–93.0 kg)	4-day food record		302 ± 48 g/d, 4.1 g/kg BW, 48% total energy,	107 ± 17g, 1.5 g/kg BW, 17% total energy	35% total energy
Grandjean 1989	275 athletes (10 male wrestlers), 13–35 years	3-day food record	2154 ± 716 kcal/d	54 ± 6% total energy	12 ± 4% total energy	34 ± 7% total energy
Heinemann and Zerbes 1989	20 male wrestlers, 19–22 years, BW = 85 kg (range 53–89 kg)	3-day food record	~56 kcal/kg BW	~44% total energy	~18% total energy	~38% total energy
Horswill et al. 1990	18 male wrestlers, BW = 16.0 ± 18.1 years Time 1: BW = 66.0 ± 11.9 kg Time 2: BW = 63.7 ± 12.7 kg Time 3: BW = 63.3 ± 12.3 kg Time 4: BW = 62.6 ± 12.3 kg	Four 7-day food records	Time 1: ~40 kcal/kg BW Time 2: ~36 kcal/kg BW Time 3: ~ 36 kcal/kg BW Time 4: ~36 kcal/kg BW	Time 1: ~5.6 g/kg BW Time 2: ~3.2 g/kg BW Time 3: ~1.0 g/kg BW Time 4: ~1.1 g/kg BW	Time 1: ~1.5 g/kg BW Time 2: ~3.4 g/kg BW Time 3: ~1.0 g/kg BW Time 4: ~1.1 g/kg BW	

(Continued)

TABLE 7.9 (Continued)
Studies Investigating Reported Dietary Intakes of Wrestlers

Ref.	Participants	Dietary Assessment Method	Energy	Carbohydrate	Protein	Fat
McCargar and Crawford 1992	14 male wrestlers Group 1 (n = 8) (weight-cyclers), 20 ± 3 years, BW = 72.4 ± 11.9 kg Group 2 (n = 6) (non-weight cyclers), 20 ± 2 years, BW = 78.2 ± 10.1 kg	3-day food record	Group 1: 2304 ± 678 kcal/d, 30.6 ± 8.8 kcal/kg BW Group 2: 3270 ± 740 kcal/d, 44.2 ± 11.0 kcal/kg BW	Group 1: 54 ± 7% total energy Group 2: 53 ± 11% total energy	Group 1: 16 ± 3% total energy Group 2: 16 ± 3% total energy	Group 1: 29 ± 6% total energy Group 2: 28 ± 6% total energy
McMurray et al. 1991	12 male wrestlers Group 1: 20.0 ± 0.6 years, BW = 79.4 ± 10.3 kg Group 2: 20.6 ± 0.6 years, BW = 73.1 ± 8.8 kg	24-h dietary recall	32.0 ± 6.9 kcal/kg BW	52% total energy	1.4 ± 0.5 g/kg BW	
Rankin et al. 1996	12 male wrestlers Group 1 (n = 6), 21.2 ± 1.2 years, BW = 72.7 ± 14.2 kg Group 2 (n = 6), 19.8 ± 1.2 years, BW = 70.0 ± 8.1 kg	2-day food record	Group 1: 3205 ± 1083 kcal/d, 44.0 kcal/kg BW Group 2: 2187 ± 710 kcal/d, 31.0 kcal/kg BW	Group 1: 61 ± 15% total energy Group 2: 60 ± 6% total energy	Group 1: 13 ± 6% total energy Group 2: 13 ± 4% total energy	Group 1: 26 ± 11% total energy Group 2: 24 ± 8% total energy

(Continued)

TABLE 7.9 (Continued)
Studies Investigating Reported Dietary Intakes of Wrestlers

Ref.	Participants	Dietary Assessment Method	Energy	Carbohydrate	Protein	Fat
Roemmich and Sinning 1997	9 male wrestlers (during the season): 15.7 ± 0.3 years, BW = 58.0 ± 3.5 kg	7-day food record	24.7 ± 3.5 kcal/kg BW	61 ± 2% total energy	0.9 g/kg BW	24 ± 2% total energy
Rokitzki et al. 1994a	13 male wrestlers, 20.6 ± 9.7 years, BW = 77.8 ± 33.5 kg	7-day weighed food record	2691 ± 3446 kcal/d, 34.6 kcal/kg BW	310 ± 292 g/d, 4.0 g/kg BW, 46% total energy		
Rokitzki et al. 1994b	13 male wrestlers, 20.6 ± 9.7 years, BW = 77.8 ± 33.5 kg	7-day weighed food record	3450 ± 3440 kcal/d, 44.3 kcal/kg BW		101 ± 107 g/d, 1.3 g/kg BW	
Short and Short 1983	114 male wrestlers Group 1 (n = 15) Group 2 (n = 12) Group 3 (n = 13) Group 4 (n = 19) Group 5 (n = 6) Group 6 (n = 7)	1- to 14-day food record	Group 1: 3887 kcal/d (range 880–14,962 kcal/d) Group 2: 1964 kcal (range 1109–3582 kcal/d) Group 3: 3667 kcal/d (range 1694–6444 kcal/d)	Group 1: 416 g/d (range 129–1632 g/d) Group 2: 880 g/d (range 118–377 g/d), 48% total energy (range 35–70% total energy) Group 3: 363 g/d (range 176–826 g/d), 40% total energy (range 24–55% total energy)	Group 1: 160 g/d (range 14–419 g/d) Group 2: 82 g/d (range 34–169 g/d), 16% total energy (range 10–26% total energy) Group 3: 169 g/d (range 63–294 g/d), 19% total energy (range 10–28% total energy)	Group 1: 176 g/d (range 14–785 g/d) Group 2: 81 g/d (range 45–158g/d), 36% total energy (range 20–45% total energy) Group 3: 166 g/d (range 47–314 g/d), 39% total energy (range 24–58% total energy)

(Continued)

TABLE 7.9 (Continued)
Studies Investigating Reported Dietary Intakes of Wrestlers

Ref.	Participants	Dietary Assessment Method	Energy	Carbohydrate	Protein	Fat
			Group 4: 2634 kcal/d (range 1246–6339 kcal/d) Group 5: 965 kcal/d (range 412–1470 kcal/d) Group 6: 3845 (range 1531–6709 kcal/d)	Group 4: 281 g/d (range 122–649 g/d), 43% total energy (range 31–58% total energy) Group 5: 104 g/d (range 60–176 g/d), 50% total energy (range 27–83% total energy) Group 6: 586 g/d (range 201–1492 g/d), 53% total energy (range 43–65% total energy)	Group 4: 133 g/d (range 40–230 g/d), 20% total energy (range 12–25% total energy) Group 5: 56 g/d (range 10–103 g/d), 21% total energy (range 7–31% total energy) Group 6: 108 g/d (range 51–166 g/d), 14% total energy (range 11–17% total energy)	Group 4: 104 g/d (range 38–287 g/d), 36% total energy (range 26–47% total energy) Group 5: 36 g/d (range 9–59 g/d), 30% total energy (range 10–41% total energy) Group 6: 105 g/d (range 48–160 g/d), 29% total energy (range 17–39% total energy)
Widerman and Hagan 1982	1 male wrestler, 21 years, BW = 43.0 kg	45-day weighed food record	2006 kcal/d, 46.7 kcal/ kg BW	61% total energy	20% total energy	19% total energy

Note: All values are means or mean ± SD. BMI = body mass index, BW = body weight, FFQ = food frequency questionnaire.

reported dietary intake patterns vary widely, depending on the time period in which the dietary surveys are measured, with lower self-reported energy intakes observed closer to competition. Overall, the reported average energy intakes of wrestlers ranged from approximately 24.7 to 56.0 kcal/kg body weight. Reported carbohydrate intakes ranged from approximately 1.0 to 5.6 g/kg body weight (40% to 61% of total daily energy intake) and protein intakes ranged from approximately 0.9 to 3.4 g/kg body weight (12% to 21% of total daily energy intake). Dietary fat ranged from approximately 19% to 39% of total energy intake.

While a large number of studies have observed the dietary patterns of wrestlers, one study is especially notable. Although this study was published in 1987, before the new NCAA weight regulations, it highlights the tremendous changes in energy intake that occur during the competitive wrestling season. Enns and colleagues (1987) examined reported dietary intakes of male collegiate wrestlers (n = 26; age: 18 to 21 years) using two 3-day food records. At the beginning of the competitive season, wrestlers reported an average energy intake of 3074 ± 959 kcal (37.5 kcal/kg body weight). The average reported energy intake decreased dramatically throughout the season. By the end of the competitive season, the wrestlers reported an energy intake of 2125 ± 1035 kcal (27.3 kcal/kg body weight). The researchers also observed changes in body weight throughout the season, ranging from –7.7 to +0.5 kg, most likely due to the substantial decline in energy intake.

DIETARY SUPPLEMENTS OF AESTHETIC AND WEIGHT-CLASS SPORTS

Similar to other athletes, aesthetic and weight-class athletes may use dietary supplements and ergogenic aids as a way to promote health, aid recovery, prevent illness, compensate for a poor diet, and enhance overall performance (Maughan et al. 2004, 2011; Sobal and Marquart 1994). These athletes may also rely on supplements to improve body composition and support quick weight loss. For example, Sobal and Stensland (1992) examined the dietary practices of ballet, jazz, and modern dancers. Sixty percent of the dancers reported taking nutrition supplements, and 84% took them daily. The dancers reported that they used dietary supplements as a way to feel healthier, prevent muscle cramps or bruising, improve recovery, prevent colds, and suppress appetite. In another study, Ziegler et al. (2003) examined the prevalence of dietary supplements use in elite figure skaters. Sixty-five percent of the male and 76% of the female figure skaters reported using dietary supplements. The three main reasons that male figure skaters used dietary supplements were to provide energy, prevent illness or disease, and enhance performance. Female figure skaters reported using supplements in order to prevent illness or disease, provide more energy, and compensate for an inadequate diet.

Unfortunately, many aesthetic and weight-class athletes are not properly educated or informed regarding dietary supplements. For example, Zenic et al. (2010) examined the use of supplements in ballet dancers, other dancers, and synchronized swimmers. The participants reported that they did not rely on the opinions of coaches or physicians when deciding to use supplements. In another study focused entirely on professional ballet dancers, 25% reported that they would use a "doping" substance if it would ensure a successful ballet performance, regardless of negative health consequences (Sekulic et al. 2010). These results are even more troubling considering the lack of formal supervision or policy regarding the use of dietary supplements and ergogenic aids in dance.

Only limited research has examined the efficacy and safety of dietary supplements and ergogenic aids in aesthetic and weight-class sport athletes. Creatine supplementation has become a popular dietary supplement among many athletes, including aesthetic and weight-class athletes. Research has examined the impact of creatine supplementation on exercise performance in wrestlers and rowers and found mixed results (Chwalbińska-Moneta 2003; Kocak and Karli 2003; Syrotuik et al. 2001). For example, a high dose of creatine (20 g) in wrestlers for 5 days resulted in a significant increase in average and peak power on a Wingate anaerobic test. Similarly, Chwalbińska-Moneta (2003) found that a daily ingestion of 20 g creatine monohydrate for 5 days improved both endurance (as measured by lactate threshold) and anaerobic performance in elite male rowers. However, Syrotuik et al. (2001) reported that a 5-day load creatine dose (0.3 g/kg body weight) followed by a 5-week maintenance dose (0.03 g/kg body weight) in rowers did not improve performance after 5 days and 5 weeks.

Additional studies have examined the role of dietary supplements on health in weight-class athletes. In one study, researchers assigned wrestlers to either a zinc supplement (5 mg/kg body weight/day) or no supplement for 8 weeks (Kara et al. 2010). At the end of the 8 weeks, the wrestlers that supplemented with zinc had higher blood concentrations of zinc and zinc-antioxidant enzymes. Furthermore, blood malondialdehyde concentrations were higher at the end of the study in the wrestlers not taking zinc, demonstrating the role of zinc in protection against free-radical formation and oxidative stress. Unfortunately, dietary intake and exercise performance measures were not included in this study.

The impact of omega-3-fatty acids has been studied in both wrestlers and judo athletes and conflicting results were reported (Filaire et al. 2010; Tartibian et al. 2010). Tartibian et al. (2010) found that supplementing for 12 weeks with 1000 mg omega-3-fatty acids (180 mg eicosapentaenoic acid [EPA] and 120 mg docosahexaenoic acid [DHA]) improved markers of pulmonary function. However, Filaire et al. (2010) found that supplementing for 6 weeks with a higher dose of omega-3-fatty acids (600 mg EPA and 400 mg DHA) resulted in an elevated level of oxidative stress after a judo-training session, thus showing a negative effect of the supplement for these athletes.

Aesthetic and weight-class athletes may use weight-loss dietary supplements as a way to improve body composition and reach body weight goals. However, most research only supports minimal results (<2 kg) at best and some of these supplements are associated with adverse side effects (Manore 2012). For example, after 14 weeks of supplementation with chromium (200 μg/day), wrestlers found no improvements in body composition or any performance measures (Walker et al. 1998). Additionally, Kern and Robinson (2011) examined the impact of β-alanine (4 g) supplementation on collegiate wrestlers in a double-blind, placebo-controlled study. Although the results were not statistically significant, the participants taking the β-alanine did improve performance in tests of anaerobic power and increased lean body mass compared to those taking the placebo.

One study did find a benefit after using a dietary supplement. Stroescu et al. (2001) examined the impact of a soy protein supplement on body composition and blood biochemical markers in elite female gymnasts. Fourteen gymnasts were randomized to receive either a soy protein supplement or a placebo twice daily for 4 months. All other aspects of their training was identical (training, dietary intake, and vitamin/mineral supplements). The gymnasts receiving the soy protein supplement had an increase in lean body mass compared to those on the placebo.

Due to the intense drive to lose weight, aesthetic and weight-class sport athletes may consider using dietary supplements that contain ephedra and other stimulants. However, many of these stimulants are banned in sport and have adverse side effects. For example, a 28-year-old male mixed martial arts athlete experienced a heart attack after using an ephedra-containing supplement in order to lose weight (Forte et al. 2006). This athlete had no prior risk factors for cardiovascular disease.

Aesthetic and weight-class sport athletes, like all athletes, should be educated on the risks and benefits of popular dietary supplements and ergogenic aids. Sports dietitians, health care providers, clinicians, and coaches should be cautious when recommending the use of dietary supplements for these athletes. Because research has not historically included children and adolescents, the age of the athlete should be considered. Aesthetic and weight-class athletes may consider using sports drinks and bars to help refuel and rehydrate during training and competition. Vitamin and mineral supplements may be used when athletes are not able to meet nutrition goals from food alone. However, more research is needed to examine the safety and efficacy of additional dietary supplements for aesthetic and weight-class sport athletes before evidence-based recommendations can be established.

CONCLUSIONS

Aesthetic and weight-class athletes face tremendous body image concerns and often report energy intakes and extreme or dangerous weight loss methods in order to meet a desired body shape or weight. Due to these pressures, few athletes participating in aesthetic and weight-class sports meet the existing dietary recommendations, and researchers have observed reported energy intakes <25 kcal/kg body weight in both male and female aesthetic and weight-class athletes. Similarly, a number of studies have reported suboptimal macronutrient consumption, including carbohydrate intake ≤4 g/kg body weight, protein intake ≤1 g/kg body weight, and fat intake ≤20% of total energy by aesthetic and weight-class athletes. The available literature suggests many of these athletes are not consuming adequate energy or macronutrients for optimal performance and overall health. If continued over a long period of time, athletes following a hypo energy, low carbohydrate, low protein, or low fat diet are at risk of weight loss, muscle atrophy, fatigue, deficiencies in essential fatty acids or other vitamins/minerals, and impaired immunity. These concerns should be taken into consideration when educating or counseling aesthetic or weight-class sport athletes, especially young or adolescent athletes. Future research is necessary to develop sport-specific, evidence-based dietary recommendations, including general nutrition, pre-competition nutrition, recovery nutrition, and appropriate supplement recommendations for aesthetic and weight-class sport athletes. In addition, education programs should be developed that focus on healthy eating behaviors, positive body image, and appropriate weight loss methods.

REFERENCES

Alderman, B.L., D.M. Landers, J. Carlson, and J.R. Scott. 2004. Factors related to rapid weight loss practices among international-style wrestlers. *Med Sci Sports Exerc* 36(2):249–252.

American College of Sports Medicine, American Dietetic Association, and Dietitians of Canada. 2009. Joint position statement: Nutrition and athletic performance. *Med Sci Sports Exerc* 41(3):709–731.

Anderson, C., and T.A. Petrie. 2012. Prevalence of disordered eating and pathogenic weight control behaviors among NCAA division I female collegiate gymnasts and swimmers. *Res Q Exerc Sport* 83(1):120–124.

Anderson, V. 1997. Female gymnasts: Older and healthier. *Phys Sportsmed* 25(3):1–3.

Artioli, G.G., B. Gualano, E. Franchini, R.N. Batista, V.O. Placow, and A.H. Lancha. 2009. Physiological, performance, and nutritional profile of the Brazilian Olympic Wushu (kung-fu) team. *J Strength Cond Res* 23(1):20–25.

Artioli, G.G., E. Franchini, H. Nicastro, S. Sterkowicz, M.Y. Solis, and A.H. Lancha. 2010a. The need of a weight management control program in judo: A proposal based on the successful case of wrestling. *J Int Soc Sports Nutr* 7(15):1–5.

Artioli, G.G., B. Gualano, E. Franchini et al. 2010b. Prevalence, magnitude, and methods of rapid weight loss among judo competitors. *Med Sci Sports Exerc* 42(3):436–442.

Artioli, G.G., R.T. Iglesias, E. Franchini et al. 2010c. Rapid weight loss followed by recovery time does not affect judo-related performance. *J Sports Sci* 28(1):21–32.

Bachner-Melman, R., A.H. Zohar, R.P. Ebstein, Y. Elizur, and N. Constantini. 2006. How anorexic-like are the symptom and personality profiles of aesthetic athletes? *Med Sci Sports Exerc* 38(4):628–636.

Benardot, D. 2000. Gymnastics. In *Nutrition in Sport*, R.J. Maughan, Ed. Oxford: Blackwell Science, 588–608.

Benardot, D., M. Schwarz, and D.W. Heller. 1989. Nutrient intake in young, highly competitive gymnasts. *J Am Diet Assoc* 89(3):401–403.

Benson, J., D.M. Gillien, K. Bourdet, and A.R. Loosli. 1985. Inadequate nutrition and chronic calorie restriction in adolescent ballerinas. *Phys Sportsmed* 13(10):79–90.

Benson, J.E., Y. Allemann, G.E. Theintz, and H. Howald. 1990. Eating problems and calorie intake levels in Swiss adolescent athletes. *Int J Sports Med* 11(4):249–252.

Bonbright, J.M. 1989. The nutritional status of female ballet dancers 15–18 years of age. *Dance Res J* 21(2):9–14.

Brito, C.J., A.F.C. Roas, I.S.S. Brito, J.C.B. Marins, C. Córdova, and E. Franchini. 2012. Methods of body-mass reduction by combat sport athletes. *Int J Sport Nutr Exerc Metab* 22:89–97.

Brooks-Gunn, J., C. Burrow, and M.P. Warren. 1988. Attitudes toward eating and body weight in different groups of female adolescent athletes. *Int J Eat Disord* 7(6):749–757.

Brownell, K.D., S.N. Steen, and J.H. Wilmore. 1987. Weight regulation practices in athletes: Analysis of metabolic and health effects. *Med Sci Sports Exerc* 19(6):546–556.

Burke, L.M. 2001. Energy needs of athletes. *Can J Appl Physiol* 26(Suppl 1):S202–S219.

Burke, L.M., B. Kiens, and J.L. Ivy. 2004. Carbohydrates and fat for training and recovery. *J Sport Sci* 22(1):15–30.

Burke, L.M., J.A. Hawley, S.H.S. Wong, and A.E. Jeukendrup. 2011. Carbohydrates for train-ing and competition. *J Sports Sci* 29(Suppl 1):S17–S27.

Carter, J.M., A.E. Jeukendrup, and D.A. Jones. 2004. The effect of carbohydrate mouth rinse on 1-h cycle time trial performance. *Med Sci Sports Exerc* 36(12):2107–2111.

Caufield, M.J., and C.I. Karageorghis. 2008. Psychological effects of rapid weight loss and attitudes towards eating among professional jockeys. *J Sports Sci* 26(9):877–883.

Centers for Disease Control and Prevention. 1998. Hyperthermia and dehydration-related deaths associated with intentional rapid weight loss in three collegiate wrestlers—North Carolina, Wisconsin, and Michigan, November-December 1997. *MMWR Morb Mortal Wkly Rep* 47(6):105–108.

Chen, J.D., J.F. Wang, K.J. Li et al. 1989. Nutritional problems and measures in elite and amateur athletes. *Am J Clin Nutr* 49:1084–1089.

Choma, C.W., G.A. Sforza, and B.A. Keller. 1998. Impact of rapid weight loss on cognitive function in collegiate wrestlers. *Med Sci Sports Exerc* 30(5):746–749.

Chwalbińska-Moneta, J. 2003. Effect of creatine supplementation on aerobic performance and anaerobic capacity in elite rowers in the course of endurance training. *Int J Sport Nutr Exerc Metab* 13:173–183.

Cotugna, N., O.S. Snider, and J. Windish. 2011. Nutrition assessment of horse-racing athletes. *J Community Health* 36(2):261–264.

Cupisti, A., C. D'Alessandro, S. Castrogiovanni, A. Barale, and E. Morelli. 2000. Nutrition survey in elite rhythmic gymnasts. *J Sports Med Phys Fitness* 40(4):350–355.

Dahlström, M., E. Jansson, E. Nordevang, and L. Kaijser. 1990. Discrepancy between esti-mated energy intake and requirement in female dancers. *Clin Physiol* 10(1):11–25.

Dahlström, M., E. Jansson, M. Ekman, and L. Kaijser. 1995. Do highly physically active females have a lowered basal metabolic rate? *Scand J Med Sci Sports* 5(2):81–87.

D'Alessandro, C., E. Morelli, I. Evangelisti et al. 2007. Profiling the diet and body composi-tion of subelite adolescent rhythmic gymnasts. *Pediatr Exerc Sci* 19(2):215–227.

Daneshvar, P., M. Hariri, R. Ghiasvand et al. 2013. Dietary behaviors and nutritional assess-ment of young male Isfahani wrestlers. *Int J Prev Med* 4(Suppl 1):S48–S52.

de Bruin, A.P., R.R.D. Oudejans, and F.C. Bakker. 2007. Dieting and body image in aesthetic sports: A comparison of Dutch female gymnasts and non-aesthetic sport participants. *Psychol Sport Exerc* 8:507–520.

Degoutte, F., P. Jouanel, and E. Filaire. 2003. Energy demands during a judo match and recovery. *Br J Sports Med* 27(3):245–249.

Degoutte, F., P. Jouanel, R.J. Bégue et al. 2006. Food restriction, performance, biochemical, psychological, and endocrine changes in judo athletes. *Int J Sports Med* 27(1):9–18.

Delistraty, D.A., E.J. Reisman, and M. Snipes. 1992. A physiological and nutritional profile of young female figure skaters. *J Sports Med Phys Fitness* 32(2):149–155.

Desgorces, F.D., M. Chennaoui, C. Drogou, C.Y. Guezennec, and D. Gomez-Merino. 2008. Relationships between leptin levels and carbohydrate intake during rowing training. *J Sports Med Phys Fitness* 48(1):83–89.

de Wijn, J.F., J. Leusink, and G.B. Post. 1979. Diet, body composition and physical condition of champion rowers during periods of training and out of training. *Bibl Nutr Dieta* 27:143–148.

Dolan, E., H. O'Connor, A. McGoldrick, G. O'Loughlin, D. Lyons, and G. Warrington. 2011. Nutritional, lifestyle, and weight control practices of professional jockeys. *J Sport Sci* 29(8):791–799.

Douka, A., E. Skordilis, D. Koutsouki, and Y. Theodorakis. 2008. Prevalence of eating disor-ders among elite female athletes in aquatic sports. *Inquires Sport Phys Ed* 6(1):87–96.

Doyle-Lucas, A.F., J.D. Akers, and B.M. Davy. 2010. Energetic efficiency, menstrual irregu-larity, and bone mineral density in elite professional female ballet dancers. *J Dance Med Sci* 14(4):146–154.

Doyle-Lucas, A.F., and B.M. Davy. 2011. Development and evaluation of an educational intervention program for pre-professional adolescent ballet dancers: Nutrition for optimal performance. *J Dance Med Sci* 15(2):65–75.

Ebine, N., J.Y. Feng, M. Homma, S. Saitoh, and P.J.H. Jones. 2000. Total energy expenditure of elite synchronized swimmers measured by the doubly labeled water method. *Eur J Appl Physiol* 83(1):1–6.

Economos, C.D., S.S. Bortz, and M.E. Nilson. 1993. Nutritional practices of elite athletes: Practical recommendations. *Sports Med* 16(6):381–399.

Enns, M.P., A. Drewnowski, and J.A. Grinker. 1987. Body composition, body size estimation, and attitudes towards eating in male college athletes. *Psychosom Med* 49(1):56–64.

Ersoy, G. 1991. Dietary status and anthropometric assessment of child gymnasts. *J Sports Med Phys Fitness* 31(4):577–580.

Ferrand, C., C. Magnan, and R.A. Philippe. 2005. Body-esteem, body mass index, and risk for disordered eating among adolescents in synchronized swimming. *Percept Mot Skills* 101(3):877–884.

Ferrand, C., C. Magnan, M. Rouveix, and E. Filare. 2007. Disordered eating, perfectionism and body-esteem of elite synchronized swimmers. *Eur J Sport Sci* 7(4):223–230.

Filaire, E., and G. Lac. 2002. Nutritional status and body composition of juvenile elite female gymnasts. *J Sport Med Phys Fitness* 42(1):65–70.

Filaire, E., A. Massart, H. Portier et al. 2010. Effect of 6 weeks of n-3 fatty acid supplementation on oxidative stress in judo athletes. *Int J Sport Nutr Exerc Metab* 20(6):496–506.

Finaud, J., F. Degoutte, V. Scislowski, M. Rouveix, D. Durand, and E. Filaire. 2006. Competition and food restriction effects on oxidative stress in judo. *Int J Sports Med* 27(10):834–841.

Fogelholm, G.M., R. Koskinen, J. Laakso, T. Rankinen, and I. Ruokonen. 1993. Gradual and rapid weight loss: Effects on nutrition and performance in male athletes. *Med Sci Sports Exerc* 25(3):371–377.

Fogelholm, G.M., T.K. Kukkonen-Harjula, S.A. Taipale, H.T. Sievänen, P. Oja, and I.M. Vuori. 1995. Resting metabolic rate and energy intake in female gymnasts, figure-skaters and soccer players. *Int J Sports Med* 16(8):551–556.

Food and Nutrition Board. Institute of Medicine. 2002. *Dietary Reference Intakes for Energy, Arbohydrate, Fiber, Fat, Fatty Acids, Cholesterol, Protein, and Amino Acids.* Washington, DC: National Academy Press.

Forte, R.Y., D. Precoma-Neto, N.C. Neto, F. Maia, and J.R. Faria-Neto. 2006. Myocardial infarction associated with the use of a dietary supplement rich in ephedrine in a young athlete. *Arq Bras Cardiol* 87(5):e179–e181.

Friedman, J.E., and P.W.R. Lemon. 1989. Effect of chronic endurance exercise on retention of dietary protein. *Int J Sport Med* 10(2):118–123.

Frusztajer, N.T., S. Dhuper, M.P. Warren, J. Brooks-Gunn, and R.P. Fox. 1990. Nutrition and the incidence of stress fractures in ballet dancers. *Am J Clin Nutr* 51(5):779–783.

Grandjean, A.D. 1989. Macronutrient intake of US athletes compared with the general population and recommendations made for athletes. *Am J Clin Nutr* 49(5 Supp):1070–1076.

Gropper, S.S., L.M. Sorrels, and D. Blessing. 2003. Copper status of collegiate female athletes involved in different sports. *Int J Sport Nutr Exerc Metab* 13(3):343–357.

Hall, C.J., and A.M. Lane. 2001. Effects of rapid weight loss on mood and performance among amateur boxers. *Br J Sports Med* 35(6):390–395.

Hargreaves, M., J.A. Hawley, and A. Jeukendrup. 2004. Pre-exercise carbohydrate and fat ingestion: Effects on metabolism and performance. *J Sports Sci* 22(1):31–38.

Hassapidou, M.N., and A. Manstrantoni. 2001. Dietary intakes of elite female athletes in Greece. *J Hum Nutr Diet* 14(5):391–396.

Heinemann, L., and H. Zerbes. 1989. Physical activity, fitness, and diet: Behavior in the population compared with elite athletes in the GDR. *Am J Clin Nutr* 49(5 Supp):1007–1016.

Hickson, J.F., J. Schrader, and L.C. Trischler. 1986. Dietary intakes of female basketball and gymnastics athletes. *J Am Diet Assoc* 86(2):251–253.

Hill, R.J., and P.S.W. Davies. 1999. The validity of a four day weighed food record for measuring energy intake in female classical ballet dancers. *Eur J Clin Nutr* 53(9):752–754.

Hill, R.J., and P.S.W. Davies. 2001. The validity of self-reported energy intake as determined using the doubly labelled water technique. *Br J Nutr* 85(4):415–430.

Hill, R.J., and P.S.W. Davies. 2002. Energy intake and energy expenditure in elite lightweight female rowers. *Med Sci Sports Exerc* 34(11):1823–1829.

Hincapié, C.A., and J.D. Cassidy. Disordered eating, menstrual disturbances, and low bone mineral density in dancers: A systematic review. 2010. *Arch Phys Med Rehabil* 91(11):1777–1789.

Horswill, C.A., S.H. Park, and J.N. Roemmich. 1990. Changes in the protein nutritional status of adolescent wrestlers. *Med Sci Sports Exerc* 22(5):599–604.

Howat, P.M., M.L. Carbo, G.Q. Mills, and P. Wozniak. 1989. The influence of diet, body fat, menstrual cycling, and activity upon the bone density of females. *J Am Diet Assoc* 89(9):1305–1307.

Ihle, R., and A.B. Loucks. 2004. Dose-response relationships between energy availability and bone turnover in young exercising women. *J Bone Miner Res* 19(8):1231–1240.

Jeukendrup, A.E., and E.S. Chambers. 2010. Oral carbohydrate sensing and exercise performance. *Curr Opin Clin Nutr Metab Care* 13(4):447–451.

Jonnalagadda, S.S., D. Bernadot, and M. Nelson. 1998. Energy and nutrient intakes of the United States National Women's Artistic Gymnastics Team. *Int J Sport Nutr* 8(4):331–344.

Jonnalagadda, S.S., D. Benardot, and M.N. Dill. 2000. Assessment of under-reporting of energy intake by elite female gymnasts. *Int J Sport Nutr Exerc Metab* 10(3):315–325.

Jonnalagadda, S.S., P.J. Ziegler, and J.A. Nelson. 2004. Food preferences, dieting behaviors, and body image perceptions of elite figure skaters. *Int J Sport Nutr Exerc Metab* 14(5):594–606.

Kara, E., M. Gunay, I. Cicioglu et al. 2010. Effect of zinc supplementation on antioxidant activity in young wrestlers. *Bio Trace Elem Res* 134:55–63.

Karelis, A.D., J.W. Smith, D.H. Passe, and F. Peronnet. 2010. Carbohydrate administration and exercise performance: What are the potential mechanisms involved? *Sports Med* 40(9):747–763.

Kaufman, B.A., M.P. Warren, J.E. Dominguez, J. Wang, S.B. Heymsfield, and R.N. Pierson. 2002. Bone density and amenorrhea in ballet dancers are related to a decreased resting metabolic rate and lower leptin levels. *J Clin Endocrinol Metab* 87(6):2777–2783.

Kazemi, M., H. Shearer, and Y.S. Choung. 2005. Pre-competition habits and injuries in Taekwondo athletes. *BMC Musculoskelet Disord* 27:6–26.

Kern, B., and T.L. Robinson. 2011. Effects of β-alanine supplementation on performance and body composition in collegiate wrestlers and football players. *J Strength Cond Res* 25(7):1804–1815.

King, M.B., and G. Mezey. 1987. Eating behavior of male racing jockeys. *Psychol Med* 17(1):249–253.

Kirchner, E.M., R.D. Lewis, and P.J. O'Connor. 1995. Bone mineral density and dietary intake of female college gymnasts. *Med Sci Sports Exerc* 27(4):543–549.

Kocak, S., and U. Karli. 2003. Effects of high dose oral creatine supplementation on anaerobic capacity of elite wrestlers. *J Sports Med Phys Fitness* 43(4):488–492.

Koral, J., and F. Dosseville. 2009. Combination of gradual and rapid weight loss: Effects on physical performance and psychological state of elite judo athletes. *J Sports Sci* 27(2):115–120.

Koutedakis, Y., and A. Jamurtas. 2004. The dancer as a performing athlete: Physiological considerations. *Sports Med* 34(10):651–661.

Krentz, E.M., and P. Warshburger. 2011. A longitudinal investigation of sports-related risk factors for disordered eating in aesthetic sports. *Scand J Med Sci Sports* 23(3):303–310.

Krieger, J.W., H.S. Sitren, M.J. Daniels, and B. Langkamp-Henken. 2006. Effects of variation in protein and carbohydrate intake of body mass and composition during energy restriction: A meta-regression. *Am J Clin Nutr* 83(2):260–274.

Labadarios, D., J. Kotze, D. Momberg, and W. Kotze. 1993. Jockeys and their practices in South Africa. *World Rev Nutr Diet* 71:97–114.

Lemon, P.W., M.A. Tarnopolsky, J.D. MacDougall, and S.A. Atkinson. 1992. Protein requirements and muscle mass/strength changes during intensive training in novice body builders. *J Appl Phys* 73(2):767–775.

Leydon, M.A., and C. Wall. 2002. New Zealand jockeys' dietary habits and their potential impact on health. *Int J Sport Nutr Exerc Meab* 12(2):220–237.

Lindholm, C., K. Hagenfeldt, and U. Hagman. 1995. A nutrition study in juvenile elite gymnasts. *Acta Pediatr* 84(3):273–277.

Loosli, A.R., and J. Benson. 1990. Nutritional intake in adolescent athletes. *Pediatr Clin North Am* 37(5):1143–1152.

López-Varela, S., A. Montero, R.K. Chandra, and A. Marcos. 2000. Nutritional status of young female elite gymnasts. *Int J Vitam Nutr Res* 70(4):185–190.

Loucks, A.B. 2004. Energy balance and body composition in sports and exercise. *J Sport Sci* 22(1):1–14.

Loucks, A.B., B. Kiens, and H.H. Wright. 2011. Energy availability in athletes. *J Sport Sci* 29(Suppl 1):S7–S15.

Lundy, B. 2011. Nutrition for synchronized swimming: A review. *Int J Sport Nutr Exerc Metab* 21(5):436–445.

Magkos, F., and M. Yannakoulia. 2003. Methodology of dietary assessment in athletes: Concepts and pitfalls. *Curr Opin Clin Nutr Metab Care* 6(5):539–549.

Manore, M.M. 2012. Dietary supplements for improving body composition and reducing body weight: Where is the evidence? *Int J Sport Nutr Exerc Metab* 22(2):139–154.

Maughan, R.J., D.S. King, and T. Lea. 2004. Dietary supplements. *J Sports Sci* 22(1):95–113.

Maughan, R.J., P.L. Greenhaff, and P. Hespel. 2011. Dietary supplements for athletes: Emerging trends and recurring themes. *J Sports Sci* 29(Suppl):S57–S66.

McCargar, L.J., and S.M. Crawford. 1992. Metabolic and anthropometric changes with weight cycling in wrestlers. *Med Sci Sports Exerc* 24(11):1270–1275.

McCargar, L.J., D. Simmons, N. Craton, J.E. Taunton, and C.L. Birmingham. 1993. Physiological effects of weight cycling in female lightweight rowers. *Can J Appl Physiol* 18(3):291–303.

McMurray, R.G., C.R. Proctor, and W.L. Wilson. 1991. Effect of caloric deficit and dietary manipulation on aerobic and anaerobic exercise. *Int J Sports Med* 12(2):167–172.

Mettler, S., N. Mitchell, and K.D. Tipton. 2010. Increased protein intake reduces lean body mass loss during weight loss in athletes. *Med Sci Sports Exerc* 42(2):326–337.

Michopoulou, E., A. Avloniti, A. Kambas, D. Leontsini, and M. Michalopoulo. 2011. Elite premenarcheal rhythmic gymnasts demonstrate energy and dietary intake deficiencies during periods of intense training. *Pediatr Exerc Sci* 23(4):560–572.

Moffatt, R.J. 1984. Dietary status of elite female high school gymnasts: Inadequacy of vitamin and mineral intake. *J Am Diet Assoc* 84(11):1361–1363.

Morris, F.L., and W.R. Payne. 1996. Seasonal variations in the body composition of lightweight rowers. *Br J Sports Med* 30(4):301–304.

Morris, F.L., W.R. Payne, and J.D. Wark. 1999. Prospective decrease in progesterone concentrations in female lightweight rowers during the competitive season compared with the off season: A controlled study examining weight loss and intensive exercise. *Br J Sports Med* 33(6):417–422.

Mountjoy, M. 2009. Injuries and medical issues in synchronized Olympic sports. *Curr Sports Med Rep* 8(5):255–261.

National Collegiate Athletic Association. 2000. *2001 NCAA Wrestling Rules and Interpretations*. Indianapolis: National Collegiate Athletic Association.

Nattiv, A., A.B. Loucks, M.M. Manore, C.F. Sanborn, J. Sundgot-Borgen, and M.P. Warren. 2007. The female athlete triad. *Med Sci Sports Exerc* 39(10):1867–1882.

O'Connor, P., R.D. Lewis, E.M. Kirchner, and D.B. Cook. 1996. Eating disorder symptoms in former female college gymnasts: Relations with body composition. *Am J Clin Nutr* 64(6):840–843.

Ohta, S., S. Nakaji, K. Suzuki, M. Totsuka, T. Umeda, and K. Sugawara. 2002. Depressed humoral immunity after weight reduction in competitive judoists. *Luminescence* 17(3):150–157.

Oppliger, R.A., S.A.N. Steen, and J.R. Scott. 2003. Weight loss practices of college wrestlers. *Int J Sport Nutr Exerc Metab* 13(1):29–46.

Pettersson, S., M.P. Ekström, and C.M. Berg. 2012. The food and weight combat. A problematic fight for the elite combat sports athlete. *Appetite* 59(2):234–242.

Pettersson, S., M.P. Ekström, and C.M. Berg. 2013. Practices of weight regulation among elite athletes in combat sports: A matter of mental advantage? *J Athl Train* 48(1):99–108.

Phillips, S.M., and L.J.C. Van Loon. 2011. Dietary protein for athletes: From requirements to optimum adaptation. *J Sports Sci* 29(Suppl 1):S29–S38.

Quintas, M.E., R.M. Ortega, A.M. López-Sobaler, G. Garrido, and A.M. Requejo. 2003. Influence of dietetic and anthropometric factors and of the type of sport practiced on bone density in different groups of women. *Eur J Clin Nutr* 57(Suppl 1):S58–S62.

Rankin, J.W., J.V. Ocel, and L.L. Craft. 1996. Effect of weight loss and refeeding diet composition on anaerobic performance in wrestlers. *Med Sci Sports Exerc* 28(10):1292–1299.

Rankinen, T., S. Lyytikainen, E. Vanninen, I. Penttila, R. Rauramaa, and M. Uusitupa. 1998. Nutritional status of the Finnish elite ski jumpers. *Med Sci Sports Exerc* 30(11):1592–1597.

Reading, K.J., L.J. McCargar, and V.J. Harber. 2002. Energy balance and luteal phase progesterone levels in elite adolescent aesthetic athletes. *Int J Sport Nutr Exerc Metab* 12(1):93–104.

Reggiani, E., G.B. Arras, S. Trabacca, D. Senarega, and G. Chiodini. 1989. Nutritional status and body composition of adolescent female gymnasts. *J Sports Med Phys Fitness* 29(3):285–288.

Roemmich, J.N., and W.E. Sinning. 1997. Weight loss and wrestling training: Effects on nutrition, growth, maturation, body composition, and strength. *J Appl Physiol* 82(6):1751–1759.

Rokitzki, L., A. Sagredos, E. Keck, B. Sauer, and J. Keul. 1994a. Assessment of vitamin B2 status in performance athletes of various types of sports. *J Nutr Sci Vitaminol* 40(1):11–22.

Rokitzki, L., A.N. Sagredos, F. Reuss, D. Cufi, and J. Keul. 1994b. Assessment of vitamin B6 status of strength and speed power athletes. *J Am Coll Nutr* 13(1):87–94.

Rosendahl, J., B. Bormann, K. Aschenbrenner, and B. Strauss. 2009. Dieting and disordered eating in German high school athletes and non-athletes. *Scand J Med Sci Sports* 19(5):731–739.

Rucinski, A. 1989. Relationship of body image and dietary intake of competitive ice skaters. *J Am Diet Assoc* 89(1):98–100.

Sansone, R.A., and R. Sawyer. 2005. Weight loss pressure on a 5-year-old wrestler. *Br J Sports Med* 39:E2.

Sekulic, D., M. Peric, and J. Rodek. 2010. Substance use and misuse among professional ballet dancers. *Subst Use Misuse* 45(9):1420–1430.

Short, S.H., and W.R. Short. 1983. Four-year study of university athletes' dietary intake. *J Am Diet Assoc* 82(6):632–645.

Slater, G.J., A.J. Rice, K. Sharpe, I. Mujika, D. Jenkins, and A.G. Hahn. 2005. Body-mass management of Australian lightweight rowers prior to and during competition. *Med Sci Sports Exerc* 37(5):860–866.

Slater, G.J., A.J. Rice, D. Jenkins, J. Gulbin, and A.G. Hahn. 2006. Preparation of former heavyweight oarsmen to complete as lightweight rowers over 16 weeks: Three case studies. *Int J Sport Nutr Exerc Metab* 16(1):108–121.

Smith, M., R. Dyson, T. Hale, M. Hamilton, J. Kelly, and P. Wellington. 2001. The effects of restricted energy and fluid intake on simulated amateur boxing performance. *Int J Sport Nutr Exerc Metab* 11(2):238–247.

Smolak, L., S.K. Murnen, and A.E. Ruble. 2000. Female athletes and eating problems: A meta-analysis. *Int J Eat Disord* 27(4):371–380.

Sobal, J., and S.H. Stensland. 1992. Dietary practices of ballet, jazz, and modern dancers. *J Am Diet Assoc* 92(3):319–324.

Sobal, J., and L.F. Marquart. 1994. Vitamin/mineral supplement use among athletes: A review of the literature. *Int J Sport Nutr* 4:320–334.

Soric, M., M. Misigoj-Durakovic, and Z. Pedisic. 2008. Dietary intake and body composition of prepubescent female aesthetic athletes. *Int J Sport Nutr Exerc Metab* 18(3):343–354.

Steen, S.N., and K.D. Brownell. 1990. Patterns of weight loss and regain in wrestlers: Has the tradition changed? *Med Sci Sports Exerc* 22(6):762–768.

Steen, S.N., K. Mayer, K.D. Brownell, and T.A. Wadden. 1995. Dietary intake of female collegiate heavyweight rowers. *Int J Sport Nutr* 5(3):225–231.

Stellingwerff, T., R.J. Maughan, and L.M. Burke. 2011. Nutrition for power sports: Middle-distance running, track cycling, rowing, canoeing/kayaking, and swimming. *J Sport Sci* 29(Suppl 1):S79–S89.

Stroescu, V., I. Dragen, L. Simionescu, and O.V. Stroescu. 2001. Hormonal and metabolic response in elite female gymnasts undergoing strenuous training and supplementation with Supro® brand isolated soy protein. *J Sport Med Phys Fitness* 41(1):89–94.

Sundgot-Borgen, J. 1994. Risk and trigger factors for the development of eating disorders in female elite athletes. *Med Sci Sports Exerc* 26(4):414–419.

Sundgot-Borgen, J. 1996. Eating disorders, energy intake, training volume, and menstrual function in high-level modern rhythmic gymnasts. *Int J Sport Nutr* 6(2):100–109.

Sundgot-Borgen, J., and M.K. Torstveit. 2004. Prevalence of eating disorders in elite athletes is higher than in the general population. *Clin J Sports Med* 14:25–32.

Sundgot-Borgen, J., and M.K. Torstveit. 2010. Aspects of disordered eating continuum in elite high-intensity sports. *Scand J Med Sci Sports* 20(Suppl 2):S112–S121.

Sundgot-Borgen, J., and I. Garthe. 2011. Elite athletes in aesthetic and Olympic weight-class sports and the challenge of body weight and body compositions. *J Sports Sci* 29(Suppl 1):S101–S114.

Syrotuik, D.G., A.B. Game, E.M. Gillies, and G.J. Bell. 2001. Effects of creatine monohydrate supplementation during combined strength and high intensity rowing training on performance. *Can J Appl Phsiol* 26(6):527–542.

Talbott, S.M., and S.A. Shapses. 1998. Fasting and energy intake influence bone turnover in lightweight male rowers. *Int J Sports Nutr* 8(4):377–387.

Tartibian, B., B.H. Maleki, and A. Abbasi. 2010. The effects of omega-3 supplementation on pulmonary function of young wrestlers during intensive training. *J Sci Med Sport* 13(2):381–386.

Teshima, K., H. Imamura, Y. Yoshimura et al. 2002. Nutrient intake of highly competitive male and female collegiate karate players. *J Physiol Anthropol Appl Human Sci* 21(4):205–211.

Thompson, J.L. 1998. Energy balance in young athletes. *Int J Sport Nutr.* 8(2):160–174.

Tipton, C.M., and T.K. Tcheng. 1970. Iowa wrestling study. Weight loss in high school students. *JAMA* 214(7):1269–1274.
Torstveit, M.K., and J. Sundgot-Borgen. 2005. Participation in leanness sports but not training volume is associated with menstrual dysfunction: A national survey of 1,276 elite
   athletes and controls. *Br J Sports Med* 39(3):141–147.
Tuttle, W.W. 1943. The effect of weight loss by dehydration and the withholding of food on the
   physiologic responses of wrestlers. *Res Q* 14(2):158–166.
Umeda, T., S. Nakaji, T. Shimoyama, Y. Yamamoto, M. Totsuka, and K. Sugawara. 2004.
   Adverse effects of energy restriction on myogenic enzymes in judoists. *J Sports Sci*
   22(4):329–338.
van Erp-Baart, A.M.J., W.H.M. Saris, R.A. Binkhorst, J.A. Vos, and J.W.H. Elvers. 1989.
   Nationwide survey on nutritional habits in elite athletes. Part I. Energy, carbohydrate,
   protein, and fat intake. *Int J Sport Med* 10(Suppl 1):S3–S10.
Van Marken Lichtenbelt, W.D., M. Fogelholm, R. Ottenheijm, and K.R. Westerterp. 1995.
   Physical activity, body composition and bone density in ballet dancers. *Br J Nutr*
   74(4):439–451.
Walker, L.S., M.G. Bemben, D.A. Bemben, and A.W. Knehans. 1998. Chrominum picolinate
   effects on body composition and muscular performance in wrestlers. *Med Sci Sport
   Exerc* 30(12):1730–1737.
Warren, M.P., J. Brooks-Gunn, R.P. Fox, C.C. Holderness, E.P. Hyle, and W.G. Hamilton.
   2002. Osteopenia in exercise-associated amenorrhea using ballet dancers as a model:
   A longitudinal study. *J Clin Endocrinol Metab* 87(7):3162–3168.
Weimann, E., C. Witzel, S. Schwidergall, and H.J. Böhles. 2000. Peripubertal perturbations
   in elite gymnasts caused by sport specific training regimes and inadequate nutritional
   intake. *Int J Sports Med* 21(3):210–215.
Widerman, P.M., and R.D. Hagan. 1982. Body weight loss in a wrestler preparing for competition: A case report. *Med Sci Sports Exerc* 14(6):413–418.
Wilson, G., N. Chester, M. Eubank et al. 2012. An alternative dietary strategy to make weight
   while improving mood, decreasing body fat, and not dehydration: A case study of a
   professional jockey. *Int J Sport Nutr Exerc Metab* 22(3):225–231.
Xia, G., M.K. Chin, R.N. Girandola, and R.Y.K. Liu. 2001. The effects of diet and supplements
   on a male world champion lightweight rower. *J Sports Med Phys Fitness* 41(2):223–228.
Yannakoulia, M., A. Keramopoulos, and A.L. Matalas. 2004. Bone mineral density in young
   active females: The case of dancers. *Int J Sport Nutr Exerc Metab* 14(3):279–291.
Zenic, N., M. Peric, N.G. Zubcevic, Z. Ostojic, and L. Ostojic. 2010. Comparative analysis of
   substance use in ballet, dance sport, and synchronized swimming: Results of a longitudinal study. *Med Probl Perform Art* 25(2)75:81.
Ziegler, P., S. Hensley, J.B. Roepke, S.H. Whitaker, B.W. Craig, and A. Drewnowski.
   1998a. Eating attitudes and energy intakes of female skaters. *Med Sci Sports Exerc*
   30(4):583–586.
Ziegler, P.J., C.S. Khoo, P.M. Kris-Etherton, S.S. Jonnalagadda, B. Sherr, and J.A. Nelson.
   1998b. Nutritional status of nationally ranked junior US figure skaters. *J Am Diet Assoc*
   98(7):809–811.
Ziegler, P.J., C.S. Khoo, B. Sheer, J.A. Nelson, W.M. Larson, and A. Drenowski. 1998c. Body
   image and dieting behaviors among elite figure skaters. *Int J Eat Disord* 24(4):421–427.
Ziegler, P.J., J.A. Nelson, and S.S. Jonnalagadda. 1999. Nutritional and physiological status of
   U.S. national figure skaters. *Int J Sport Nutr* 9(4):345–360.
Ziegler, P., J.A. Nelson, A. Barratt-Fornell, L. Fiveash, and A. Drenowski. 2001. Energy and
   macronutrient intakes of elite figure skaters. *J Am Diet Assoc* 101(3):319–325.
Ziegler, P.J., S.S. Jonnalagadda, J.A. Nelson, C. Lawrence, and B. Baciak. 2002a. Contribution
   of meals and snacks to nutrient intake of male and female elite figure skaters during
   peak competitive season. *J Am Coll Nutr* 21(2):114–119.

Ziegler, P.J., R. Sharp, V. Hugher, W. Evans, and C.S. Khoo. 2002b. Nutritional status of teen-age female competitive figure skaters. *J Am Diet Assoc* 102(3):374–379.

Ziegler, P.J., J.A. Nelson, and S.S. Jonnalagadda. 2003. Use of dietary supplements by elite figure skaters. *Int J Sport Nutr Exerc Metab* 13(3):266–276.

Ziegler, P.J., S. Kannan, S.S. Jonnalagadda, A. Krishnakumar, S.E. Taksali, and J.A. Nelson. 2005a. Dietary intake, body image perceptions, and weight concerns of female US international synchronized figure skating teams. *Int J Sport Nutr Exerc Metab* 15(5):550–556.

Ziegler, P.J., J.A. Nelson, C. Tay, B. Bruemmer, and A. Drenowski. 2005b. A comparison of three methods of determination of energy density of elite figure skaters. *Int J Sport Nutr Exerc Metab* 15(5):537–549.

Zucker, N.L., L.G. Womble, D.A. Williamson, and L.A. Perrin. 1999. Protective factors for eating disorders in female college athletes. *Eat Disord* 7(3):207–218.

8 Dietary Supplement (and Food) Safety for Athletes

Ronald J. Maughan, PhD, FACSM

School of Sport, Exercise and Health Sciences,
Loughborough University, Leicestershire, United Kingdom

CONTENTS

The use of dietary supplements is widespread in all sports and at all levels of sport, reflecting the prevalence of use in the wider society. It is estimated that about half of the U.S. population uses dietary supplements (Bailey et al. 2011) and a similar prevalence is likely in many other countries. There are many reasons individuals choose to use supplements (Fennell 2004): maintenance of good health and prevention of illness are commonly cited reasons for use, even though health claims regulations in most countries prevent the promotion of supplements for these purposes. More specific uses of supplements include increased alertness, weight loss, alleviation of muscle and joint pain, etc. Some of these effects are attractive to athletes, but there is an additional focus on supplements that have the potential to improve performance, either during training or in competition. With such widespread use of supplements in the general population and with the specific focus of athletes on both physical and mental performance, it is perhaps not surprising that a high prevalence of supplement use is reported in most surveys of athletes (Maughan et al. 2007).

Athletes who take supplements, however, should only do so after carrying out a careful cost-benefit analysis. On one side of the balance are the potential rewards, and on the other side are the costs and risks (Maughan 2013). Vitamin and mineral supplements are generally perceived as being harmless, and the one-a-day multivitamin tablet is often seen as an insurance policy "just in case" of an inadequate dietary intake. Although these supplements are mostly benign, this is not always the case. Routine iron supplementation, for example, can do more harm than good, and the risk of iron toxicity is very real (Papanikolaou and Pantopoulos 2005). It has been estimated that, among the population of industrialized countries, twice as many men suffer from iron overload due to excessive use of iron supplements as suffer from iron deficiency (Eichner 2000). Similarly, there is disagreement as to whether excessive use of antioxidant supplements can impair the metabolic adaptations to training by blunting the signaling pathways that are normally activated by increased free radical activity (Gross et al. 2011; Sachdev and Davies 2008).

More exotic supplements, many of which have names that suggest an anabolic or stimulant action and with promotional material to match, have become a prominent feature on the shelves of sports nutrition stores in the last decade or two. Some of these products make extravagant claims about building bigger, stronger, and faster muscles, repairing the damage caused by hard training, resisting infections and illnesses, and preventing chronic fatigue. They usually come with a price tag to match, too, but for the athlete who is training to the limits, no price seems too high. This may be true in a strictly financial sense, but there is ever-growing evidence of the potential for adverse effects resulting from indiscriminate supplement use. These effects include serious and occasionally fatal effects on health, adverse effects on performance, and the risk of a positive result if an athlete is tested for drugs that are prohibited in sport.

Dietary supplements on sale in the United States are not subject to premarket review for safety or efficacy by the Food and Drug Administration (FDA) unless they contain new dietary ingredients. Manufacturers are not required to secure FDA approval before producing or selling dietary supplements (Food and Drug Administration 2015), thus limiting the checks on products that are offered for sale to the public. Similar regulation (or lack thereof) applies in most countries, although local regulations do vary and some products that are classified as medicines in one country are classified as dietary supplements in another country. Elite athletes are regular international travelers, whether for training camps or for competition, and they are well aware of the opportunities to purchase supplements that are not legally available in their home countries. Internet selling has also eliminated many of the limitations on the supplements that an athlete can obtain and has removed most of the checks on the quality of supplements that are on sale by preventing opportunities for inspection of manufacturing, packaging, and storage premises.

SUPPLEMENTS AS FOODS

Because dietary supplements are classified as foods rather than as drugs, the legal requirements that govern their production and distribution are less strict, and are less strictly enforced, than those related to pharmaceuticals are. Government food inspectors publish regular reports of breaches of food safety regulations, often covering issues such as the presence of undeclared allergens, bacterial and fungal organisms, foreign objects (glass, metal, etc.), heavy metals, and other potentially hazardous substances. The websites of the FDA and the U.K. Food Standards Agency (FSA) contain daily notices of food product recalls because of manufacturing issues. In a 14-day period in January 2013, the FDA issued recall notices for food products because of undeclared milk (two products from different companies), peanuts and eggs, the presence of metal fragments (two products from different companies), and the presence of *Listeria* (two products from different companies) and *E. coli* (http://www.fda.gov/Safety/Recalls/ucm2005683.htm). In the corresponding period, the FSA notified recalls of products because of the presence of *salmonella* and *Bacillus cereus* and because of inspections that revealed poor standards of hygiene in two separate factory premises (http://www.food.gov.uk/news-updates/news/food-alerts?keyword=&page=8).

It is not unusual to find cases of poor hygiene in the manufacture, storage, and provision of foodstuffs to the public, so it should not be surprising that some dietary supplement manufacturers fail to follow good manufacturing practice. A 2012 report by the FDA revealed that violations of manufacturing rules were found in half of the nearly 450 dietary supplement firms it had inspected in the previous four years. In 2012, FDA inspectors found violations of good manufacturing practices during two-thirds of the 204 inspections they conducted in nearly 200 supplement firms' facilities, with 70 of these inspections resulting in the agency's most serious rating (Tsouderos 2012). Some supplement products have been shown to contain impurities (lead, broken glass, animal feces, etc.) because of poor quality control during manufacture or storage. The risk of gastrointestinal upset because of poor hygiene during the production and storage of products is a concern to athletes. At best, this may be nothing more than a minor inconvenience, but it may cause the athlete to miss a crucial competition.

This same lax approach to quality assurance can lead to large variations in the content of the active ingredients in supplements. Some investigations have shown that some products do not contain any measurable amount of the substances identified on the label, while others may contain up to 150% of the stated dose (Gurley et al. 2000; Parasrampuria et al. 1998). Where relatively expensive ingredients are involved, it seems that some products contain little or no active ingredient (Green et al. 2001). In a survey of the caffeine content of supplements on sale in military bases, Cohen et al. (2013) analyzed the caffeine content of 31 products that are known to have added caffeine or herbal ingredients that naturally contain caffeine. Eleven of the supplements listed herbal ingredients; these products had either no caffeine or only trace levels. Nine of the other 20 products had labels with accurate caffeine information. Another five had varying caffeine contents that were either much lower or higher than the amount listed on the label. The remaining six products did not have caffeine levels on their labels, but each of these had a high caffeine content of between 210 and 310 mg per serving. For the athlete who plans to use caffeine as part of a competition strategy, this variability is rather alarming.

A recent analysis of commercially available herbal products used DNA analysis to assess the identity of herbal species present in those products (Newmaster et al. 2013). More than half (59%) of the herbal products tested contained species of plants that were not listed on the label, and one-third (33%) of the authenticated herbal products also contained contaminants or fillers not listed on the label. They also found that several products contained materials from plants that are known to be toxic, to have adverse side effects, or to interact negatively with other herbs, supplements, or medications. This is clearly a public health issue rather than a specific problem for athletes, but all consumers are at risk of adverse reactions.

In addition, in January 2013, the Food Safety Authority of Ireland (FSAI) announced that beef burgers on sale in the United Kingdom and Ireland showed evidence of the presence of horse and pig DNA (http://www.fsai.ie/news_centre/press _releases/horseDNA15012013.html). Of 27 beef burger products analyzed, 10 (37%) tested positive for horse DNA and 23 (85%) tested positive for pig DNA. In 9 of the 10 beef burger samples, horse DNA was found at very low levels, but analysis of one sample indicated that horsemeat accounted for approximately 29% of the total meat content of the burger. While there was no suggestion that these products would be harmful to health, many consumers would wish to know if they were eating horsemeat. Those whose religious beliefs require them to avoid any contact with pigs would be seriously alarmed to know that they have been eating pig—even if only in trace amounts. There must also be a concern that disregard of regulations relating to sourcing of the meat included in products suggests that compliance with hygiene regulations is unlikely.

In 2012, the FSA identified eight cases where samples of horsemeat collected at abattoirs tested positive for the presence of phenylbutazone (http://www.food.gov.uk /news-updates/news/2013/jan/bute-horsemeat-update). Phenylbutazone, often referred to as bute, is a nonsteroidal anti-inflammatory drug (NSAID) that is commonly used for the short-term treatment of pain and fever in animals, though it is not approved for use in humans. Five of the animals where bute was detected were exported for entry into the food chain.

These reports follow the recognition of the widespread presence in the human food chain of clenbuterol, which is widely used to promote growth of lean muscle tissue in food animals in some countries. Clenbuterol is also used by some athletes for the same reasons. The presence of residues in meat, however, may give rise to a positive doping outcome in athletes who consume meat from animals that have been injected with prohibited compounds. In 2011, the Manfred Donike Institute for Doping Analysis at the German Sports University in Cologne reported that it had detected clenbuterol in the urine of 22 of 28 travelers who had returned from a short visit to China (Guddat et al. 2011). Later that summer, it was reported that traces of clenbuterol were detected in 109 of the 208 urine samples provided by players at the FIFA Under-17 World Cup in Mexico, and again, this was attributed to the ingestion of meat products from animals that had been treated with clenbuterol. In spite of the evidence that a doping offense had been committed, under the principle of strict liability that is normally applied no sanctions were imposed on these players or on other senior players who also tested positive for clenbuterol (FIFA 2011).

These findings indicate that false-positive doping outcomes may result from contaminated food as well as from contaminated dietary supplements. The principle of strict liability places the onus on the athlete, even where there was no deliberate intent to commit an offense. The offense lies in the presence of the substance in the athlete's sample rather than in the intent to take a performance-enhancing substance. The potential problems that can result from use of contaminated supplements can be managed by avoiding supplements or by taking great care in the choice of supplements used. The problem of contaminated foods is less easily managed and raises new concerns for athletes and doping authorities alike.

SUPPLEMENT CONTAMINATION

Athletes who are liable to testing for the use of drugs that are prohibited in sport—and those who advise these athletes—should be aware of the possibility that a supplement may contain something that will cause a positive doping test (Maughan 2005). Only a very small number of individuals are tested for evidence of the use of doping agents, but these are invariably the most successful performers. For these athletes, a failed drug test may mean the loss of medals won or records set, as well as temporary suspension from competition. It also leads to damage to the athlete's reputation and perhaps to permanent loss of employment and income. Where there has been deliberate cheating, such penalties seem entirely appropriate, but it is undoubtedly true that some failed doping tests can be attributed to the innocent ingestion of dietary supplements. The strict liability principle applied by the World Anti-Doping Agency (WADA) does not distinguish between deliberate cheating and inadvertent doping, so athletes must accept personal responsibility for all supplements (and medications) that they use. Where the athlete can establish that a positive test was the result of inadvertent ingestion rather than deliberate doping, there may be some relaxation of the sanctions imposed, but the athlete will still be guilty of a doping offense.

Numerous published studies show that contamination of dietary supplements with prohibited substances is not uncommon (Maughan 2005). A wide range of stimulants, steroids, and other agents that are included on WADA's prohibited list has been identified in otherwise innocuous supplements. These instances are quite distinct from the legitimate sale of some of these substances, as their presence is not declared on the product label. In some cases, these adulterated products are even labeled as being safe for use by athletes. In some, but not all, cases, the extraneous additions have actions that are linked to the intended use of the product. Thus, anabolic agents have been found in supplements sold as muscle growth promoters, stimulants in herbal tonics, and anorectic agents in herbal weight loss supplements. These observations suggest that this is either a deliberate act to add active ingredients to otherwise ineffective products or that the manufacturers have allowed some mixing of separate products at the manufacturing facility. This might occur in the preparation of the raw ingredients or in the formulation of the finished product. In some cases, the amount of supplement present may be high, even higher than the normal therapeutic dose. Geyer et al. (2002) purchased a "body building" supplement in England and upon analysis found it to contain methandieneone (commonly known as Dianabol) in an amount substantially higher than the therapeutic dose. This drug was present in high amounts, enough to have an anabolic effect, but also enough to produce serious side effects, including liver toxicity and carcinogenicity. Unlike many of the earlier cases involving steroids related to nandrolone and testosterone, these are not trivial levels of contamination, which raises the probability of deliberate adulteration of the product with the intention of producing a measurable effect on muscle strength and muscle mass (Geyer et al. 2008). The prospect of adverse health effects at these high doses also raises real concerns.

PHARMACEUTICALS SOLD AS SUPPLEMENTS

Because of the blurring of the boundaries that distinguish between pharmaceutical drugs and dietary supplements, it is hardly surprising that many consumers fail to pay attention to some important differences. Most effective pharmaceutical agents are not without side effects; their use is based on a careful weighing of the benefits against the risk and the medicines regulatory agencies decide whether the evidence of a benefit is sufficient to warrant use in specific situations. Where there is no clinical need, however, the balance is shifted. Likewise, where the evidence of a performance benefit is not strong, the athlete should require compelling evidence of safety before risking the use of a supplement. Not only is there limited evidence on the safety and efficacy of many of the supplements that are sold to athletes, loose control of labeling requirements means that the consumer cannot always be certain of what exactly a supplement contains. Many products list ingredients using abbreviations that are not recognizable as the names of either food components or chemical ingredients. The consumer cannot know what these compounds are (Geyer et al. 2008).

Many steroid-related compounds are on sale as dietary supplements; some are likely to be effective in achieving physiological effects, though many may well be ineffective in the doses contained in these products. The use of precursors of testosterone and nandrolone attracted much attention around the year 2000 when a number of high-profile athletes failed doping control tests for nandrolone. Analysis of commercial supplements on sale showed a high prevalence of contamination of testosterone-related and nandrolone-related steroid compounds (Geyer et al. 2004). At this time, androstenedione ("andro") and 19-norandrostenediol were widely sold as dietary supplements. There is no good evidence that androstenedione is effective in promoting muscle growth (Broeder et al. 2000), but it currently is banned by WADA and by most professional sports bodies but not by the U.S. National Basketball Association (NBA). Subsequently (April 11, 2004), the FDA banned the sale of androstenedione in the United States on the basis that it poses significant health risks similar to those that are normally associated with anabolic androgenic steroids.

19-Norandrostenedione is a metabolic precursor of the anabolic steroid nandrolone (19-nortestosterone); however, while nandrolone is unequivocally regarded as a drug, 19-norandrostenedione has been sold as a prohormone dietary supplement. The diagnostic metabolite measured in urine as a marker for nandrolone use is 19-norandrosterone, and this can be derived from use of either nandrolone itself or 19-norandrostenedione. Because of the widespread use of 19-norandrostenedione as a dietary supplement, and its presence as a contaminant in small amounts in a range of non-steroid supplements, a number of high-profile athletes recorded positive results for nandrolone, even where the balance of the available evidence suggested that there was no intent, and in spite of the evidence that oral administration of 19-norandrostenedione is not effective in promoting gains in skeletal muscle mass or in functional outcomes (Parr et al. 2009). Some of the uncertainties were removed by the specific identification of 19-norandrostenedione as a prohibited compound on the WADA prohibited list (WADA 2013).

In September 2010, manufacturers announced a voluntary recall of a product marketed as "Off Cycle II Hardcore." One of the ingredients that this product contained was 3,17-keto-etiochol-triene (an aromatase inhibitor), but the product was marketed as a dietary supplement (Food and Drug Administration 2010). Aromatase inhibitors block the action of the enzyme aromatase, which converts androgens into estrogens. These agents have clinical uses in the treatment of breast and ovarian cancers in women but are also used by athletes who take high doses of androgens. They reduce the formation of estrogens and the consequent development of gynecomastia. The product recall was described by the manufacturers as a voluntary recall, but it was a direct response to intervention by the FDA.

Methylhexanamine, commonly known as 1,3-dimethylamylamine or DMAA, is a stimulant that has been marketed as the primary active ingredient of many popular dietary supplements, with claims that it can promote fat loss and increase energy levels during exercise. Its widespread use attracted the attention of regulatory authorities and it is now classified as a medicine in many, but not all, countries. Methylhexanamine has been linked to a number of adverse events, including the deaths during military training of two soldiers who suffered fatal heart attacks during training in 2010 (Army Times 2011). A female marathon runner who collapsed and died near the finish of the 2012 London Marathon had been consuming a commercially available product during the race and the coroner's investigation concluded that it had likely contributed to her death (BBC News 2013).

Dinitrophenol (DNP) is used in the manufacturing process for explosives. In the early twentieth century, munitions workers reported large losses of body fat, as well as other symptoms, including headaches, dizziness, and night sweats. These observations led to the use of DNP as a weight loss agent, but adverse side effects soon appeared. This is perhaps not surprising as DNP acts by uncoupling mitochondrial respiration, leading to up to twofold increases in metabolic rate and resulting in large rises in body temperature. Its use as a dietary supplement was prohibited, but it continues to be used by some bodybuilders because of its high potency in reducing body fat levels. As recently as 2012, the death of a gym user from this supplement was reported (BBC 2012).

Elsewhere, there is growing evidence of adverse health effects resulting from inappropriate supplement use and, in most cases, these reports identify the presence of undeclared ingredients as the primary cause of harm. Several reports have documented cases of serious adverse effects on health resulting from the use of dietary supplements containing undeclared anabolic steroids, so it is clear that some products on the market remain unsafe (Krishnan 2009). A recent survey of liver injuries in hospital patients implicated the use of bodybuilding supplements as the most common cause of liver injury (Navarro et al. 2014). Using data from the Drug-Induced Liver Injury Network (DILIN), which was established in 2003 by the National Institute of Diabetes and Digestive and Kidney Diseases to collect and analyze cases, it was found that in the period from September 2004 to March 2013, 845 cases of liver injury were thought to be "definitely, highly likely, or probably" from an herbal or dietary supplement, or from prescription drugs. In 2004–2005, 7% of all liver injuries were attributed to herbal and dietary supplements, but this figure increased to 20% in 2010–2012. Although the steroid prohormone 3β-hydroxy-5α-androst-1-en-17-one is classified as a prohibited substance by WADA, it is marketed as a supplement and is available without prescription in some parts of the world. A recent report shows that even a short period of use of this supplement in healthy resistance-trained men enhances resistance-training gains relative to placebo but compromises both markers of cardiovascular health and liver function (Granados et al. 2014). Another recent report describes the case of a young man who presented with chest pain and was diagnosed with myocardial infarction. He had been ingesting a dietary supplement sold as a stimulant (declared principal ingredient, 1,3-dimethylamylamine) and a weight loss supplement (declared principal ingredient, Citrus aurantium) daily for 3 weeks before undertaking physical activity (Smith et al. 2014). After appropriate medical treatment and discontinuation of supplement use, the symptoms resolved.

QUALITY ASSURANCE SCHEMES

In spite of the various problems that have been reported, it remains true that the majority of dietary supplements is safe and will not result in either health problems or violations of the doping code. It is equally true, however, that a problem remains in that a significant minority of the products on sale to athletes do carry such risks. Many attempts are being made to address these problems, but at present there is no way in which a particular product as purchased in a retail outlet can be guaranteed to be free of any risk. In part, this is due to the difficulties that even reputable manufacturers have in controlling their supply chain and their distribution network. It is also due to the extremely small amounts of some substances that may cause a positive doping outcome. Ingestion of 19-norandrostenedione, a prohibited substance and precursor of nandrolone, will result in the appearance in the urine of 19-norandrosterone, the diagnostic metabolite for nandrolone use. If the urinary concentration of 19-norandrosterone exceeds 2 ng/nL, a doping offense is deemed to have occurred. The addition of as little as 2.5 µg of 19-norandrostenedione to a supplement can result in a urinary concentration of 19-norandrosterone in excess of this threshold in some, but not all, individuals (Watson et al. 2009). This effect is transient, and even when a larger dose (10 µg) of steroid is administered, it is likely that only the first or second urine sample after ingestion will contain enough of the steroid metabolites to give a positive test. This means that an athlete who ingests this may or may not test positive, depending on when the sample is collected in relation to consumption of the supplement. The amount of steroid added is close to the limits of detection of the analytical methods currently applied to the analysis of dietary supplements, and there is no certainty that analysis of the finished product would have detected this.

The very small amounts of extraneous doping agents that have been reported to be present in many supplements—perhaps in as many as one in four of those selected for testing—will have no effect on physiological function, even though they may result in a positive doping test (Geyer et al. 2004). New and more sensitive methods for the detection of prohibited substances allow for better detection of abuse of prohibited substances, but may also increase the likelihood of innocent ingestion of trivial amounts causing an adverse finding (Geyer et al. 2014). This problem is addressed in part by the introduction of the athlete's Biological Passport, which relies on hormonal feedback mechanisms caused by ingestion of pharmacological doses of steroid. These result in changes in the profile of urinary endogenous steroid excretion that can be detected with serial measures made over time.

It seems likely that the presence of doping substances in foods and supplements is often due to accidental contamination at some stage of the manufacture, storage, or distribution of the raw ingredients or the finished product. This may be due to cross-contamination of production lines where prohibited substances are processed alongside dietary supplements or due to poor quality control in the production of raw ingredients. Various efforts are being made to address the problems and to minimize the risk of inadvertent doping positives by athletes by identifying products that athletes may use with confidence (Judkins and Prock 2012). Several countries have quality assurance schemes where supplement manufacturers can have product samples analyzed to verify the absence of WADA-prohibited substances. As indicated previously, the amount of a contaminant may be at or below the limits of detection of the analytical method used: analysis of the supplement may give a negative finding, but ingestion of a large amount of the supplement might result in a positive test. It is also the case that some of these schemes do not test for all prohibited substances. There can be no absolute guarantee that any product is entirely safe, but such schemes do help the athlete to manage the risk.

Cases of deliberate adulteration of products with high doses of compounds that are a risk to health as well as being likely to cause a positive doping outcome may be more difficult to control. Because of the strict liability principle that applies in doping cases, inadvertent ingestion of a prohibited substance through use of a contaminated dietary supplement does not absolve the athlete of guilt. Athletes contemplating the use of dietary supplements should consider very carefully whether the potential benefits outweigh the risks of a doping offense that might end their career.

COST-BENEFIT ANALYSIS

Athletes who take supplements often have no clear understanding of the potential effects of the supplements they are using, but it seems clear that supplements should be used only after a careful cost-benefit analysis has been conducted. On one side of the balance are the rewards, the most obvious of which is an improved performance in sport, and on the other side are the costs and the risks. For several of the supplements used by athletes, there is good evidence of a performance or health benefit for some athletes in some specific situations (Maughan et al. 2007). In addition, individual athletes may respond very differently to a given supplement, with some exhibiting a beneficial effect while others experience a negative effect on performance. Hence, supplements are often used in an inappropriate way, and athletes should seek professional advice from a qualified sports nutrition expert before using any supplements. Such advice, however, is not easily available to all athletes, and much of the available information emanates from those who stand to gain from the sale of supplements.

Vitamin and mineral supplements are generally perceived as being harmless, and the one-a-day multivitamin tablet is seen as an insurance policy "just in case." Many herbal products are also used, even though there is little or no evidence to support their claimed benefits. The fact that most of these supplements enjoy only brief periods of popularity before disappearing from the marketplace suggests that any benefits perceived by athletes are not strong enough to warrant continued use or recommendation to friends and colleagues. Although these supplements are mostly benign, this is not always the case.

A cost-benefit analysis is not easily completed for most supplements, as much of the necessary information is simply not available. For many supplements, there is little or no evidence of performance effects. Of the many hundreds or even thousands of supplements on sale to athletes, only a few are supported by strong evidence for positive effects on health or performance and by evidence of absence of harm. The picture, however, continues to evolve as new evidence emerges, and many supplements experience short periods of popularity before falling out of favor. The scientific evidence often appears to have little impact on sales, so by implication, there is little incentive for those selling supplements to support scientific evaluation of their products. Even where some evidence does exist, it may not be relevant to the consumer because of limitations in the exercise tests used, in the study populations, or in the veracity of the supplements used in published research. Likewise, there is little or no evidence of safety for most supplements.

It seems sensible to exercise caution. Any compound that has the potential to alter physiological function to enhance exercise performance must also have the potential for adverse effects in some individuals. Athletes should see good evidence of a performance or other benefit before accepting the financial cost and the health or performance risks associated with any supplement.

CONCLUSION

The use of dietary supplements does not compensate for poor food choices and an inadequate diet, but supplements that provide essential nutrients may be a short-term option when food intake or food choices are restricted due to travel or other factors. Of the many different dietary ergogenic aids available to athletes, a very small number may enhance performance for some athletes when used in accordance with current evidence under the guidance of a well-informed professional. Athletes contemplating the use of supplements and sports foods should consider their efficacy, their cost, the risk to health and performance, and the potential for a positive doping test.

REFERENCES

Army Times. 2011. DMAA products pulled from base shelves. http://www.armytimes.com /offduty/health/offduty-dmma-products-pulled-from-shelves-122911/. Accessed January 31, 2013.

Bailey, R.L., J.J. Gahche, C.V. Lentino et al. 2011. Dietary supplement use in the United States, 2003–2006. *J Nutr* 141(2):261–266.

BBC. 2012. Sean Cleathero dies after taking "gym drug." http://www.bbc.co.uk/news/uk-england -beds-bucks-herts-20016068. Accessed January 30, 2013.

BBC News. 2013. Claire Squires inquest: DMAA was factor in marathon runner's death. http://www.bbc.co.uk/news/uk-england-london-21262717. Accessed January 30, 2013.

Broeder, C.E., J. Quindry, K. Brittingham et al. 2000. The Andro project: Physiological and hormonal influences of androstenedione supplementation in men 35 to 65 years old participating in a high-intensity resistance training program. *Arch Intern Med* 160:3093–3104.

Cohen, P.A., S. Attipoe, J. Travis, M. Stevens, and P.A. Deuster. 2013. Caffeine content of dietary supplements consumed on military bases. *JAMA Intern Med* 173:592–594.

Eichner, E.R. 2000. Minerals: Iron. In *Nutrition in Sport*, R.J. Maughan, Ed. Oxford: Blackwell, 326–338.

Fennell, D. 2004. Determinants of supplement usage. *Prev Med* 39(5):932–939.

FIFA. 2011. FIFA satisfied with WADA decision to withdraw CAS appeal in case of Mexican footballers. http://www.fifa.com/aboutfifa/footballdevelopment/news/newsid =1526355/. Accessed January 31, 2013.

Food and Drug Administration. 2010. Voluntary nationwide recall. http://www.fda.gov/Safety /Recalls/ucm226109.htm. Accessed September 18, 2010.

Food and Drugs Administration 2015. FDA 101: Dietary Supplements. http://www.fda.gov /ForConsumers/ConsumerUpdates/ucm050803.htm. Accessed May 4, 2015.

Geyer, H., M. Bredehoft, U. Marek, M.K. Parr, and W. Schanzer. 2002. Hohe Dosen des Anabolikums Metandienon in Nahrungserganzungsmitteln. *Deutsche Apotheke Zeitung* 142:29.

Geyer, H., M.K. Parr, U. Mareck, U. Reinhart, Y. Schrader, and W. Schänzer. 2004. Analysis of non-hormonal nutritional supplements for anabolic-androgenic steroids—Results of an international study. *Int J Sports Med* 25:124–129.

Geyer, H., M.K. Parr, K. Koehler, U. Mareck, W. Schänzer, and M. Thevis. 2008. Nutritional supplements cross-contaminated and faked with doping substances. *J Mass Spectrom* 43(7):892–902.

Geyer, H., W. Schänzer, and M. Thevis. 2014. Anabolic agents: Recent strategies for their detection and protection from inadvertent doping. *Br J Sports Med.* 48:820–826. doi:10.1136/bjsports-2014-093526.

Granados, J., T.L. Gillum, K.M. Christmas, and M.R. Kuennen. 2014. Prohormone supplement 3β-hydroxy-5α-androst-1-en-17-one enhances resistance training gains but impairs user health. *J Appl Physiol* 16:560–569.

Green, G.A., D.H. Catlin, and B. Starcevic. 2001. Analysis of over-the-counter dietary supplements. *Clin J Sports Med* 11:254–259.

Gross, M., O. Baum, and H. Hoppeler. 2011. Antioxidant supplementation and endurance training: Win or loss? *Eur J Sports Sci* 11:27–32.

Guddat, S., G. Fussholler, H. Braun et al. 2011. Clenbuterol—Regional food contamination as possible source for positive findings in doping control. 29th Cologne Workshop on Dope Analysis, February 14.

Gurley, B.J., S.F. Gardner, and M.A. Hubbard. 2000. Content versus label claims in ephedra-containing dietary supplements. *Am J Health Syst Pharm* 57:963.

Judkins, C., and P. Prock. 2012. Supplements and inadvertent doping—How big is the risk to athletes. *Med Sport Sci* 59:143–152.

Krishnan, P.V., Z.-Z. Feng, and S.C. Gordon. 2009. Prolonged intrahepatic cholestasis and renal failure secondary to anabolic androgenic steroid-enriched dietary supplements. *J Clin Gastroenterol* 43:672–675.

Maughan, R.J. 2005. Contamination of dietary supplements and positive drugs tests in sport. *J Sports Sci* 23:883–889.

Maughan, R.J. 2013. Quality assurance issues in the use of dietary supplements, with special reference to protein supplements. *J Nutr* 143:1843–1847.

Maughan, R.J., F. Depiesse, and H. Geyer. 2007. The use of dietary supplements by athletes. *J Sports Sci* 25:S103–S113.

Navarro, V.J., H. Barnhart, H.L. Bonkovsky et al. 2014. Liver injury from herbals and dietary supplements in the U.S. Drug-Induced Liver Injury Network. *Hepatology* 60(4):1399–1408. doi: 10.1002/hep.27317.

Newmaster, S.G., M. Grguric, D. Shanmughanandhan, S. Ramalingam, and S. Ragupathy. 2013. DNA barcoding detects contamination and substitution in North American herbal products. *BMC Med* 11:222. doi:10.1186/1741-7015-11-222.

Papanikolaou, G., and K. Pantopoulos. 2005. Iron metabolism and toxicity. *Toxicol Appl Pharmacol* 202:199–211.

Parasrampuria, M., K. Schwartz, and R. Petesch. 1998. Quality control of dehydroepiandrosterone dietary supplement products. *JAMA* 280:1565.

Parr, M.K., U. Laudenbach-Leschowsky, N. Höfer, W. Schänzer, and P. Diel. 2009. Anabolic and androgenic activity of 19-norandrostenedione after oral and subcutaneous administration—Analysis of side effects and metabolism. *Toxicol Lett* 188(2):137–141.

Sachdev, S., and K.J. Davies. 2008. Production, detection, and adaptive responses to free radicals in exercise. *Free Radic Biol Med* 44:215–223.

Smith, T.B., B.A. Staub, G.M. Natarajan, D.M. Lasorda, and I.G. Poornima. 2014. Acute myocardial infarction associated with dietary supplements containing 1,3-dimethylamylamine and citrus aurantium. *Tex Heart Inst J* 41:70–72.

Tsouderos, T. 2012. Dietary supplements: Manufacturing troubles widespread, FDA inspections show. *Chicago Tribune*. http://articles.chicagotribune.com/2012-06-30/news/ct-met-sup plement-inspections-20120630_1_dietary-supplements-inspections-american-herbal -products-association. Accessed January 29, 2013.

WADA. 2013. The 2013 Prohibited List World Anti-Doping Code. https://wada-main-prod.s3 .amazonaws.com/resources/files/WADA-Prohibited-List-2013-EN.pdf. Accessed January 31, 2013.

Watson, P., C. Judkins, E. Houghton, C. Russell, and R.J. Maughan. 2009. Supplement contamination: Detection of nandrolone metabolites in urine after administration of small doses of a nandrolone precursor. *Med Sci Sports Exerc* 41:766–772.

9 Drug, Nutrient, and Exercise Interactions

Adam M. Persky, PhD, FACSM
Mariana Lucena, PharmD Candidate
Jayme Hostetter, PharmD Candidate
Eshelman School of Pharmacy, University of North
Carolina at Chapel Hill, Chapel Hill, North Carolina

CONTENTS

INTRODUCTION

The highly competitive athlete must optimally train and maintain a diet to facilitate performance and promote recovery. While some high-level athletes may use pharmacologic agents to help in both these areas, it is more common for athletes to require medications for non-performance reasons. Imagine a hockey team prophylaxing with a flu medication to prevent an outbreak during the playoffs. Now imagine those players skating upward of 30 miles per hour experiencing dizziness because of a side effect of the medication. On the other hand, imagine a player is being treated with antibiotics and potentially being sub-therapeutic because the rate and extent of metabolism of the highly trained athlete is not taken into account. Finally, imagine an athlete drinking grapefruit juice with his or her allergy medication or consuming a high protein diet while taking warfarin—both situations can alter drug effects by modulating drug concentration. These are the issues of the health care team.

Drug effects are determined by pharmacodynamics (PD), the relationship between drug concentration and effect, and pharmacokinetics, the relationship between time and drug concentration. By understanding both the pharmacokinetics and pharmacodnaymics of medications, we are able to make reasonable predictions and adjustments to achieve optimal medication therapy for the athlete while minimizing any detrimental effects. This chapter will focus on exercise-drug interactions and nutrient-drug interactions.

PHARMACOKINETIC BASICS

Pharmacokinetics is the study of how a drug behaves in the body or the study of "what the body does to a drug." Pharmacokinetics is described by the acronym "ITE"—I stands for input into the body, T for transfer within the body, and E for elimination from the body.

The goal of pharmacokinetics is to obtain the desired drug concentration in the body by optimizing the dosage regimen (i.e., dose and frequency of dosing) and dosage form. The problem with attaining this goal lies in the determination of the optimum target drug concentration, which is addressed by the field of PD, or the study of the relationship between the drug concentration at the site of action and the pharmacologic response. Within PD, a correlation often exists between the drug concentration at the site of action and pharmacologic response. Unfortunately, we typically do not know the drug concentration at the site of action, so we estimate it based on plasma concentrations.

TERMINOLOGY

Within pharmacokinetics, there are several terms that are used to describe the primary pharmacokinetic parameters of the system: clearance, volume of distribution, fraction absorbed, and the rate of absorption. Clearance is defined as a flow parameter—the volume of blood (or plasma) irreversibly removed of drug per unit time. Volume of distribution describes the total distributional space of a drug. Drugs with a higher volume of distribution typically accumulate more in tissues than the blood, and drugs with smaller volumes of distributions tend to stay in blood and total body water. Bioavailability refers to the rate and extent to which a drug is absorbed and available at the site of action. The fraction absorbed is defined as the fraction of the administered dose that enters systemic circulation, and the rate of absorption describes the rate at which that fraction enters the systemic circulation; both fraction absorbed and rate of absorption are components of the bioavailability of a drug.

There are several secondary parameters used to describe drug behavior: AUC, half-life, C_{max}, and t_{max}. These parameters are derived from the primary parameters just discussed. The area-under-the-concentration-time curve (AUC) is a measure of systemic exposure and is proportional to the administered dose and the fraction absorbed (e.g., the larger the dose, the larger the AUC) and inversely proportional to the drug's clearance (e.g., the higher the drug clearance, the lower the AUC). A drug's half-life is the time required to remove half of the drug concentration from the body. Half-life is proportional to the volume of distribution (e.g., the higher the volume of distribution, the longer the half-life) and inversely proportional to the clearance (e.g., the higher the clearance, the shorter the half-life). Other parameters often reported are the maximal drug concentration (C_{max}) and the time of maximal concentration (t_{max}). A drug's effects may be related to systemic exposure (AUC) or its peaks (C_{max}) or even its minimal concentrations (C_{min}).

INPUT

Drugs can be introduced into the body through a variety of pathways including orally, subcutaneously, intramuscularly, inhalation, or intravenously. Drugs administered intravenously directly enter systemic circulation, but drugs given extravascularly must be absorbed from the site of administration into the systemic circulation. We will limit this discussion to oral agents, as this is the most common route of administration.

Drugs administered extravascularly now depend on the rate and extent of absorption of the drug product. Rate, of course, means how fast the drug is absorbed and extent refers to how much of the dose enters systemic circulation. Drugs administered by any extravascular (non-IV) route must travel from the site of administration (e.g., muscle, mouth) to the systemic circulation; thus, the potential for loss of drug prior to entry into the systemic circulation is increased. Examples of approximate bioavailability values for various drugs and factors that impact bioavailability are shown in Tables 9.1 and 9.2.

Consider a drug tablet administered orally. The drug enters the stomach and subsequently moves through the small intestine, colon, etc. The amount of time for this transit process is referred to as gastrointestinal transit time. Once the tablet is in the gastrointestinal tract, it must undergo disintegration and must dissolve into solution (dissolution).

Returning to the example of oral administration, after dissolution, the drug is in solution and must pass through or around the cells that line the intestine before it

TABLE 9.1
Examples of Drug Bioavailabilities

Drug	Bioavailability
Caffeine	1.0
Nicotine (inhaled)	0.90
Acetylsalicylic acid (aspirin)	0.88
Ibuprofen	0.80
Codeine	0.57
Nicotine (oral)	0.30
Morphine	0.24
Lovastatin	<0.05

TABLE 9.2

Examples of Factors That Impact the Rate of Absorption or the Fraction Absorbed

Factors Impacting Drug Absorption Rate	Factors Impacting Drug Absorption Extent
Transit time	Enzyme degradation
Disintegration	pH-dependent degradation
Dissolution	CYP P450 metabolism (intestinal)
Mechanism of absorption/diffusion	P-glycoprotein
P-glycoprotein	First-pass metabolism (liver metabolism)
	Entero-hepatic recirculation

can enter the blood supply. Absorption can occur via diffusion (a passive process) or active transport. A growing body of evidence suggests that drugs also can be pumped back into the intestine by transporters like P-glycoprotein (PGP) and that drugs can be metabolized by enzymes associated with intestinal cells. Finally, the proportion of drug that makes it through the intestinal wall intact will reach the portal vein leading into the liver. Once in the liver, the drug can be taken up by hepatocytes and metabolized, transported into bile or transported back into the blood to enter systemic circulation.

Next, we will discuss factors that influence the extent to which a given drug dose will enter systemic circulation. During the absorption process, a drug is exposed to various changes in pH, degradative enzymes, and drug efflux transporters such as PGP. The acidic environment of the stomach can degrade certain drugs (e.g., beta-lactam antibiotics). Within the gastrointestinal tract are cytochrome P450 enzymes, which can metabolize drugs before they have a chance to be systemically absorbed. In addition, intestinal cells contain the efflux transport protein, PGP, which can decrease the amount of drug entering the systemic circulation. If a drug survives these processes, it can be absorbed by intestinal cells or continue down the gastrointestinal tract and be eliminated in the feces. These same types of processes may also be relevant for other drug administration modalities. For example, insulin tends to degrade in the muscle; enzymes, immune cells, or muscle pH may also degrade a drug, thus limiting the amount that eventually enters into the systemic circulation. While we are focusing on orally administered drugs, parallels can be drawn for other routes; for example, following intramuscular administration, absorption time could be dependent on factors such as muscle size, blood flow, or amount of adipose tissue.

Absorption can occur through a variety of mechanisms but generally falls into two categories: transcellular and paracellular. In the transcellular pathway, a drug passes through the cell and its membranes through passive diffusion, facilitative transport, or active transport. In the paracellular pathway, the drug moves in between cells, not through them. If a drug requires transporters to be absorbed, then the capacity of these transporters to move the drug will be yet another determining factor of how much of the drug eventually reaches the blood. Some drugs that utilize endogenous transport proteins include methyldopa, valcyclovir, certain cephalosporins, and salicylic acid. Drugs that depend on active transport may be subject to drug interactions by various nutrients because transporters absorb many nutrients.

Drugs will eventually reach the portal circulation, providing exposure to the liver, where a large amount of cytochrome P450 enzymes resides. Following transit through the liver, the remaining fraction of the drug will enter the systemic circulation. The liver's ability to clear the drug from the body after oral administration is called the "first-pass effect" because the first passage of the drug through the liver (i.e., before entry into the systemic circulation and subsequent additional passages through the liver) can remove a significant amount of drug from circulation.

TRANSFER

Once a drug enters systemic circulation, it will be distributed throughout the body, accumulating in different tissues to different extents and at different rates. The extent of distribution depends on the lipophilicity and charge of the drug, with uncharged, lipophilic drugs typically having larger distributional volumes. The rate of distribution also can depend on lipophilicity and charge of the molecule but also the tissue membrane and perfusion of the organ. The final distribution will ultimately depend on protein binding within the blood and the protein binding within the tissue space.

The volume of drug distribution refers to the extent to which the drug penetrates various body tissues but it does not have a true physiological meaning. When we talk about distribution, we often talk about the rate of distribution and the concentration within tissue compartments. Both the rate and amount of drug that accumulates in a tissue is determined by physicochemical properties of the drug molecule, blood flow, extent of protein binding in the plasma and tissue, and the presence of transporter proteins that may move a drug across membranes.

The rate of drug distribution can be important as it can dictate the onset of pharmacologic effect. The distribution of a drug into blood and highly perfused organs (e.g., kidneys, liver) is typically very fast, but it may take time to enter tissues that are less well-perfused (e.g., fat) or tissues that have protective barriers (e.g., the brain). As such, there may be a disconnect between drug concentration in the blood and effect because it takes time for a drug to accumulate sufficient drug quantities to elicit the effect.

The extent, like the rate, is impacted by the ability of drugs to cross biologic membranes. Most hydrophilic drugs have difficulty passing through biological membranes, but are able to distribute within the extracellular fluid unless they are too large to pass through fenestrations in capillaries (e.g., heparin). They tend to have lower protein bindings to both plasma proteins and tissues. As such, we tend to think of hydrophilic drugs as having volumes of distribution on the smaller side, typically under total body weight. Lipophilic substances, on the other hand, are able to distribute throughout the body because they can pass through biological membranes more easily than hydrophilic drugs can. Again, biologic membranes can determine both the rate and extent of distribution.

The first situation we will discuss, called *perfusion-limited distribution*, concerns a membrane situated between blood and tissue, with very high permeability for a given drug (i.e., lipophilic drugs, or cell membranes, which are loosely knitted like muscle). Essentially, the membrane provides *no barrier* for the drug and results in fast uptake of the drug into tissues until unbound drug levels in blood and tissues are in equilibrium. In this case, the faster the blood flow through that organ, the faster the distribution into tissue; hence, distribution is essentially only limited by the rate of perfusion. The second situation is called *permeability-limited distribution*. In this case, the membrane is not very permeable to the drug (e.g., the blood–brain barrier), functioning as a barrier between blood and tissue. The drug will enter permeability-limited tissue very slowly, and blood flow is not important for rate of uptake. Here, distribution is only limited by the rate at which the drug is able to permeate the membrane. The movement of the drug into the tissue in this case is determined by Fick's law of diffusion, which is a function of the surface area of a membrane, membrane thickness, concentration gradient, partition coefficient, and ionization.

At the molecular level, the ability of a drug to travel outside of plasma is determined by how strongly it binds to plasma proteins vs. tissue proteins. If tissue has a higher drug-binding affinity than blood, then the drug will be "pulled" into tissues and the distributional volume will be larger, but if plasma pulls harder than tissue, the drug will remain in the vasculature and the volume will be smaller.

When a drug interacts with plasma proteins, only a portion of the drug in the plasma is bound to protein at a given time. Thus, there are always two pools of drug: unbound drug and bound drug. As in the blood, there are both bound and unbound drug in the tissue. Only the unbound drug in the plasma is in equilibrium with unbound drug in tissue. The fraction of unbound drug is the ratio of the unbound concentration and the total drug concentration. This unbound concentration is important because the unbound concentration drives pharmacologic effect.

Albumin, lipoproteins, immunoglobulins (e.g., IgG), erythrocytes, and α_1-acid glycoprotein can and will bind various drugs. Albumin is distributed in plasma and extracellular water, and will transport various endogenous compounds and exogenous compounds, especially weak acids (e.g., salicylic acid, penicillin). Albumin levels will change with certain diseases such as renal failure. Levels of α_1-acid glycoprotein, which predominantly binds weak bases (e.g., propranolol, imipramine), are known to be altered in various pathologic states as well, especially inflammatory diseases. Drugs also bind to tissue components (e.g., proteins, DNA, bone, fat). Unfortunately, tissue binding cannot easily be measured directly, but binding to

TABLE 9.3

Example Drugs and Their Volumes of Distribution

Drug	Indication of Use	Apparent Volume of Distribution (L)
Aspirin	Analgesia, anti-platelet	10
Lithium	Manic-depression	46
Codeine	Cough suppressant, analgesia	182
Cyclosporine	Immunosuppressant	280
Digoxin	Heart failure	660
Desipramine	Antidepressant	1400
Chloroquine	Anti-malarial	8050

plasma protein can be measured easily. See Table 9.3 for examples of drugs and their apparent volumes of distribution.

ELIMINATION

Two major organs remove the majority of drugs from system circulation: the kidney and the liver. The kidney utilizes three processes that influence a drug's clearance: passive filtration, active tubular secretion, and reabsorption (passive or active). The liver relies predominantly on metabolic biotransformation and less on excretion into the bile of unchanged drug. Approximately 70% of medications on the market are metabolically transformed by the liver, primarily by the action of cytochrome P450 enzymes. Three factors dictate extent of medication removal by the liver: protein binding, hepatic blood flow, and the intrinsic ability of the enzymes.

The topic of P450 reactions has become increasingly complex with the discovery of various subclasses and polymorphs of the enzymes in this family. In addition, many of these enzymes may be induced or inhibited by drugs (e.g., phenobarbital, fluoxetine), dietary supplements (e.g., St. John's Wort), foods (e.g., high protein diet), and exercise (e.g., higher in trained individuals). Since so many factors can potentially modulate hepatic function, it is important to understand the basic principles of hepatic clearance and how factors like enzyme function can impact systemic exposure to a drug. In the following sections, a basic model of hepatic function will be introduced, followed by a discussion of important components of this model.

When a drug molecule enters the liver, two possible routes are available: one route is to leave the liver unchanged, and a second route is to undergo metabolism and elimination. The mass of drug that will eventually enter the systemic circulation depends on the fraction of drug that moves by each route. The fraction that is metabolized and eliminated from the liver is termed the extraction ratio. The extraction ratio reflects the ability of the liver to extract drug from the systemic circulation on a single pass through the liver. For example, an extraction ratio of 0.25 indicates that 25% of the drug in the blood will be extracted on a single pass through the liver.

Various models have been developed to describe the liver's ability to clear drugs. The *venous equilibrium model* or the *well-stirred model* is the most commonly used model. This model incorporates the hepatic blood flow rate, enzyme activity, and the unbound fraction of drug. Blood flow influences clearance because it dictates the rate of presentation of drug to drug metabolizing enzymes. The inherent activity of enzymes determines clearance, as they are the responsible party for the conversion of the drug. Lastly, only unbound drug is accessible to enzymes, and thus the unbound fraction determines the proportion of drugs able to be metabolized.

Next, we can discuss how the physiologic parameters of hepatic blood flow, protein binding, and enzyme activity serve as underpinnings that determine the hepatic clearance of a drug. First, we will discuss the case of a low extraction ratio drug (E < 0.3). Low extraction ratio drugs are extracted inefficiently by the liver and therefore alterations in the expression level of enzymes (e.g., enzyme induction), the function of existing enzymes (e.g., enzyme inhibition), and changes in the fraction of unbound drug (i.e., resulting in more "free" drug to metabolize) will alter systemic clearance. For a high extraction ratio (E > 0.7), the metabolic efficiency of the enzymes is high and therefore the only way to increase hepatic clearance is to increase the rate of presentation of drug via hepatic blood flow. When discussing the impact of exercise or nutrition on the pharmacokinetics of drugs, we will revisit these factors.

As stated earlier, the two organs responsible for the majority of drug elimination from the body are the liver and the kidneys. Renal clearance processes, which are generally lower in efficiency than hepatic clearance processes, reflect the net movement of a drug and metabolites from blood into urine via four types of mechanisms. These mechanisms include glomerular filtration, active tubular secretion, tubular reabsorption, and metabolism. The impact of metabolism, however, is often ignored, because of its very minor contribution to renal drug clearance.

There are two mechanisms by which a drug can enter the urine. One mechanism is filtration and the other is secretion. Solutes in blood are passively filtered through the glomerulus, with hydrostatic pressure constituting the primary driving force for this passive movement. The rate at which solute is filtered through the glomerulus depends on (1) the mass of the molecule, (2) the number of functional nephrons, (3) the rate of plasma flow, and (4) the extent of protein binding. Small molecules (MW ≤ 500 Da) can undergo glomerular filtration; however, large molecules (MW ≥ 60,000 Da; the mass of albumin and other plasma proteins) cannot, as they are too large to enter the glomerulus. Only unbound drug is filtered, again,

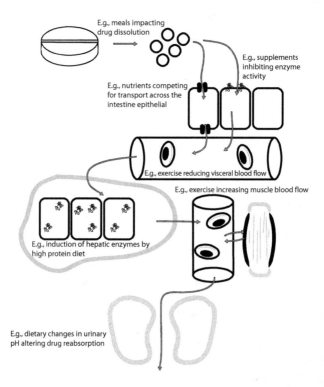

FIGURE 9.1 The pathway a drug can take from mouth (ingestion and dissolution) through out of the body through the kidneys and how exercise or nutrients may impact the various processes.

because proteins are typically too large to enter the glomerulus (the presence of protein in urine is usually an indicator of kidney damage). While filtration is passive, secretion of drugs is an active process dependent on transporters. Many of the same factors that influence hepatic disposition according to the well-stirred model also influence the process of active tubular secretion. These factors include (1) blood flow, (2) protein binding, and (3) the intrinsic activity of the transporter (i.e., intrinsic clearance).

Reabsorption removes the drug from the urine and can occur as either a passive or an active process. Passive reabsorption is dependent on (1) urine pH (as ionized molecules will not be passively reabsorbed), (2) the pKa of the drug, (3) the rate of urine flow, and (4) lipophilicity of the drug. Ionized drugs have a difficult time passing through membranes compared to their non-ionized counterparts. Increases in urine flow decrease the contact time of the drug with the tubule, thus reducing the opportunity for reabsorption and increasing the amount of drug that is eliminated from the body in urine. Like the liver, exercise and nutrition can impact drug filtration, secretion, and/or reabsorption. Figure 9.1 depicts various areas where the pharmacokinetics of a drug can be altered by either exercise or nutrition.

ACUTE EXERCISE–DRUG INTERACTION

A single, acute bout of exercise can impact the pharmacokinetics of drugs, but its impact will be determined predominately by the timing of exercise relative to the time of drug administration and length of exercise session relative to half-life of the drug. The mechanism by which acute exercise can impact drug behavior is dominated by changes in tissue blood flow and potentially other acute changes. Only drugs whose distribution or clearance is flow dependent (i.e., high extraction-ratio drugs) would be most subject to changes during acute exercise. Examples of drugs and their impact during acute exercise are summarized in Table 9.4.

We assume it takes approximately five half-lives to eliminate a drug from the body. If a single bout of exercise is short relative to the drug half-life, the relative impact on the drug concentrations could be small. For example, if an athlete were taking a non-sedating, over-the-counter antihistamine for seasonal allergies that has a half-life of several hours (e.g., loratadine, fexofenadine), a 30- to 60-min run would have minimal impact on drug concentrations. However, this would depend, in part, on timing. If the drug is administered right before exercise, exercise could slow absorption or change the fraction absorbed due to changes in gastrointestinal motility or redistribution of blood away from the viscera.

ABSORPTION

As discussed earlier, drug properties, such as lipophilicity and charge, can determine how well a drug is absorbed (i.e., the fraction absorbed) as well as the rate of absorption. The physiologic limits of lipophilic drugs being absorbed may be due to blood flow, while for less lipophilic drugs the rate-limiting step may be the diffusional barrier (i.e., the cell membranes). During acute exercise, blood flow is altered, resulting in a reduction in splanchnic blood flow of 20% to 80% (Somani 1996) depending on

TABLE 9.4
Synopsis of Drugs and Acute Exercise Interactions

Drug	Route	Indication of Use	Exercise Intensity	Impact on Concentration	Ref.
Atenolol	IV	Hypertension	Moderate	No change	van Baak et al. (1992)
Propranolol	IV	Hypertension	Moderate	Increase	van Baak et al. (1992)
Propranolol	IV	Hypertension	Moderate	No change	Arends et al. (1986)
Verapamil	IV	Hypertension	Moderate	Increase	van Baak et al. (1992)
Propranolol	IV/PO	Hypertension	Moderate	No change	Frank et al. (1990)
Verapamil	IV/PO	Hypertension, angina	Moderate	No change	Mooy et al. (1986)
Acebutolol	PO	Hypertension	Moderate	Increase	Henry et al. (1981)
Atenolol	PO	Hypertension	Moderate	No change	van Baak et al. (1992)
Atenolol	PO	Hypertension	Stress test	No change	Mason et al. (1980)
Caffeine	PO	Headache	Moderate	No change	Collomp et al. (1991)
Caffeine	PO	Headache	Moderate	No change	Haller et al. (2008)
Caffeine	PO	Headache	Moderate	No change	McLean and Graham (2002)
Carvedilol	PO	Hypertension	Moderate	No change	Stoschitzky et al. (2002)
Digoxin	PO	Heart failure	Moderate	Decrease	Pedersen et al. (1983)
Indomethacin	PO	Analgesia	Moderate	No change	Henry et al. (1981)
Prednisolone	PO	Anti-inflammatory	Moderate	Decrease	Chien et al. (2012)
Propranolol	PO	Hypertension	Moderate	Increase	van Baak et al. (1992)
Propranolol	PO	Hypertension	Moderate	Decrease	Arends et al. (1986)
Propranolol	PO	Hypertension	Moderate	Increase	Henry et al. (1981)
Quinidine	PO	Arrythmia	Moderate	Decrease	Aslaksen and Aanderud (1980)
Salicyclate	PO	Analgesia	Moderate	No change	Aslaksen and Aanderud (1980)
Synephrine	PO	Stimulant, weight loss	Moderate	No change	Haller et al. (2008)
Theophylline	PO	Asthma	Light/Moderate	Increase	Schlaeffer et al. (1984)
Insulin	SQ	Diabetes	Moderate	Increase	Koivisto and Felig (1978)

Note: IV = intravenous; PO = oral; SQ = subcutaneous injection.

exercise intensity. As an example, when participants were administered oral prednisolone and exercised, lower peak concentrations were noted but there was no effect on systemic exposure or the drug's half-life. This suggests the impact was on the rate of the absorption more so than the fraction absorbed, clearance, or the volume of distribution (Chien et al. 2012). If we look at the intramuscular route and use insulin as an example, one study showed an increase in absorption of insulin when injected into a leg that was exercised (Koivisto and Felig 1978).

DISTRIBUTION

Changes in the distribution of drugs during acute exercise could be due to changes in protein binding, blood flow, fluid shifts, body temperature, or pH. The latter two factors may not be particularly strong under physiologic conditions due to relatively tight control of these systems. There are small fluid shifts during exercise, mainly due to a shift of plasma water into the interstitial space. However, this shift is generally small and may not impact distribution significantly (Khazaeinia et al. 2000). While some studies have shown changes in the volume of distribution of drugs (Somani 1996), some are difficult to interpret because studies were conducted with orally administered medications. Estimates of the volume of distribution can be confounded by changes in the oral bioavailability. Changes in the volume of distribution could impact the peak concentration and the drugs' half-life but would not change the overall systemic exposure (i.e., the area under the curve). It is difficult to predict the clinical importance of these changes. In one example, digoxin's volume of distribution was increased because of the increase in blood flow to skeletal or cardiac muscle (Joreteg and Jogestrand 1983). During acute exercise, there is an increase in muscle blood flow of 3.5 to 21 times (Somani 1996) depending on exercise intensity, and this large change can provide more drug to bind to cardiac tissue.

ELIMINATION

The most important contributor to differences in drug concentration during exercise is the clearance of the drug because acute exercise modifies blood flow to both major clearing organs. It is unlikely that acute exercise would cause significant changes in enzyme activity, although these effects cannot be ruled out due to increases in metabolic rate associated with exercise.

During exercise, there is a reduction in renal blood flow caused by changes to the sympathetic nervous system and the renin-angiotensin system. Atenolol is predominately cleared by the kidney; however, one study found an increase in atenolol concentrations during acute exercise (Stoschitzky et al. 2002) while others found no change in atenolol concentration. Digoxin is also predominately cleared by the kidneys, and several studies have found digoxin concentrations were decreased during exercise, indicating a reduction in absorption, an increase in the volume of distribution, or an increase in renal clearance. Evidence suggests a change in volume, not clearance, explains these findings as shunting of blood to the muscles and heart increases tissue binding of the digoxin.

During exercise, hepatic blood flow also tends to decrease with increasing exercise intensity. This would most likely impact high extraction ratio drugs; that is, drugs that are efficiently cleared by the liver. Propranolol is an example of such a drug, and most studies seem to show an increase in concentration of the drug during exercise, reflecting reduced hepatic clearance (see Table 9.4). Low extraction ratio drugs are minimally impacted by changes in hepatic blood flow and generally show little to no change in concentration during exercise. These drugs would include caffeine, carvedilol, indomethacin, salicyclate, and verapamil.

EXERCISE TRAINING ADAPTATION
ON DRUG PHARMACOKINETICS

We have just discussed how an acute bout of exercise may impact drug behavior. The other consideration is the behavior of a drug within the body of elite athletes or highly trained individuals compared to the sedentary individual. We again must consider some of the physiologic changes that occur during training (e.g., cardiovascular system, metabolism).

ABSORPTION

Overall, there is a paucity of data reporting if highly trained individuals absorb drugs substantially differently than their sedentary counterparts do, especially for oral medications. There is some evidence that trained individuals have slower gastrointestinal transit time, but there is a lack of evidence that this impacts drug absorption to a clinically important degree. The increase in capillary density associated with training could increase the absorption of drugs administered intramuscularly, but again there is no substantial data to suggest that this is clinically significant.

DISTRIBUTION

The distributional behavior of a drug can be impacted by changes in body composition and protein binding. With training, fat mass can be reduced and the fat-free mass increased. In addition, there are increases in plasma water and total amount of protein in the blood. The reduction in fat mass can decrease the volume of distribution of more lipophilic compounds (e.g., sedatives like propofol). Likewise, the increase in lean body mass could increase the volume of distribution for more hydrophilic drugs. One study utilized the beta-blocker propranolol and found no changes in the volume of distribution between sedentary and trained individuals (Panton et al. 1995).

ELIMINATION

Drug elimination tends to be the most impactful pharmacokinetic process. For drugs cleared predominately by the liver, drugs that are considered low extraction ratio drugs tend to demonstrate higher clearance in trained individuals than in the sedentary (Persky et al. 2003) because low extraction ratio drugs are impacted primarily by changes in enzyme activity. Most of the studies in humans used the probe drug, antipyrine, an early non-steroidal anti-inflammatory that is metabolized by multiple P450 enzymes, although CYP3A4 may be the predominate enzyme (Engel et al. 1996). These studies make it unclear as to what specific enzymes are more impacted by exercise. In these studies, antipyrine clearance is enhanced by 20% to 40% (Persky et al. 2003), which can be clinically significant. In one study, propranolol pharmacokinetics were unchanged in trained individuals, which suggests that CYP2D6 (the major enzyme of propranolol metabolism) may not be enhanced by exercise training.

There is less evidence exercise training impacts drugs that are renally cleared. In one clinical study, subjects were trained for 16 weeks and the pharmacokinetics of digoxin were examined; there was no change in the pharmacokinetics. To date, it appears training does not significantly alter renal elimination of drugs.

NUTRITION–DRUG INTERACTION

To ensure optimal performance, the athlete focuses on exercise/training and proper nutrition. Optimal diets provide the fuel and energy to sustain the level of exercise and facilitate recovery. Although lifestyle and time constraints may impede the athlete's ability to meet the necessary nutritional requirements, drugs also have a significant impact on this aspect. Nutrient-drug interactions can lead to changes in the bioavailability or clearance of drugs, resulting in sub-therapeutic drug concentrations or unwanted adverse events. We will discuss the nutrient drug interaction in terms of individual nutrients and foods, meal composition, and dietary supplements.

NUTRIENTS AND MEAL COMPOSITION

As with changes with exercise, nutrients and diet can impact pharmacokinetics in several areas. Some of these interactions are more defined than with exercise, and nutrient-drug interactions has been a growing area of interest, especially in the areas of dietary supplement–drug and fruit juice–drug interactions. We will start with a more general discussion of nutrients, meals, and meal composition.

The first area of interest is drug absorption and some examples are summarized in Table 9.5. We assume meals stimulate gastric and intestinal secretions, slow gastrointestinal motility, and increase bile salts, which can impact the dissolution of a drug and potentially impact drug stability. For example, the immunosuppressant cyclosporine has enhanced bioavailability and clearance when given with a high fat meal (Gupta et al. 1990; Tan et al. 1995) and the antiviral zidovudine has a slowing of absorption and reduced C_{max} (Moore et al. 1999; Yuen et al. 2001) when taken with a high fat meal. Individual components within the meals can complex or bind drugs, which would interfere with the drug moving across intestinal membranes.

TABLE 9.5
Nutrient–Drug Interactions for Absorption Examples

Drug	Indication of Use	Interaction	Impact on Bioavailability	Ref.
Gabapentin	Seizure, analgesia	Protein	Increase	Gidal et al. (1998)
Tetracycline	Antibiotic	Dairy/minerals	Decrease	Jung et al. (1997)
Ciprofloxacin	Antibiotic	Dairy/minerals	Decrease	Marchbanks (1993)
Amitriptyline	Antidepressant	Fiber	Decrease	Stewart (1992)
Cyclosporine	Immunosuppresant	High fat meal	Increase	Gupta et al. (1990)
Zidovudine	Antiviral (HIV)	High fat meal	Decrease	Moore et al. (1999)

Antibiotics such as tetracycline (Jung et al. 1997) and ciprofloxacin (Frost et al. 1989; Sahai et al. 1993) chelate with dietary calcium, resulting in a reduction of drug absorbed. For these reasons, package inserts recommend separating meals with these medications. Certain drugs utilize nutrient transport proteins to cross the intestinal barriers. The anticonvulsant and neuropathic pain agent gabapentin utilizes the L-amino acid transport system. There is some evidence that a high protein meal taken with gabapentin might increase drug exposure through a trans-stimulatory mechanism (Gidal et al. 1996), although these results are equivocal (Benetello et al. 1997; Gidal et al. 1998).

The second area of interest is the distributional behavior of medications. The main mechanism of interactions is displacement or altered binding by dietary agents. For example, the anticonvulsant valproic acid can be displaced from its binding sites on albumin by free fatty acids (Levy and Koch 1982). Some antidepressants can bind to lipoproteins, which could alter their plasma protein binding. Still other drugs, like the beta-blocker propranolol, bind to alpha-acid glycoprotein, which could be up- or down-regulated by inflammatory processes (De Paepe et al. 2002), some of which might occur during recovery from exercise. Displacement of a drug could theoretically increase the volume of distribution and lower the peak drug concentrations; increased binding could have lowered the drug's volume of distribution and increased peak concentrations. It should be noted that a change in protein binding also would change the drug's clearance; thus, it can be difficult to make firm conclusions on the net impact.

The largest and potentially most important area of research is the impact of nutrition on the clearance of drugs. High protein intake (40% of kcal) has been associated with an increase in metabolic enzymes that clear drugs, while a low protein intake (10% of kcal) decreases these proteins (Burton 2006). In addition, changes in total calories ingested seem to reduce metabolism of drugs (Burton 2006). Charbroiled beef has led to a 29% to 147% increase in CYP1A2 activity using a caffeine probe (Kall and Clausen 1995); thus, eating a high quantity of this type of food could reduce concentrations of drugs like caffeine, theophylline, and some antidepressants. Ingestion of cruciferous vegetables (Brussels sprouts, cabbage) has similar effects and changes caffeine metabolic ratio 19% (500 g/d broccoli) (Kall et al. 1996).

In a case report, the anticoagulant warfarin started a high protein intake that ultimately negatively impacted their coagulation status. When the patient returned to a less protein-rich diet, her coagulation status improved. A high protein, low carbohydrate diet has shown to decrease TNF-α and IL-6 (Forsythe et al. 2008) and has a positive relationship with P450 activity (Anderson and Kappas 1991). TNF-α has an inverse relationship with P450 activity (Miyoshi et al. 2005); that is, the lower the TNF-α concentration, the higher the metabolic activity and IL-6 inverse relationship with P450 activity. The modulation of metabolic enzymes (i.e., the P450s) is complex and can be impacted by numerous factors (Monostory and Dvorak 2011).

In addition to changes in metabolism caused by nutritional factors, there could also be changes in the renal clearance of medications. The two most notable areas are drugs that are actively secreted into the urine and drugs that are reabsorbed from the urine back into systemic circulation. There is a relationship between the role of the liver and kidney in drug removal. The role of drug metabolism within the liver is to convert a lipophilic compound into a more hydrophilic compound so the kidney can remove it. As such, some drugs are glucuronidated or sulfated. These compounds, as with some drugs, are actively secreted by organic acid or organic base transport proteins in the urine.

Once in the urine, some drugs can be passively or actively reabsorbed. Drugs that are passively reabsorbed depend on diffusion, and as such, drugs that are charged are not readily reabsorbed. An important determinant of reabsorption is the drug's pKa (the pH at which it is neutral) relative to the urine pH. Weak bases (e.g., amphetamines, antihistamines) will be ionized under acidic conditions— conditions brought about by a high protein diet, for example—and will have enhanced clearance. Conversely, weak acids (e.g., aspirin, penicillin) will be ionized under basic conditions—for example, brought about by a high carbohydrate diet or dietary supplements like sodium bicarbonate—and again, their clearance will be enhanced.

In one study, an isocaloric, high protein diet (26% vs. 13% of calories from protein) decreased urinary pH (6.45 vs. 5.79) and increased the glomerular filtration rate (GFR) (141 vs. 125 mL/min) but not renal plasma flow (Frank et al. 2009) demonstrating, at least, the theoretical implications of dietary changes. One study examined the renal clearance of conjugates of acetaminophen and oxazepam (Pantuck et al. 1991). Acetaminophen is metabolized to a glucuronide and sulfate metabolite and oxazepam is metabolized to glucuronide conjugate. Subjects on a high protein, low carbohydrate diet had significantly higher renal clearance of the glucuronide and sulfate conjugates compared to the low protein, high carbohydrate group. This increase could be due to a stimulation of secretion via the organic acid transport protein responsible for the secretion of these conjugates, the potential increase in GFR noted from high protein diets, or a decrease in reabsorption of the conjugates. As for the latter process, some conjugates are reabsorbed in the kidney, but this is usually an active process; thus, there could be competition between dietary components and drug conjugates for these transport proteins. As noted previously, high protein diets can impact cytokines like TNF-α and IL-6, which also impact organic acid transport protein expression. A decrease in TNF-α and IL-6 will increase organic anion transporting polypeptide (OATP) activity and thus may be responsible for the increase in renal clearance of these organic acid conjugates (Svoboda et al. 2011).

Supplements

Dietary supplements sold on the market are usually tailored toward building lean muscle mass, improving recovery, enhancing endurance performance, or causing weight loss. These supplements, especially herbals, are known to have a variable impact on drug pharmacokinetics and pharmacodynamics. Even non-herbal products, such as sodium bicarbonate, could impact drug disposition. This section will briefly explore some of these interactions.

Sodium bicarbonate is utilized to help offset acidic changes associated with prolonged endurance exercise. As a base, bicarbonate will increase urinary pH causing basic drugs to become unionized and thus reabsorbed to a greater extent. Conversely, bicarbonate ingestion can cause acidic drugs to ionize and be reabsorbed to a lesser extent. For example, amphetamine, a weak base, is excreted as unchanged amphetamine ~1% in alkaline urine to ~75% in acidic urine (Anonymous 2013).

Various reviews have been published regarding herb-drug interactions (Gouws et al. 2012; Yang and Pan 2012). While athletes do not use many of these supplements for performance enhancement, a brief synopsis is warranted. From a pharmacokinetic perspective, herbs can inhibit or induce drug-metabolizing enzymes in the liver or gastrointestinal tract or they can inhibit or induce active transport of drugs in the liver, gastrointestinal tract, or kidney. From a pharmacodynamic standpoint, this could cause an augmentation or reduction of therapeutic effects. Goldenseal increased the immunosuppressant cyclosporine concentrations by inhibiting enzymes that clear the drug (Wu et al. 2005). St. John's Wort will reduce the concentrations of the sedative midazolam by inducing its metabolism (Dresser et al. 2003). St. John's Wort will also reduce the bioavailability of the allergy medication fexofenadine by inhibiting p-glycoprotein, an efflux transport protein in the gut (Wang et al. 2002). The supplement fish oil has anticoagulant properties and can have additive effects with warfarin (Buckley et al. 2004) and non-steroidal anti-inflammatory drugs (McClaskey and Michalets 2007). The banned supplement ephedra increased heart rate and blood pressure and could negate the effects of drugs like beta-blockers, which serve to decrease blood pressure. Athletes need to be careful when taking dietary supplements and medications (either over-the-counter or prescription), as there is growing documentation of cases of supplement-drug interactions.

Fruit Juice

One of the biggest areas of drug-nutrient interaction is with fruit juices. Fruit juice contains various polyphenols that can inhibit or induce drug metabolizing enzymes in the gut or liver and some transport proteins in the gastrointestinal tract. One common element appears to be drugs that are metabolized by cytochrome P450 3A4. See Tables 9.6 and 9.7 for some documented fruit juice-drug interactions.

Extensive research and studies on grapefruit juice have concluded that it specifically inhibits cytochrome P450 3A4 enzyme, one of the major drug metabolizing systems. Compounds called furanocoumarins found in grapefruit juice have been established as the culprit of this inhibition. Because of the inhibition, drug concentrations can increase more than fivefold and lead to adverse reactions and events. However, drugs formulated as prodrugs would have a decreased active concentration because metabolism is required to activate the drug.

Additional issues arise as calcium-fortified juices have a significant effect on the bioavailability of drugs, specifically fluoroquinolone antibiotics. The calcium ion (and other divalent cations) has been found to interact with the chemical composition of drugs such as floxacins, thereby inhibiting the absorption process and leading to low drug plasma concentrations. For instance, ciprofloxacin has a warning label emphasizing that it should not be taken with any dairy products or calcium-fortified juices to prevent any potential interactions (Huang et al. 2004).

TABLE 9.6
Impact of Grapefruit Juice (GFJ) on Various Medications

Drug	Indication	Potential GFJ Effect
Midazolam (Versed)	Sedative/hypnotic	Prolonged sedation
Lovastatin (Mevacor)	Hyperlipidemia	Rhabdomyolisis
Simvastatin (Zocor)	Hyperlipidemia	Rhabdomyolisis
Cyclosporine (Neoral)	Immunosuppression	Nephrotoxicity
Tacrolimus (Prograf)	Immunosuppression	Nephrotoxicity
Nifedipine (Procardia)	Hypertension	Hypotension
Felodipine (Plendil)	Hypertension	Hypotension
Terfenadine (Seldane)[a]	Allergies	QT prolongation
Astemizole (Hismanal)[a]	Allergies	QT prolongation
Cisapride (Propulsid)[a]	GERD	QT prolongation

Source: Adapted from Dresser, G.K. et al. 2000. *Clin Pharmacokinet* 38 (1):41–57.
[a] Pulled from the market.

TABLE 9.7
Examples of Other Fruit Juices That Impact Drug Pharmacokinetics

Juice	Drug	Inhibited Enteric Protein	Change in Mean AUC	Ref.
Lime	Felodipine	–	20% ↑ (ns)	Bailey et al. (2003)
Seville orange	Felodipine	CYP3A	76% ↑	Malhotra et al. (2001)
	Cyclosporine	–	–	Edwards et al. (1999)
	Saquinavir	CYP3A	70% ↑	Mouly et al. (2005)
	Indinavir	–	–	Penzak et al. (2002)
Pomelo	Cyclosporine	CYP3A/P-gp	20% ↑	Grenier et al. (2006)
Orange (sweet)	Fexofenadine	OATP	70% ↓	Dresser et al. (2002)
	Celiprolol	OATP(?)	83% ↓	Lilja et al. (2004)
	Pravastatin	P-gp/MRP-2/BCRP(?)	52% ↓	Koitabashi et al. (2006)
Cranberry	Cyclosporine	–	–	Grenier et al. (2006)
	Nifedipine	CYP3A	60% ↑	Ngo et al. (2009)
Pomegranate	Carbamazepine	CYP3A	50% ↑	Moore et al. (1999)

Note: ns = non-significant.

OTHER DRUG–EXERCISE EFFECTS

While we have discussed how exercise and nutrients can impact drug behavior, it is important to note that there is some evidence that medications can impact, sometimes negatively, adaptations to exercise. For example, one study found that the use of pain medications such as acetaminophen and ibuprofen reduced the fractional synthetic rate for protein, indicating these medications may impair recovery (Trappe et al. 2002). Another study investigated the impact of beta-blockers on various cardiovascular adaptations. The use of beta-blockers may impact adaptations to resting heart rate, stroke volume, and VO_{2MAX} (Ades et al. 1990). A final example of a negative drug-exercise adaptation is statins, which may lead to myalgia. Only 20% of professional athletes with familial hypercholestermia can tolerate statins (i.e., not have myalgia side effects) (Sinzinger and O'Grady 2004).

Little is known about how acute exercise or exercise training may impact sensitivity to medications. In a study in rats, acute exercise increased sensitivity to certain drugs that target muscarinic receptors but there was no influence of exercise training (McMaster and Carney 1985).

SUMMARY

Highly trained athletes may respond to over-the-counter or prescription medications differently than the sedentary population. While the extent of these changes varies depending on the medication and nature of the interaction (acute exercise, nutrients, etc.), it is an important consideration. Some of these interactions can be minimized by separating the time between medication administration (especially systemic administration vs. topical) and exercise or ingestion of certain dietary components or supplements. In some cases, such as exercise training or diets high in protein, alternative doses or dosing strategies may be needed to achieve favorable outcomes, but this can only be accomplished on an individual basis.

REFERENCES

Ades, P.A., P.G. Gunther, W.L. Meyer, T.C. Gibson, J. Maddalena, and T. Orfeo. 1990. Cardiac and skeletal muscle adaptations to training in systemic hypertension and effect of beta blockade (metoprolol or propranolol). *Am J Cardiol* 66(5):591–596.

Anderson, K.E., and A. Kappas. 1991. Dietary regulation of cytochrome P450. *Annu Rev Nutr* 11:141–167.

Arends, B.G., R.O. Bohm, J.E. van Kemenade, K.H. Rahn, and M.A. van Baak. 1986. Influence of physical exercise on the pharmacokinetics of propranolol. *Eur J Clin Pharmacol* 31(3):375–377.

Aslaksen, A., and L. Aanderud. 1980. Drug absorption during physical exercise. *Br J Clin Pharmacol* 10(4):383–385.

Bailey, D.G., G.K. Dresser, and J.R. Bend. 2003. Bergamottin, lime juice, and red wine as inhibitors of cytochrome P450 3A4 activity: Comparison with grapefruit juice. *Clin Pharmacol Ther* 73(6):529–537.

Benetello, P., M. Furlanut, M. Fortunato et al. 1997. Oral gabapentin disposition in patients with epilepsy after a high-protein meal. *Epilepsia* 38(10):1140–1142.

Buckley, M.S., A.D. Goff, and W.E. Knapp. 2004. Fish oil interaction with warfarin. *Ann Pharmacother* 38(1):50–52.

Burton, M.E. 2006. *Applied Pharmacokinetics & Pharmacodynamics: Principles of Therapeutic Drug Monitoring*, 4th ed. Baltimore: Lippincott Williams & Wilkins.

Chien, K.Y., T.T. Chen, J. Hsu et al. 2012. Sub-maximal exercise altered the prednisolone absorption pattern. *J Pharm Pharm Sci* 13(1):58–66.

Collomp, K., F. Anselme, M. Audran, J.P. Gay, J.L. Chanal, and C. Prefaut. 1991. Effects of moderate exercise on the pharmacokinetics of caffeine. *Eur J Clin Pharmacol* 40(3):279–282.

De Paepe, P., F.M. Belpaire, and W.A. Buylaert. 2002. Pharmacokinetic and pharmacodynamic considerations when treating patients with sepsis and septic shock. *Clin Pharmacokinet* 41(14):1135–1151.

Dresser, G.K., J.D. Spence, and D.G. Bailey. 2000. Pharmacokinetic-pharmacodynamic consequences and clinical relevance of cytochrome P450 3A4 inhibition. *Clin Pharmacokinet* 38(1):41–57.

Dresser, G.K., D.G. Bailey, B.F. Leake et al. 2002. Fruit juices inhibit organic anion transporting polypeptide-mediated drug uptake to decrease the oral availability of fexofenadine. *Clin Pharmacol Ther* 71(1):11–20.

Dresser, G.K., U.I. Schwarz, G.R. Wilkinson, and R.B. Kim. 2003. Coordinate induction of both cytochrome P4503A and MDR1 by St John's Wort in healthy subjects. *Clin Pharmacol Ther* 73(1):41–50.

Edwards, D.J., M.E. Fitzsimmons, E.G. Schuetz et al. 1999. $6',7'$-Dihydroxybergamottin in grapefruit juice and Seville orange juice: Effects on cyclosporine disposition, enterocyte CYP3A4, and P-glycoprotein. *Clin Pharmacol Ther* 65(3):237–244.

Engel, G., U. Hofmann, H. Heidemann, J. Cosme, and M. Eichelbaum. 1996. Antipyrine as a probe for human oxidative drug metabolism: Identification of the cytochrome P450 enzymes catalyzing 4-hydroxyantipyrine, 3-hydroxymethylantipyrine, and norantipyrine formation. *Clin Pharmacol Ther* 59(6):613–623.

Forsythe, C.E., S.D. Phinney, M.L. Fernandez et al. 2008. Comparison of low fat and low carbohydrate diets on circulating fatty acid composition and markers of inflammation. *Lipids* 43(1):65–77.

Frank, H., J. Graf, U. Amann-Gassner et al. 2009. Effect of short-term high-protein compared with normal-protein diets on renal hemodynamics and associated variables in healthy young men. *Am J Clin Nutr* 90(6):1509–1516.

Frank, S., S.M. Somani, and M. Kohnle. 1990. Effect of exercise on propranolol pharmacokinetics. *Eur J Clin Pharmacol* 39(4):391–394.

Frost, R.W., J.D. Carlson, A.J. Dietz, Jr., A. Heyd, and J.T. Lettieri. 1989. Ciprofloxacin pharmacokinetics after a standard or high-fat/high-calcium breakfast. *J Clin Pharmacol* 29(10):953–955.

Gidal, B.E., M.M. Maly, J. Budde, G.L. Lensmeyer, M.E. Pitterle, and J.C. Jones. 1996. Effect of a high-protein meal on gabapentin pharmacokinetics. *Epilepsy Res* 23(1):71–76.

Gidal, B.E., M.M. Maly, J.W. Kowalski, P.A. Rutecki, M.E. Pitterle, and D.E. Cook. 1998. Gabapentin absorption: Effect of mixing with foods of varying macronutrient composition. *Ann Pharmacother* 32(4):405–409.

Gouws, C., D. Steyn, L. Du Plessis, J. Steenekamp, and J.H. Hamman. 2012. Combination therapy of Western drugs and herbal medicines: Recent advances in understanding interactions involving metabolism and efflux. *Expert Opin Drug Metab Toxicol* 8(8):973–984.

Grenier, J., C. Fradette, G. Morelli, G.J. Merritt, M. Vranderick, and M.P. Ducharme. 2006. Pomelo juice, but not cranberry juice, affects the pharmacokinetics of cyclosporine in humans. *Clin Pharmacol Ther* 79(3):255–262.

Gupta, S.K., R.C. Manfro, S.J. Tomlanovich, J.G. Gambertoglio, M.R. Garovoy, and L.Z. Benet. 1990. Effect of food on the pharmacokinetics of cyclosporine in healthy subjects following oral and intravenous administration. *J Clin Pharmacol* 30(7):643–653.

Haller, C.A., M. Duan, P. Jacob, III, and N. Benowitz. 2008. Human pharmacology of a performance-enhancing dietary supplement under resting and exercise conditions. *Br J Clin Pharmacol* 65(6):833–840.

Henry, J.A., A. Iliopoulou, C.M. Kaye, M.G. Sankey, and P. Turner. 1981. Changes in plasma concentrations of acebutolol, propranolol and indomethacin during physical exercise. *Life Sci* 28(17):1925–1929.

Huang, S.M., S.D. Hall, P. Watkins et al. 2004. Drug interactions with herbal products and grapefruit juice: A conference report. *Clin Pharmacol Ther* 75(1):1–12.

Joreteg, T., and T. Jogestrand. 1983. Physical exercise and digoxin binding to skeletal muscle: Relation to exercise intensity. *Eur J Clin Pharmacol* 25(5):585–588.

Jung, H., A.A. Peregrina, J.M. Rodriguez, and R. Moreno-Esparza. 1997. The influence of coffee with milk and tea with milk on the bioavailability of tetracycline. *Biopharm Drug Dispos* 18(5):459–463.

Kall, M.A., and J. Clausen. 1995. Dietary effect on mixed function P450 1A2 activity assayed by estimation of caffeine metabolism in man. *Hum Exp Toxicol* 14(10):801–807.

Kall, M.A., O. Vang, and J. Clausen. 1996. Effects of dietary broccoli on human in vivo drug metabolizing enzymes: Evaluation of caffeine, oestrone and chlorzoxazone metabolism. *Carcinogenesis* 17(4):793–799.

Khazaeinia, T., A.A. Ramsey, and Y.K. Tam. 2000. The effects of exercise on the pharmacokinetics of drugs. *J Pharm Pharm Sci* 3(3):292–302.

Koitabashi, Y., T. Kumai, N. Matsumoto et al. 2006. Orange juice increased the bioavailability of pravastatin, 3-hydroxy-3-methylglutaryl CoA reductase inhibitor, in rats and healthy human subjects. *Life Sci* 78(24):2852–2859.

Koivisto, V.A., and P. Felig. 1978. Effects of leg exercise on insulin absorption in diabetic patients. *N Engl J Med* 298(2):79–83.

Levy, R.H., and K.M. Koch. 1982. Drug interactions with valproic acid. *Drugs* 24(6):543–556.

Lilja, J.J., L. Juntti-Patinen, and P.J. Neuvonen. 2004. Orange juice substantially reduces the bioavailability of the beta-adrenergic-blocking agent celiprolol. *Clin Pharmacol Ther* 75(3):184–190.

Malhotra, S., D.G. Bailey, M.F. Paine, and P.B. Watkins. 2001. Seville orange juice-felodipine interaction: Comparison with dilute grapefruit juice and involvement of furocoumarins. *Clin Pharmacol Ther* 69(1):14–23.

Marchbanks, C.R. 1993. Drug-drug interactions with fluoroquinolones. *Pharmacotherapy* 13(2 Pt 2):23S–28S.

Mason, W.D., G. Kochak, N. Winer, and I. Cohen. 1980. Effect of exercise on renal clearance of atenolol. *J Pharm Sci* 69(3):344–345.

McClaskey, E.M., and E.L. Michalets. 2007. Subdural hematoma after a fall in an elderly patient taking high-dose omega-3 fatty acids with warfarin and aspirin: Case report and review of the literature. *Pharmacotherapy* 27(1):152–160.

McLean, C., and T.E. Graham. 2002. Effects of exercise and thermal stress on caffeine pharmacokinetics in men and eumenorrheic women. *J Appl Physiol* 93(4):1471–1478.

McMaster, S.B., and J.M. Carney. 1985. Changes in drug sensitivity following acute and chronic exercise. *Pharmacol Biochem Behav* 23(2):191–194.

Miyoshi, M., M. Nadai, A. Nitta et al. 2005. Role of tumor necrosis factor-alpha in down-regulation of hepatic cytochrome P450 and P-glycoprotein by endotoxin. *Eur J Pharmacol* 507(1–3):229–237.

Monostory, K., and Z. Dvorak. 2011. Steroid regulation of drug-metabolizing cytochromes P450. *Curr Drug Metab* 12(2):154–172.

Moore, K.H., S. Shaw, A.L. Laurent et al. 1999. Lamivudine/zidovudine as a combined formulation tablet: Bioequivalence compared with lamivudine and zidovudine administered concurrently and the effect of food on absorption. *J Clin Pharmacol* 39(6):593–605.

Mooy, J., B. Arends, J. van Kemenade, R. Boehm, K.H. Rahn, and M. van Baak. 1986. Influence of prolonged submaximal exercise on the pharmacokinetics of verapamil in humans. *J Cardiovasc Pharmacol* 8(5):940–942.

Mouly, S.J., C. Matheny, M.F. Paine et al. 2005. Variation in oral clearance of saquinavir is predicted by CYP3A5*1 genotype but not by enterocyte content of cytochrome P450 3A5. *Clin Pharmacol Ther* 78(6):605–618.

Ngo, N., Z. Yan, T.N. Graf et al. 2009. Identification of a cranberry juice product that inhibits enteric CYP3A-mediated first-pass metabolism in humans. *Drug Metab Dispos* 37(3):514–522.

Panton, L.B., G.J. Guillen, L. Williams et al. 1995. The lack of effect of aerobic exercise training on propranolol pharmacokinetics in young and elderly adults. *J Clin Pharmacol* 35(9):885–894.

Pantuck, E.J., C.B. Pantuck, A. Kappas, A.H. Conney, and K.E. Anderson. 1991. Effects of protein and carbohydrate content of diet on drug conjugation. *Clin Pharmacol Ther* 50(3):254–258.

Pedersen, K.E., J. Madsen, K. Kjaer, N.A. Klitgaard, and S. Hvidt. 1983. Effects of physical activity and immobilization on plasma digoxin concentration and renal digoxin clearance. *Clin Pharmacol Ther* 34(3):303–308.

Penzak, S.R., E.P. Acosta, M. Turner et al. 2002. Effect of Seville orange juice and grapefruit juice on indinavir pharmacokinetics. *J Clin Pharmacol* 42(10):1165–1170.

Persky, A.M., N.D. Eddington, and H. Derendorf. 2003. A review of the effects of chronic exercise and physical fitness level on resting pharmacokinetics. *Int J Clin Pharmacol Ther* 41(11):504–516.

Sahai, J., D.P. Healy, J. Stotka, and R.E. Polk. 1993. The influence of chronic administration of calcium carbonate on the bioavailability of oral ciprofloxacin. *Br J Clin Pharmacol* 35(3):302–304.

Savarese, D, and J.M. Zand. 2015. Dextroamphetamine and amphetamine: Drug information In T. W. Post (Ed.), UpToDate. Retrieved April 27, 2015.

Schlaeffer, F., I. Engelberg, J. Kaplanski, and A. Danon. 1984. Effect of exercise and environmental heat on theophylline kinetics. *Respiration* 45(4):438–442.

Sinzinger, H., and J. O'Grady. 2004. Professional athletes suffering from familial hypercholesterolaemia rarely tolerate statin treatment because of muscular problems. *Br J Clin Pharmacol* 57(4):525–528.

Somani, S.M. 1996. *Pharmacology in exercise and sports, pharmacology and toxicology.* Boca Raton, FL: CRC Press.

Stewart, D.E. 1992. High-fiber diet and serum tricyclic antidepressant levels. *J Clin Psychopharmacol* 12(6):438–440.

Stoschitzky, K., R. Zweiker, W. Klein et al. 2002. Unpredicted lack of effect of exercise on plasma concentrations of carvedilol. *J Cardiovasc Pharmacol* 39(1):58–60.

Svoboda, M., J. Riha, K. Wlcek, W. Jaeger, and T. Thalhammer. 2011. Organic anion transporting polypeptides (OATPs): Regulation of expression and function. *Curr Drug Metab* 12(2):139–153.

Tan, K.K., A.K. Trull, J.A. Uttridge et al. 1995. Effect of dietary fat on the pharmacokinetics and pharmacodynamics of cyclosporine in kidney transplant recipients. *Clin Pharmacol Ther* 57(4):425–433.

Trappe, T.A., F. White, C.P. Lambert, D. Cesar, M. Hellerstein, and W.J. Evans. 2002. Effect of ibuprofen and acetaminophen on postexercise muscle protein synthesis. *Am J Physiol Endocrinol Metab* 282(3):E551–E556.

van Baak, M.A., J.M. Mooij, and P.M. Schiffers. 1992. Exercise and the pharmacokinetics of propranolol, verapamil and atenolol. *Eur J Clin Pharmacol* 43(5):547–550.

Wang, Z., M.A. Hamman, S.M. Huang, L.J. Lesko, and S.D. Hall. 2002. Effect of St John's wort on the pharmacokinetics of fexofenadine. *Clin Pharmacol Ther* 71(6):414–420.

Wu, X., Q. Li, H. Xin, A. Yu, and M. Zhong. 2005. Effects of berberine on the blood concentration of cyclosporin A in renal transplanted recipients: Clinical and pharmacokinetic study. *Eur J Clin Pharmacol* 61(8):567–572.

Yang, C.S., and E. Pan. 2012. The effects of green tea polyphenols on drug metabolism. *Expert Opin Drug Metab Toxicol* 8(6):677–689.

Yuen, G.J., Y. Lou, N.F. Thompson et al. 2001. Abacavir/lamivudine/zidovudine as a combined formulation tablet: Bioequivalence compared with each component administered concurrently and the effect of food on absorption. *J Clin Pharmacol* 41(3):277–288.

10 Nutrition, Exercise, and Immunology

Mary P. Miles, PhD, FACSM

Department of Health and Human Development,
Montana State University, Bozeman, Montana

CONTENTS

The immune system, like all other systems of the body, requires nutrients for energy, for biosynthesis of structural and functional molecules, to enable proper functioning of enzymes, and to protect cells from oxidative damage. Strenuous exercise contributes to the overall stress placed on the immune system. Training at high intensity or volume places demands on the body that can stress tissues such as muscle to the point of injury, increase the likelihood of acute illness, or push the athlete into a state of overreaching or overtraining (Smith 2004; Walsh et al. 2011a). These unintended consequences may compromise training and performance or knock athletes out of competition altogether. Any of these outcomes has the potential to be devastating within the ranks of highly competitive or demanding sporting endeavors. Consider the potential impact of becoming ill during Olympic competition or during a Mount Everest trek. The immune system mediates the response to tissue injury, defends against viral, bacterial, and all other pathogen infections, and it is influenced by and may play a role in the physiology of overreaching and overtraining. To that end, consideration of nutrition for elite athletes should incorporate supplying the body with all of the nutrients needed to maintain optimal immune function.

There are several mechanisms through which nutrition can modulate the interaction between exercise and the immune system in athletes, and thus influence tissue injury, susceptibility to acute illness, and the likelihood of overreaching or overtraining. Nutrients that modulate inflammation may influence the extent of muscle damage that occurs in response to exercise. For example, antioxidants modulate the production of free radicals by inflammatory cells and have the potential to mediate inflammation-induced tissue damage (Peternelj and Coombes 2011). Nutrients can modulate the degree of stress induced by exercise. For example, low carbohydrate availability during exercise can increase the physiological stress of an exercise bout and the extent to which immunological factors are impacted by the exercise (Gunzer et al. 2012; Nieman 2008). Nutrients can influence immune function and immune system status, thereby influencing the degree of readiness of the body to withstand immune challenges. For example, zinc is a mineral with a key role in many immune system functions and low zinc availability may make it more difficult for the immune system to suppress a virus (Gleeson 2006a).

ACUTE INFECTION AND ILLNESS SYMPTOMS

IMMUNE DEFENSES AGAINST INFECTION AND ACUTE ILLNESS

A brief explanation as to how the body defends itself against bacterial or viral infection is needed so that the influences of nutrition and exercise can be placed in a meaningful context. Only the briefest of explanations regarding immune defense mechanisms can be given within the present chapter; however, interested readers may find more detailed information within sources on which the information in this section is based (Gleeson 2006b; Martin et al. 2009). The immune system is designed to provide defense against a variety of foreign invaders such as bacteria and viruses, collectively referred to as pathogens. There are two arms of the immune system. The first arm, typically referred to as the innate immune system, is a non-specific, rapid response system that provides the first line of defense. The second arm, typically referred to as the acquired immune system, is an antigen-specific system that provides a delayed, but very specific and adaptive, second line of defense. Antigens are components of the pathogen that are presented to the acquired immune system by cells of the innate immune system. Thus, there is a great deal of coordination and integration between the two arms of the system, and both are needed to provide protection against the nearly infinite number of potential pathogens to which we may be exposed over the course of our lifetimes. An overview of the immune system functioning to provide defense against a viral infection is illustrated in Figure 10.1.

Components of the innate immune system may be considered barriers or obstacles that a pathogen such as a virus must overcome in order to become an established or symptomatic infection. As illustrated in Figure 10.1, the first obstacle for a pathogen to overcome is to get past the physical (skin) and mucosal immune barriers. If the pathogen passes this first hurdle, then cells of the innate immune system are an

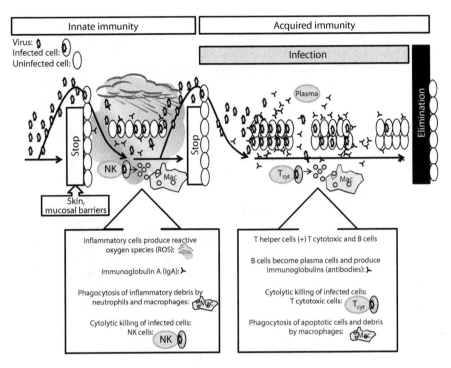

FIGURE 10.1 In defense against infections—viral infection illustrated here—the innate immune system provides barriers that may stop a virus from establishing a symptomatic state of infection. If the virus is not stopped by physical barriers, then soluble IgA may bind and neutralize virus, oxidative bursts of local inflammatory cells may create a toxic local cloud of ROS, NK cells may exert cytotoxic effects to remove infected cells, and other components of the innate immune arm of the immune system contribute to potentially stopping viral invasion. However, if the virus is not stopped by the innate immune system and a state of infection is established, then the acquired arm of the immune system will be activated. T helper lymphocytes provide stimulatory signals (cytokines) that allow T cytotoxic cells to kill infected cells and B cells to become antibody-secreting plasma cells. T and B cell actions are antigen-specific.

awaiting second barrier. The primary cells of the innate immune system include neutrophils, macrophages, and natural killer cells. When signs of a pathogen are detected, an inflammatory response that includes the action of neutrophils and macrophages is initiated. Neutrophils provide an oxidative burst to cloud the local area with toxic reactive oxygen species (ROS) to injure and kill local bacteria or cells that may be infected. The non-specific nature of the ROS produced is such that both intended and unintended targets are not distinguished, and damage to healthy as well as infected cells and tissues results. Monocytes are a precursor cell found in the circulation that can leave the circulation to infiltrate tissues and differentiate to become macrophages. Macrophages release ROS and a variety of cytokines to signal and coordinate other immune defense components. Both neutrophils and macrophages can act as phagocytes to engulf cellular and other types of debris created by the inflammatory process. Natural killer (NK) cells are more targeted in their cytotoxic actions. Using pattern recognition receptors expressed on virally infected or tumor cells, NK cells identify cells that are virally infected, adhere to them, and inject a death signal into the infected cells to induce apoptosis.

If a pathogen is not stopped by the innate immune system components and manages to establish a state of infection, for example, infection symptoms present, then the acquired immune system is needed to eliminate the infection from the system. Signals from and antigen-presentation by the cells of the innate immune system activate cells of the acquired immune system. Cytokines and chemokines produced by injured or infected cells and by cells of the innate immune system are common signal and regulatory molecules within the immune system (see Table 10.1 for specific examples). Cytokines and antigen presentation by cells of the innate immune system activate the T helper (CD4+) subclass of T lymphocytes, which activates T cytotoxic (CD8+) and B lymphocytes with specificity to the specific antigen (virus, bacteria, parasite, etc.). Activated T cytotoxic cells identify cells infected with their specific antigen, adhere to them, and inject a death signal to induce apoptosis. Activated B lymphocytes differentiate to become plasma cells that produce immunoglobulins (Ig), also known as antibodies, with specificity to the infecting antigen. Specificity within this response is derived from the matching of the antigen specific to the invading pathogen to specific T and B cells capable of recognizing that specific antigen. A

TABLE 10.1
Cytokines and Chemokines

	Source of Production	Effect
Tumor necrosis factor-α (TNF-α)	Activated innate immune system cells	Pro-inflammatory, "alarm cytokine"
Interleukin-1(α or β), IL-1	Activated innate immune system cells, for example, macrophages	Pro-inflammatory, "alarm cytokine"
Interleukin-2 (IL-2)	Th1 lymphocytes	Pro-inflammatory, promotes T cytotoxic activity against virally infected cells
Interleukin-4 (IL-4)	Activated Th2 lymphocytes	Anti-inflammatory activity and stimulation of B cell to plasma cell conversion for production of immunoglobulins
Interleukin-6	Activated innate immune system cells, contracting skeletal muscle	
Interleukin-10	Activated Th2 lymphocytes	Anti-inflammatory activity
Interleukin-12 (IL-12)	Activated innate immune system cells	Stimulates production of pro-inflammatory cytokines (IL-2, IFN-γ) by Th1 lymphocytes
Interferon-γ	Activated Th1 lymphocytes	Stimulates anti-viral activity

Source: Martin, S.A. et al. 2009. *Exerc Sport Sci Rev* 37(4):157–164. With permission.

necessary part of this process is the replication of the lymphocyte clones for the cells to be able to recognize and respond to the antigen, a process known as clonal expansion. If the system has never seen the antigen before, then initially there are few cells capable of recognizing the antigen. If the system has been previously exposed to the antigen, either through previous infection or through vaccination, then the system stores T and B lymphocytes with memory of that antigen so that the pathogen can be eliminated before establishing an active, symptomatic infection.

EXERCISE-INDUCED IMMUNOMODULATION

At rest, the immune system of an elite athlete is neither substantially weaker nor stronger than that of healthy, moderately active individuals of comparable age and body composition. There may be enhancement of NK cell activity and a slight reduction in neutrophil activity within the innate arm of the immune system, but there are no consistent differences within the acquired arm of the immune system (Nieman 2008). The immune system needs to be responsive but not overly zealous. For example, it is optimal to be able to eradicate the occasional infection but not to be so aggressive that excessive inflammation causes damage or disease, or that autoimmune disorders result, for example, rheumatoid arthritis or lupus. The general consensus of many researchers of exercise and immunology is that prolonged strenuous endurance events and high intensity or volume training cycles both have the capacity to induce transient reductions in immune defenses that may result in increased incidence of infections, particularly those of the respiratory tract (Gleeson and Walsh 2012; Walsh et al. 2011b).

There is a brief period of time from 3–24 or even up to 72 h following prolonged, strenuous exercise in which immune defenses are lowered. This time is often referred to as an "open window" in which there is opportunity for infections that might have failed otherwise to succeed in establishing a presence in the body (Gunzer et al. 2012; Walsh et al. 2011b). During intensified training periods, elite athletes may accumulate time in the "open window" state. Specific immune defenses that are lowered during the open window following strenuous exercise include lower salivary IgA concentrations, and decreased neutrophil, T, and NK cell function (Gunzer et al. 2012). It is difficult to differentiate the accumulation of time in the typical acute post-exercise state from a lengthening of that state or from a somewhat chronic state that will reverse only with a decrease in training over time. Regardless, the result is an apparent increase in susceptibility to infection during strenuous training periods leading up to competitive events.

RESPIRATORY TRACT INFECTIONS IN ATHLETES

As in the general population, respiratory tract infections (RTI) are the most common cause of illness in athletes. Respiratory tract viral infections include both the rhinovirus leading to the common cold, affecting primarily the upper respiratory tract, and the more systemic and debilitating influenza viruses (Martin et al. 2009). An average person will experience two to five RTI in a year, with most infections occurring within flu season, spanning roughly from October to April with a peak in January or February (Bishop 2006; Martin et al. 2009). Typical symptoms are cough, runny nose or nasal congestion, fever, and general achiness of the body. These symptoms of a viral infection occur when the virus is not eliminated by innate immune defenses or when a dormant virus is reactivated (Walsh et al. 2011b). Dormant viruses, such as herpes group viruses or Epstein-Barr virus, reside in an organism in an inactive and asymptomatic state but can be stimulated to become active.

There is a reasonable level of acceptance for a relationship between exercise quantity in both intensity and duration, which follows what was originally proposed by Nieman (1994) many years ago as a "J" shaped curve. This curve describes the occurrence of an average frequency of infectious episodes for sedentary or low active individuals, a decrease in frequency with activity levels that are moderate (the nadir of the curve), and an upswing and high point in frequency with volumes and intensities of training described as "high," "severe," or "very demanding" (Nieman 1994). Rather than being temporally related to the flu season, the upswing for athletes occurs when training loads are greatest and around the time of competitions, although some endurance athletes may have a higher incidence of RTI at any time in their training (Walsh et al. 2011b). Elite athletes must contend with the apparent increase in frequency of RTI by doing what they can to support optimal immune function. In addition to taking preventive actions to avoid exposure to infectious pathogens, key influences of immune function over which an athlete may exert some level of control are environmental, physiological, and psychological stresses and nutritional factors (Gleeson 2006b; Nieman 2008). However, a recent consensus statement from a panel of experts in the field of exercise and immunology asserts that decreases in salivary IgA concentration and secretion rates are the one clear, evidence-based change in immune function to associate with upper RTI symptom development (Walsh et al. 2011b).

NON-VIRAL CAUSES OF RTI SYMPTOMS IN ATHLETES

Researchers working to determine the underlying cause of upper RTI symptoms in athletes report that roughly one-third of the cases of RTI could be identified as being caused by a specific virus, about 5% were caused by bacteria, and the remaining cases were from other causes including allergy, asthma, drying of the airways due to exposure to high ventilation or cold, dry air, other stressors, or simply "unknown" causes (Martin et al. 2009; Walsh et al. 2011b). Without confirmation such as virus measurement in the blood, it is not possible to be sure of the underlying cause of the symptoms. Inflammation is a common element to many of these non-viral causes or RTI symptoms. This connection between RTI and other infection symptoms and inflammation gives rise to a very interesting and potentially emerging, yet unresearched link between nutrition and RTI symptoms. Nutrient status or availability may influence susceptibility to, duration of, and severity of RTI with nutritional countermeasures that influence inflammation.

BACTERIAL INFECTIONS

Many routes of bacterial infection are relevant to athletes. All living beings are exposed to potentially infectious bacteria at all times. For example, everything a person touches or ingests, including air, delivers a challenge to the immune system because bacteria are on or within virtually everything. Fortunately, the immune system is very good at protecting against bacterial infection. Within the innate arm of the immune system, skin, mucosal, and chemical barriers keep bacteria out or kill bacteria quickly. Additionally, neutrophils can create a hostile local environment of ROS and phagocytize bacteria. The acquired arm of the immune system also is active within mucosal barriers as one of the places where plasma, B and T lymphocytes, and immunoglobulin A (IgA) are found. These innate and acquired defenses are particularly abundant in the upper respiratory tract, the lungs, and the gastrointestinal tract. While there is less research regarding exercise and susceptibility to bacterial infections and the unique way that the immune system defends against bacterial infections, many of the underlying concepts are similar to defending against viral infections.

INFLUENCE OF ACUTE CHANGES IN STRESS HORMONES ON IMMUNE FUNCTION

The interaction among nervous, endocrine, and immune systems is extensive and complex. A great deal can be understood about both nutritional and neuroendocrine modulation of immune function by describing some of the key immune influences of catecholamines (e.g., epinephrine) and glucocorticoids (e.g., cortisol). A substantial portion of the influence of nutrition on the immune system during exercise is the influence of nutrient availability on hormone responses. When nutrient availability induces an endocrine response that exerts a change in immune function, this is an example of an "indirect effect" of a nutrient on the immune system (Table 10.2) (Walsh 2006).

As a catecholamine associated with activating physiologic and anticipatory responses for exercise and protection from harm, epinephrine has a mixture of effects that may be classified as immunosuppressive or anti-inflammatory (↓) or as increasing immune surveillance (↑). Epinephrine induces the following immune system changes: (↓) decreased neutrophil respiratory burst activity, (↓) decreased NK cell cytolytic activity, (↑) increased NK cells, T and B lymphocytes, monocytes (which differentiate to become macrophages after leaving the circulation), and neutrophils in the circulation (Blannin 2006).

As a glucocoriticoid and stress hormone, cortisol also has a mixture of effects that may be classified as immunosuppressive or anti-inflammatory (↓) or as increasing immune surveillance (↑). However, the balance of the effects of cortisol tilts heavily toward immunosuppression. Acute increases in cortisol induce the following immune system changes: (↓) a delayed (one to several hours) decrease in T, B, and NK cells in the circulation (Blannin 2006), (↓) decreased immunoglobulin production (Walsh 2006), (↓) decreased lymphocyte proliferation for clonal expansion (Walsh 2006), (↓) decreased NK cell cytolytic activity (Walsh 2006), and (↑) a delayed (one to several hours) increase in monocytes and neutrophils in the circulation (Blannin 2006).

MODULATION OF THE ACUTE IMMUNE RESPONSE
WITH CARBOHYDRATE SUPPLEMENTATION

Researchers have not identified specific nutritional strategies that athletes can employ to decrease their risk of RTI. However, there is a great deal of evidence

TABLE 10.2
Direct and Indirect Effects of Nutrient Availability on the Immune System

Insufficient Availability	Direct Effect	Indirect Effect
Water		↑ Cortisol
Energy		↑ Cortisol
Glucose	↓ Neutrophil, macrophage, and lymphocyte function; ↓ IL-6 production in exercising skeletal muscle	↑ Cortisol
Protein	↓ Lymphocyte quantity and function; ↓ macrophage phagocytosis and production of pro-inflammatory cytokines (IL-1β)	↑ Catecholamines
Glutamine	↓ Energy and nucleotide synthesis (influences proliferation capacity) in leukocytes	↓ Levels of glutathione (endogenous antioxidant)
Fat in the diet (<15% of energy)		↑ Oxidative stress owing to low intake of fat (soluble antioxidants)
n-6 Fatty acids		↓ Synthesis of eicosanoids derived from arachadonic acid, for example, prostaglandin E_2 (generally immunosuppressive or anti-inflammatory)
n-3 Fatty acids		↑ Synthesis of eicosanoids derived from arachadonic acid, for example, prostaglandin E_2 (generally immunosuppressive or anti-inflammatory)

(Continued)

TABLE 10.2 (Continued)
Direct and Indirect Effects of Nutrient Availability on the Immune System

Insufficient Availability	Direct Effect	Indirect Effect
Zinc	↓ Lymphocyte quantity and function; ↓ IL-2 production; ↓ NK cell cytolytic activity; ↓ ROS production by macrophages and neutrophils	None reported
Iron[a]	↓ IL-1 production by macrophages; ↓ lymphocyte proliferation; ↓ NK cell cytolytic activity	None reported
Magnesium	↑ Inflammation	None reported
Copper	↓ Antibody formation; ↓ inflammation; ↓ phagocytosis; NK and T lymphocyte cytolytic activity	None reported
Selenium	↓ Glutathione peroxidase/reductase activity (↓ antioxidant defenses)	None reported
Manganese	↓ Superoxide dismutase activity (↓ antioxidant defenses)	None reported
Cobalt/B12	↓ Leukocyte count; ↓ neutrophil bactericidal activity; ↓ lymphocyte proliferation	None reported

Source: Reprinted from *Immune Function in Sport and Exercise*, M. Gleeson, Ed., Walsh, N. P., 161–182, Copyright 2006, with permission from Elsevier; Reprinted with permission from *Immune Function in Sport and Exercise*, M. Gleeson, Ed., Gleeson, M., 183–204, Copyright 2006, with permission from Elsevier; Gunzer, W. et al. 2012. *Nutrients* 4(9):1187–1212. With permission.

Note: ↑ = increase; ↓ = decrease.

[a] One important note with respect to iron is that low iron availability is beneficial with respect to making it more difficult for bacterial growth.

to demonstrate that the stress hormone responses, that is, cortisol and the catecholamines (epinephrine and norepinephrine) and a variety of related neutrophil, monocyte, and cytokine responses (IL-6, IL-10, IL-1 receptor antagonist) are decreased when carbohydrate is consumed during prolonged endurance exercise (Nieman 2008; Walsh 2006). Carbohydrate ingestion has the greatest benefit in reducing immune system changes when the exercise is of sufficient intensity and duration to increase stress hormones, typically above 75% VO_{2max} for 90 min or more (Nieman 2008; Walsh 2006). The amount of carbohydrate used in placebo-controlled studies to reduce stress hormone and immune responses is typically around 60 g of carbohydrate per hour (1 L of a 6% carbohydrate drink). While there is almost no evidence to suggest that carbohydrate ingestion changes risk of RTI following prolonged and strenuous exercise events (Nieman 2008), these research findings do link glucose availability during exercise to stress hormone responses, particularly cortisol.

In addition to lowering cortisol and its immunosuppressive actions, other mechanisms for carbohydrate intake during exercise to attenuate the exercise-induced immune response may include a decrease in (1) the production and release of IL-6 by skeletal muscle, (2) pro- and anti-inflammatory cytokine gene expression and plasma levels (IL-6, IL-10, IL-1ra), and (3) circulating neutrophils, and an increase in (a) salivary IgA, (b) plasma glutamine, and (c) energy for immune cell function and synthetic processes (Gunzer et al. 2012; Nieman 2008; Walsh 2006). A mechanism linking these changes to RTI incidence has not been established, but one possible explanation to be researched is that carbohydrate ingestion during exercise decreases inflammation, and this decreases the anti-inflammatory and generally immunosuppressive responses to counter the inflammation.

NUTRITION RECOMMENDATIONS TO SUPPORT THE IMMUNE SYSTEM

While our defenses against a nearly infinite array of potential infections are impressive, a healthy underlying immune system is needed to provide this impressive protection. Effects of a variety of nutrients on immune function are described in Table 10.2. Athletes in training, like any other individual, may benefit from nutritional practices that support the immune system by experiencing fewer or less severe infections. Maintaining a healthy immune system may help athletes avoid loss of training time or competition performance due to illness, infection, or poor healing of injuries. The same underlying basic nutrition principles apply to the immune system as to all systems of the body. Fortunately, for athletes, all that needs to be done to provide the immune system with the nutrients needed for optimal function is to follow the same nutrition recommendations for optimal training, performance, and recovery, as described in Chapters 2, 4, 6, 7, 11, and 12. Specifically, the immune system functions best when the following dietary needs are adequately met (Gleeson 2006a; Gleeson and Walsh 2012; Walsh 2006):

- Sufficient energy, particularly in the form of carbohydrate, on a dietary basis and during exercise (a minimum of 8–10 g of carbohydrate per kilogram of body mass per day)

- Consumption of 30–60 g of carbohydrate per hour during prolonged exercise
- Availability of amino acids for cellular maintenance and protein synthesis (a minimum of 1.6 g of protein per kilogram of body mass per day)
- Availability of both n-6 and n-3 fatty acids to maintain optimal cellular membrane fluidity and for the production of eicosanoids (at least 20% of energy intake)
- Sufficient vitamin and mineral availability to support enzyme functions and biosynthesis (eating a varied diet that includes vegetables and fruits)
- Sufficient fluids (fluid intake greater than fluid loss)

In addition to the same basic nutritional requirements of all cells and organ systems, the immune system has some unique functions that are particularly dependent on vitamin C (ascorbic acid), vitamin E (α-tocopherol), vitamin A, vitamin B12, folic acid, iron, zinc, selenium, copper, magnesium, and manganese (Gleeson 2006a). It is generally accepted that this increased need is covered by an increase in dietary intake to match caloric needs (Gleeson 2006a). However, this means that athletes in a caloric deficit are less likely to be meeting their nutrient demands, and may be more likely to have suboptimal immune function and increased incidence of infections. Additionally, greater intake of many of the minerals (particularly electrolytes and iron) may be needed in athletes who have substantial sweat losses during training or competition (Gleeson 2006a).

NUTRITION AND MUSCLE DAMAGE

EXERCISE-INDUCED MUSCLE DAMAGE (EIMD)

Intense training often places metabolic or mechanical stresses on skeletal muscle that can cause damage to this tissue. In contrast to a muscle pull or muscle tear generally felt to be an acute injury, exercise-induced muscle damage (EIMD) is a subcellular phenomenon that is initiated during exercise, without noticeable pain, and with no symptoms other than fatigue. A hallmark characteristic of EIMD is a prolonged, post-exercise decrease in force production capacity (Faulkner et al. 1993). In the days following the exercise, varying levels of delayed onset muscle soreness (DOMS), swelling, range of motion decrease, and efflux of intramuscular proteins to the circulation are common "indirect" or secondary indicators of EIMD (Miles and Clarkson 1994; Miles et al. 2008). Strategies to minimize the loss of function and discomfort may be beneficial to athletes, in which case examination of the influence of nutrition on the mechanisms underlying and outcomes of EIMD and DOMS is important. However, the term "adaptive microtrauma" has been used to describe processes associated with EIMD (Smith and Miles 2000), and the question often arises as to whether short-term modulation of cellular events is beneficial or detrimental to long-term adaptations to training. More research evidence is needed on this evolving issue.

Several different metabolic processes are capable of triggering EIMD. Metabolically stressful exercise increases oxidative stress to produce reactive oxygen and nitrogen species (RONS) and induce cellular damage. During prolonged or intense exercise, the production of energy and related metabolism results in the production of RONS from a small fraction (estimated at ~0.15%) of electrons that are lost from the electron transport chain, and increases in the activity of several enzymes including the inducible form of nitric oxide synthase, xanthine oxidase, and nicotinamide adenine dinucleotide phosphate oxidase (NADPH) (Peternelj and Coombes 2011). The RONS produced act as cellular signals to increase performance and to promote cellular adaptations to increase oxygen consumption capacity and antioxidant defenses (Peternelj and Coombes 2011; Radak et al. 2012). To this end, RONS play a key role in the process of beneficial cellular adaptations resulting from exercise training. While RONS are desirable and increased production during exercise is unavoidable, high levels of these molecules damage cellular components to the point of eliciting an inflammatory response by the immune system.

The triggering event during mechanically stressful activities, typically including high-force eccentric muscle actions, is microscopic tearing of the cytoskeleton within a skeletal muscle fiber. Individuals not accustomed to this type of exercise are most vulnerable to EIMD, so this mechanism is most likely to occur at the onset of training or after training that includes more high force work than an athlete typically performs, for example, a great deal of downhill running or heavy weight lowering. Electron micrographs of muscle injured with high-force eccentric muscle actions show that the z-disc is the weak link that is vulnerable to tearing and EIMD results from the accumulation of multiple disrupted sarcomeres dispersed at many anatomically independent sites within a damaged muscle (Friden and Lieber 1998).

INFLAMMATION RESPONSE TO EIMD

While there are several mechanisms to elicit EIMD, tissue damage invariably causes an inflammation response that includes a series of events beginning with local initiation, followed in some cases by systemic amplification, and culminating in resolution of inflammation and healing of injured tissue (Smith and Miles 2000). As shown in Figure 10.2, the following is a typical sequence of inflammation events:

1. Activation of resident macrophages to release pro-inflammatory cytokines, for example, IL-1β and TNF-α
2. Increases in chemotactic agents and adhesion molecules to attract inflammatory leukocytes to the location of injury
3. Infiltration by neutrophils and then macrophages
4. Production of additional inflammatory cytokines and RONS
5. Production of cytokines with anti-inflammatory effects, for example, IL-1ra, IL-6, or IL-10
6. Eventual removal of inflammatory cells via apoptosis, regeneration of sarcomere and myofibrillar order, and termination

The response may include systemic elements including increases in cortisol and acute phase proteins such as C-reactive protein (CRP). The resulting changes in the indirect markers of muscle damage including loss of strength/function and DOMS take several days to resolve (Miles and Clarkson 1994); however, full resolution

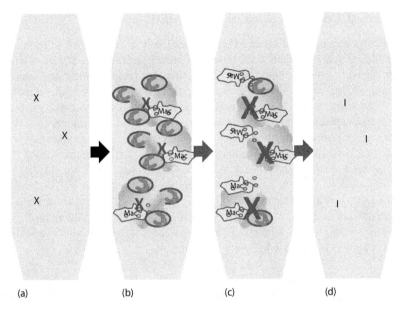

(a)   (b)   (c)   (d)

FIGURE 10.2 (a) EIMD starts with microscopic, focal disruptions of the cytoskeleton within sarcomeres interspersed throughout a muscle. (b) Resident macrophages respond to the microscopic points of injury by secreting "alarm cytokines" and chemokines to attract additional inflammatory cells, including neutrophils, to the point of damage. Inflammatory cells produce ROS, which stimulates additional inflammatory activity and increases the extent of cellular injury. This process stimulates DOMS, strength loss, and loss of strength. (c) Macrophages become more abundant and ROS continue to be produced. The extent of cellular injury continues to increase. Factors to terminate inflammatory cell activity and promote regeneration of cellular structures gain momentum. (d) Inflammatory cells are eventually cleared and tissue regeneration is completed.

including apoptotic removal of inflammatory cells and regeneration of cytoskeletal and contractile proteins takes several weeks (Paulsen et al. 2012).

The inflammation response to EIMD is aseptic and severity is influenced by the local production of RONS. With EIMD, there is no pathogen to be eliminated and the amount of intracellular damage is influenced by RONS-generating processes that occur either during the exercise or from oxidative burst activity of inflammatory cells (neutrophils and macrophages). RONS stimulate adaptation, removal of damaged proteins, and inflammation (Radak et al. 2012). Thus, the underlying questions of most interest for many researchers are (1) whether it is beneficial to reduce the inflammatory response, and (2) whether there are nutritional strategies effective for influencing the extent of inflammation and EIMD. While the questions of whether reducing inflammation limits exercise-induced adaptations for athletes is quite interesting and important, it remains a provocative question at this point in time. Regardless, nutritional strategies to limit inflammation and EIMD have been investigated.

NUTRITIONAL COUNTERMEASURES TO REDUCE EIMD

The use of nutrients to influence EIMD is most likely to be effective when the function and timing are matched to the processes underlying the development of damage or the recovery process. There is an association between inflammation biomarkers and both DOMS and swelling (Miles et al. 2008). Further, there is direct evidence of inflammatory cell infiltration into damaged muscle (MacIntyre et al. 1996). Thus, there is evidence associating underlying inflammation and indirect markers of muscle damage. Consequently, most of the research on nutritional countermeasures has focused on potentially anti-inflammatory nutrients, and indirect markers of EIMD are measured to determine efficacy. Alternatively, carbohydrate, protein, and nutrients with anabolic properties have been widely used to limit protein breakdown or to promote recovery and adaptation. For the purposes of this chapter, the former is most directly related to the immune system and will be given the most attention.

Dietary strategies and supplements to reduce EIMD have been widely researched. These strategies involve the following mechanisms:

1. Protection against RONS
2. Reducing metabolic stress by making energy nutrients available during exercise
3. Providing nutrients that stimulate protein synthesis during recovery

The immune system is linked to RONS as activators of and participants in the inflammatory process, and this aspect of EIMD is an important topic within the area of nutrition, exercise, and immunology. Energy availability also influences the immune response to exercise, as discussed in the previous section on "Modulation of the Acute Immune Response with Carbohydrate Supplementation." Nutrients to stimulate recovery are discussed briefly next.

The role of RONS in converting focal, pinpoint disruptions of skeletal muscle ultrastructure to large areas of inflammatory destruction is widely recognized as a factor potentially influencing the magnitude of EIMD. Anti-inflammatory nutrients, nutrient cocktails, or foods have been extensively investigated as a means of reducing EIMD. As noted previously, whether short-term reduction of EIMD is beneficial, neutral, or detrimental to long-term training outcomes is not known. This issue is well documented and analyzed in a recent review by Peternelj and Coombes (2011), in which these researchers concluded that (1) evidence to support the use of antioxidants to decrease EIMD is lacking, and (2) the possibility that antioxidant supplements may undermine beneficial adaptations to training is gaining support. However, having measured similar training adaptations in placebo and vitamin E and C supplemented groups of reasonably well-trained individuals prior to onset of training, other researchers have proposed the idea that blunting of training adaptations by antioxidant supplements may be more likely in unfit or low fit individuals (Yfanti et al. 2010). One important point to note is that most investigations of EIMD focus on indirect markers of muscle damage (DOMS, strength, efflux of intramuscular proteins such as creatine kinase or myoglobin, range of motion, swelling) or biomarkers of inflammation, and they do not directly assess muscle damage (electron micrographs of muscle) or oxidative stress (Peternelj and Coombes 2011). With these limitations in mind, there have been studies to show inflammation and/or EIMD decreases in response to the following nutritional countermeasures:

- Consumption of cherry juice (Bowtell et al. 2011)
- Consumption of blueberries (McLeay et al. 2012)
- Supplementation with vitamin E (Silva et al. 2010)
- Supplementation with vitamins E and C plus selenium (Bloomer et al. 2004)

There have been studies to show inflammation and EIMD are not affected by the following nutritional countermeasures:

- Supplementation with vitamins C and or E (Theodorou et al. 2011)
- Supplementation with quercetin (O'Fallon et al. 2012)
- Supplementation with fish oil and isoflavones (Lenn et al. 2002)
- Supplementation with coenzyme Q10 (Ostman et al. 2012)

Finally, there have been studies to show that inflammation and/or EIMD may be made worse by the following nutritional countermeasures:

- Vitamin C and N-acetyl-cysteine (Childs et al. 2001) or N-acetyl-cysteine alone (Cobley et al. 2011)
- Vitamin E (Nieman et al. 2004)
- Antioxidant cocktail of alpha-tocopherol, vitamin C, beta-carotene, lutein, selenium, zinc, and magnesium (Teixeira et al. 2009)

For the sake of brevity, the above lists do not include all of the studies or all of the nutritional countermeasures that have been investigated, and only studies based on human participants are reported, those with trained participants when possible. Regardless, the reported research is sufficient to illustrate that there is little in the way of nutritional countermeasures that consistently reduce EIMD or related inflammation. Dosing and time course differences across studies make comparisons and interpretation difficult. There are no clear recommendations to be made regarding use of antioxidants to decrease EIMD or related inflammation.

While evidence to support recommendations of supplemental nutrition is not convincing, there is some evidence that dietary intake of some foods or recommended intakes of antioxidant nutrients may be more consistently beneficial. For example, a comparison of female professional soccer (football) players who met vs. those who did not meet Dietary Reference Intakes (DRI) for macro- and micronutrients found higher levels of intramuscular protein efflux after a match in the players who were below the DRI for carbohydrate and vitamin E (Gravina et al. 2012). Trained runners ingesting tart cherry juice for one week prior to a long distance relay race (26.3 ± 2.5 km average distance run) had lower post-race soreness than those consuming placebo (Kuehl et al. 2010). In contrast, a recent study including a fruit and vegetable juice containing 230 mg of flavonoids consumed before and immediately after swim workouts in elite level swimmers did not elicit a measurable anti-inflammatory benefit; however, levels of inflammation were low throughout the study (Knab et al. 2013). In combination with the lowering of muscle damage and inflammation with cherry juice and blueberries, it does seem that athletes can safely focus on consumption of an antioxidant-rich diet, as this is one area in which beneficial or neutral, but not detrimental, findings are consistent. Additional research to clarify the doses, timing, and situations to which supplements may provide protection against EIMD appears warranted.

Having identified RONS and inflammation as important issues related to nutrition and immunology for elite athletes, it is important to describe other nutritional influences on EIMD related to the roles of carbohydrate and protein. Rather than influencing the immune system, protein, essential amino acids, branched chain amino acids, amino acid metabolites, and carbohydrate have been used to decrease post-exercise protein degradation and stimulate anabolic processes. There is the usual assortment of studies showing either no effect or a benefit, but few if any reports of detrimental effects to EIMD indicators and anabolic responses. Thus, following the sports nutrition guidelines for macronutrient intake composition, amounts, and timing (Kerksick et al. 2008; Rodriguez et al. 2009) is likely to be the wisest course of action for athletes. It is worth noting that a recent review concluded that supplementation of the leucine metabolite beta-hydroxy-beta-methylbutyrate (HMB) is safe and effective for reducing and enhancing recovery from EIMD in trained athletes when a dose of approximately 3 g/day is taken for at least two weeks (Molfino et al. 2013).

NUTRITION AND OVERREACHING OR OVERTRAINING

Diagnosis of overreaching or overtraining is complicated by the wide variety of signs and symptoms associated with these states. A decrease in exercise performance ability despite intense training efforts is the primary symptom associated with conditions of either overreaching or overtraining. A period of rest restores performance in overreaching but is not sufficient to restore performance capacity when overtraining syndrome occurs (Smith 2004). Other common symptoms include a perception by an athlete of "staleness" or "burnout." Beyond these central symptoms and perceptions, there is an extensive list of signs and symptoms that are common occurrences associated with and resulting in the designation of overreaching and overtraining as syndromes. According to a review and hypothesis paper by Smith (2004), the signs or symptoms of overtraining syndrome that involve the immune system are constant fatigue, muscle and joint aches and pains, headaches, nausea, gastrointestinal disturbances, muscle soreness or tenderness, increased incidence and severity of illnesses, infections and allergy symptoms, and lymph gland enlargement.

The factors that influence the likelihood of an athlete developing overtraining syndrome are unclear and several hypotheses have been proposed. Insufficient recovery relative to the stress of exercise training is a generally agreed on component of the mechanism (Smith 2004). To that end, the influence of nutrition on overtraining may include the influence of nutrient availability on the stress response during exercise, the recovery process, and possibly a more general influence of nutrition on the immune system.

Immune function measures in athletes during increased training periods or with overtraining are consistent with increased infection risk. There are small but potentially significant shifts in some measures of innate immunity that occur as well-trained athletes increase training volumes or intensities (Moreira et al. 2009). In the acquired arm of the immune system, lower circulating concentrations of type 1 T helper (Th1) lymphocytes responsible for promoting cellular immune responses, lower T cell proliferation responses, and lower levels of Ig production by stimulated B cells all have been measured in well-trained athletes when increased training loads were undertaken (Walsh et al. 2011b). Consistent with lower Ig production by stimulated B cells, a decrease in salivary IgA is a commonly measured phenomenon across severely stressful challenges, such as military training that may include various combinations of insufficient energy intake, high physical demands, sleep deprivation, environmental extremes, and psychological stress (Gleeson and Robson-Ansley 2006). A decrease in Th1 lymphocytes results in a decrease of the Th1/type 2 T helper (Th2) lymphocyte ratio. This reflects a shift to fewer cells producing IL-2 and IFN-γ and to more cells producing IL-4, IL-6, and IL-10. Some researchers have proposed that this shift or skewing toward Th2 may be in response to increased influence of glucocorticoids and catecholamines and leave athletes more susceptible to RTI (Martin et al. 2009; Smith 2004). In these situations, it is likely that the cumulative stress is the key factor, and nutrition is one of many factors to be considered when training is intensified. Poor nutrition may increase and optimal nutrition may decrease the level of stress for an athlete.

SUPPLEMENTS

Overconsumption of some nutrients may reduce immune function. As noted earlier in the chapter, there is debate as to whether suppression of the inflammatory response to tissue injury may limit the ability to repair and regenerate. Further, anti-inflammatory nutrients may also be immunosuppressive. Thus, athletes are cautioned against n-3 fatty acid intakes greater than 2.5 g/day (Walsh 2006). Additionally, high intakes of the micronutrients iron, zinc, and vitamin E (>200 mg/day) are capable of reducing immune defenses and increasing incidence of RTI (Chandra 1997; Gleeson 2006a). Consistent with most other physiologic systems, immune system performance will only be enhanced by intake of nutrient supplements when the supplement reverses a malnutrition deficiency. Thus, in the absence of known nutrient deficiencies, it may be better to avoid potential detrimental effects of supplements by discouraging indiscriminate use of n-3 fatty acid, iron, zinc, and vitamin E supplements.

It is important to be aware that high doses of some micronutrients, doses that can only occur with the intake of supplements, can inhibit certain immune functions. For example, high doses of both zinc and iron can decrease aspects of immune function and increase susceptibility to infection (Gleeson 2006a). Thus, where there is concern for adequate intake of one of these micronutrients, the recommendation is for athletes to be aware of foods that are rich sources and target their food intake to ensure intakes at or above recommended levels.

There is a great deal of interest in dietary supplements that may help athletes boost immunity. Table 10.3 lists some of the key supplements that have been researched

TABLE 10.3

Dietary Supplements and Their Influence on RTI Incidence for Exercising Humans

Supplement	Dose and Timing	Effect
Glutamine	5 g during exercise	Mixed findings, but typically viewed as having no effect
Vitamin C	600–1000 mg/day vs. placebo for 3 weeks to 2 months prior to marathon/ultramarathon competitions	Mixed findings of either a decrease in upper RTI symptoms/incidence or no effect
β-Glucan	5.6 g/day vs. placebo for 2 weeks prior to a 3-day challenge of 3 h exercise per day	No effect
Quercetin	1000 mg/day vs. placebo for 3 weeks prior to 3 days of exhaustive exercise	Decrease in upper RTI symptoms/incidence but no change in direct measures of immune function
Lactobacillus probiotics	1–2 daily doses for 11–16 weeks	Possible benefit, but more research is needed
Bovine serum colostrum	25 g·d⁻¹ (no change) to 60 g·d⁻¹ (decrease in upper RTI symptoms)	Possible benefit, but more research is needed

Source: Walsh, N.P. et al. 2011. *Exerc Immunol Rev* 17:64–103; Reprinted from *Immune Function in Sport and Exercise*, M. Gleeson, Ed., Walsh, N.P., 161–182, Copyright 2006, with permission from Elsevier; Nieman, D.C. 2008. *Nutr Rev* 66(6):310–320; Gunzer, W. et al. 2012. *Nutrients* 4(9):1187–1212; Akerstrom, T.C., and B.K. Pedersen. 2007. *Sports Med* 37(4–5):416–419. With permission.

regarding their influence on exercise-induced immune responses and RTI incidence. A current area of research interest is to address the hypotheses that (1) a "cocktail" approach to supplements containing several active elements may be effective in reducing RTI rates, for example, quercetin, fish oil, and green tea in combination, and (2) supplements that enhance the innate immune system may be the most effective for reducing RTI rates (Walsh et al. 2011a). However, given the potential negative effects of supplement use, recommendations linked to these hypotheses will have to wait until further evidence is available.

SUMMARY

There are a number of ways for athletes to influence immune function, including nutritional strategies. A wide array of nutrients supports immune system function. Carbohydrate intake and availability during exercise has a profound impact on the magnitude of exercise-induced stress hormone responses and related immune changes. Nutritional recommendations to maintain immune health are consistent with nutritional recommendations to support high training intensities and volumes. Some supplements may offer a degree of protection to lower risk of RTI, but further research is needed. There is evidence that inclusion of antioxidant-rich foods in the diet may be a safe strategy to reduce ROS and lower EIMD, but findings relating to antioxidant supplements are inconsistent. The pathology of overtraining is likely to include the immune system, but research on nutritional strategies to lower risk of RTI is limited. Available research is supportive of following sports nutrition guidelines for sufficient energy, carbohydrate, protein, fats, vitamins, minerals, and fluids, as well as timing of nutrient intake as a means of providing optimal support for the immune system.

REFERENCES

Akerstrom, T.C., and B.K. Pedersen. 2007. Strategies to enhance immune function for marathon runners: What can be done? *Sports Med* 37(4–5):416–419.
Bishop, N.C. 2006. Exercise and infection risk. In *Immune Function in Sport and Exercise Science*, M. Gleeson, Ed. Edinburgh: Churchill Livingstone Elsevier, 1–14.
Blannin, A.K. 2006. Acute exercise and innate immune function. In *Immune function in sport and exercise*, M. Gleeson, Ed. Edinburgh: Churchill Livingstone Elsevier, 67–90.
Bloomer, R.J., A.H. Goldfarb, M.J. McKenzie, T. You, and L. Nguyen. 2004. Effects of antioxidant therapy in women exposed to eccentric exercise. *Int J Sport Nutr Exerc Metab* 14(4):377–388.
Bowtell, J.L., D.P. Sumners, A. Dyer, P. Fox, and K.N. Mileva. 2011. Montmorency cherry juice reduces muscle damage caused by intensive strength exercise. *Med Sci Sports Exerc* 43(8):1544–1551.
Chandra, R.K. 1997. Nutrition and the immune system: An introduction. *Am J Clin Nutr* 66(2):460S–463S.
Childs, A., C. Jacobs, T. Kaminski, B. Halliwell, and C. Leeuwenburgh. 2001. Supplementation with vitamin C and N-acetyl-cysteine increases oxidative stress in humans after an acute muscle injury induced by eccentric exercise. *Free Radic Biol Med* 31(6):745–753.
Cobley, J.N., C. McGlory, J.P. Morton, and G.L. Close. 2011. N-Acetylcysteine's attenuation of fatigue after repeated bouts of intermittent exercise: Practical implications for tournament situations. *Int J Sport Nutr Exerc Metab* 21(6):451–461.
Faulkner, J.A., S.V. Brooks, and J.A. Opiteck. 1993. Injury to skeletal muscle fibers during contractions: Conditions of occurrence and prevention. *Phys Ther* 73(12):911–921.
Friden, J., and R.L. Lieber. 1998. Segmental muscle fiber lesions after repetitive eccentric contractions. *Cell Tissue Res* 293(1):165–171.
Gleeson, M. 2006a. Exercise, nutrition and immune function. II. Micronutrients, antioxidants and other supplements. In *Immune Function in Sport and Exercise*, M. Gleeson, Ed. Edinburgh: Churchill Livingstone Elsevier, 183–204.
Gleeson, M. 2006b. Introduction to the immune system. In *Immune function in sport and exercise*, M. Gleeson, Ed. Edinburgh: Churchill Livingstone Elsevier, 15–44.
Gleeson, M., and P. Robson-Ansley. 2006. Immune responses to intensified training and overtraining. In *Immune Function in Sport and Exercise*, M. Gleeson, Ed. Edinburgh: Churchill Livingstone Elsevier, 115–138.
Gleeson, M., and N.P. Walsh. 2012. The BASES expert statement on exercise, immunity, and infection. *J Sports Sci* 30(3):321–324.
Gravina, L., F. Ruiz, E. Diaz et al. 2012. Influence of nutrient intake on antioxidant capacity, muscle damage and white blood cell count in female soccer players. *J Int Soc Sports Nutr* 9(1):32.
Gunzer, W., M. Konrad, and E. Pail. 2012. Exercise-induced immunodepression in endurance athletes and nutritional intervention with carbohydrate, protein and fat—What is possible, what is not? *Nutrients* 4(9):1187–1212.

Kerksick, C., T. Harvey, J. Stout et al. 2008. International Society of Sports Nutrition position stand: Nutrient timing. *J Int Soc Sports Nutr* 5:17.

Knab, A.M., D.C. Nieman, N.D. Gillitt et al. 2013. Effects of a flavonoid-rich juice on inflammation, oxidative stress, and immunity in elite swimmers: A metabolomics-based approach. *Int J Sport Nutr Exerc Metab* 23(2):150–160.

Kuehl, K.S., E.T. Perrier, D.L. Elliot, and J.C. Chesnutt. 2010. Efficacy of tart cherry juice in reducing muscle pain during running: A randomized controlled trial. *J Int Soc Sports Nutr* 7:17.

Lenn, J., T. Uhl, C. Mattacola et al. 2002. The effects of fish oil and isoflavones on delayed onset muscle soreness. *Med Sci Sports Exerc* 34(10):1605–1613.

MacIntyre, D.L., W.D. Reid, D.M. Lyster, I.J. Szasz, and D.C. McKenzie. 1996. Presence of WBC, decreased strength, and delayed soreness in muscle after eccentric exercise. *J Appl Physiol* 80(3):1006–1013.

Martin, S.A., B.D. Pence, and J.A. Woods. 2009. Exercise and respiratory tract viral infections. *Exerc Sport Sci Rev* 37(4):157–164.

McLeay, Y., M.J. Barnes, T. Mundel, S.M. Hurst, R.D. Hurst, and S.R. Stannard. 2012. Effect of New Zealand blueberry consumption on recovery from eccentric exercise-induced muscle damage. *J Int Soc Sports Nutr* 9(1):19.

Miles, M.P., and P.M. Clarkson. 1994. Exercise-induced muscle pain, soreness, and cramps. *J Sports Med Phys Fitness* 34(3):203–216.

Miles, M.P., J.M. Andring, S.D. Pearson et al. 2008. Diurnal variation, response to eccentric exercise, and association of inflammatory mediators with muscle damage variables. *J Appl Physiol* 104(2):451–458.

Molfino, A., G. Gioia, F. Rossi Fanelli, and M. Muscaritoli. 2013. Beta-hydroxy-beta-methylbutyrate supplementation in health and disease: A systematic review of randomized trials. *Amino Acids* 45(6):1273–1292.

Moreira, A., L. Delgado, P. Moreira, and T. Haahtela. 2009. Does exercise increase the risk of upper respiratory tract infections? *Br Med Bull* 90:111–131.

Nieman, D.C. 1994. Exercise, infection, and immunity. *Int J Sports Med* 15(Suppl 3):S131–S141.

Nieman, D.C. 2008. Immunonutrition support for athletes. *Nutr Rev* 66(6):310–320.

Nieman, D.C., D.A. Henson, S.R. McAnulty et al. 2004. Vitamin E and immunity after the Kona Triathlon World Championship. *Med Sci Sports Exerc* 36(8):1328–1335.

O'Fallon, K.S., D. Kaushik, B. Michniak-Kohn, C.P. Dunne, E.J. Zambraski, and P.M. Clarkson. 2012. Effects of quercetin supplementation on markers of muscle damage and inflammation after eccentric exercise. *Int J Sport Nutr Exerc Metab* 22(6):430–437.

Ostman, B., A. Sjodin, K. Michaelsson, and L. Byberg. 2012. Coenzyme Q10 supplementation and exercise-induced oxidative stress in humans. *Nutrition* 28(4):403–417.

Paulsen, G., U.R. Mikkelsen, T. Raastad, and J.M. Peake. 2012. Leucocytes, cytokines and satellite cells: What role do they play in muscle damage and regeneration following eccentric exercise? *Exerc Immunol Rev* 18:42–97.

Peternelj, T.T., and J.S. Coombes. 2011. Antioxidant supplementation during exercise training: Beneficial or detrimental? *Sports Med* 41(12):1043–1069.

Radak, Z., Z. Zhao, E. Koltai, H. Ohno, and M. Atalay. 2012. Oxygen consumption and usage during physical exercise: The balance between oxidative stress and ROS-dependent adaptive signaling. *Antioxid Redox Signal* 18(10):1208–1246.

Rodriguez, N.R., N.M. DiMarco, and S. Langley. 2009. Position of the American Dietetic Association, Dietitians of Canada, and the American College of Sports Medicine: Nutrition and athletic performance. *J Am Diet Assoc* 109(3):509–527.

Silva, L.A., C.A. Pinho, P.C. Silveira et al. 2010. Vitamin E supplementation decreases muscular and oxidative damage but not inflammatory response induced by eccentric contraction. *J Physiol Sci* 60(1):51–57.

Smith, L.L. 2004. Tissue trauma: The underlying cause of overtraining syndrome? *J Strength Cond Res* 18(1):185–193.

Smith, L.L., and M.P. Miles. 2000. Exercise-induced muscle injury and inflammation. In *Exercise and sport science*, W.E. Garrett, and D.T. Kirkendall, Eds. Philadelphia, PA: Lippincott Williams & Wilkins, 401–411.

Teixeira, V.H., H.F. Valente, S.I. Casal, A.F. Marques, and P.A. Moreira. 2009. Antioxidants do not prevent postexercise peroxidation and may delay muscle recovery. *Med Sci Sports Exerc* 41(9):1752–1760.

Theodorou, A.A., M.G. Nikolaidis, V. Paschalis et al. 2011. No effect of antioxidant supplementation on muscle performance and blood redox status adaptations to eccentric training. *Am J Clin Nutr* 93(6):1373–1383.

Walsh, N.P. 2006. Exercise, nutrition, and immune function. I. Macronutrients and amino acids. In *Immune Function in Sport and Exercise*, M. Gleeson, Ed. Edinburgh: Churchill Livingstone Elsevier, 161–182.

Walsh, N.P., M. Gleeson, D.B. Pyne et al. 2011a. Position statement. Part two: Maintaining immune health. *Exerc Immunol Rev* 17:64–103.

Walsh, N.P., M. Gleeson, R.J. Shephard et al. 2011b. Position statement. Part one: Immune function and exercise. *Exerc Immunol Rev* 17:6–63.

Yfanti, C., T. Akerstrom, S. Nielsen et al. 2010. Antioxidant supplementation does not alter endurance training adaptation. *Med Sci Sports Exerc* 42(7):1388–1395.

11 Hydration for High-Level Athletes

Douglas J. Casa, PhD, ATC, FACSM, FNATA

Lawrence E. Armstrong, PhD, FACSM
Korey Stringer Institute, Department of Kinesiology,
University of Connecticut, Storrs, Connecticut

Mathew S. Ganio, PhD

Stavros A. Kavouras, PhD, FACSM
Department of Health, Human Performance and
Recreation, University of Arkansas, Fayetteville, Arkansas

Rebecca L. Stearns, PhD, ATC
Korey Stringer Institute, Department of Kinesiology,
University of Connecticut, Storrs, Connecticut

Jonathan E. Wingo, PhD
Department of Kinesiology, University of Alabama,
Tuscaloosa, Alabama

CONTENTS

Numerous factors can influence the performance outcome for elite athletes. Whether it be training, equipment, nutrition, heat acclimatization, or a myriad of other possibilities, the athlete faces a laundry list of items for which to develop a plan in order to optimize performance outcomes. One of the factors that high-level athletes in a wide variety of sports must consider is a hydration strategy that is specific to the confines of the sport, environmental conditions, and individual considerations. The aim of this chapter is to show how hydration plays a role in physiological function and to offer practical solutions on how to best develop an individualized hydration strategy to optimize performance during training and competition.

PHYSIOLOGICAL CONSIDERATIONS OF HYDRATION, DEHYDRATION, AND REHYDRATION

Adequate fluid balance is paramount for optimal physiological function in elite athletes. An important part of achieving adequate fluid balance is understanding the physiological responses related to hydration, dehydration, and rehydration. Accordingly, the following subsections will address the physiological considerations related to these processes.

HYDRATION

Hydration is the process of adding water to body tissues and herein refers to the period of fluid intake prior to starting exercise. This process results in several physiological responses; the response most related to elite athletic performance is optimization of intravascular fluid volume because arguably this fluid compartment has the greatest impact on athletic performance, at least in endurance-type events. Additionally, this fluid compartment is heavily defended during dynamic exercise, which provides further evidence of its relevance to elite athletic performance. Accordingly, the hydration goal of elite athletes, at least those competing in events that could be negatively affected by hypohydration (e.g., endurance athletes), should be to ensure euhydration combined with normal plasma electrolyte levels. "Topping off" the intravascular fluid compartment with adequate pre-exercise hydration will optimize cardiovascular stability and temperature regulation during subsequent exercise.

As fluid is ingested, fluid balance is achieved as the various fluid compartments (intracellular, extracellular) equilibrate. Urine output increases with elevated fluid intake (Sawka et al. 2007), so a prolonged period (e.g., 8–12 h) may be necessary to optimize pre-exercise hydration. Sodium ingestion in the form of meals, snacks, and beverages will augment fluid retention. A prolonged hydration period may not be feasible in circumstances in which repeated practices or competitions occur in close chronological proximity to one another. In such instances, a more aggressive pre-exercise hydration strategy may be needed.

Interestingly, inadequate pre-exercise hydration (i.e., voluntary dehydration) is offset by increased thirst-driven drinking during subsequent exercise (Maresh et al. 2004). This results in plasma volume, plasma osmolality, and fluid regulatory hormone responses that are comparable to those encountered if exercise is begun in a euhydrated state and fluid is ingested *ad libitum* during exercise (Maresh et al. 2004). That said, increased thirst-driven drinking during exercise requires greater fluid availability in order to avoid negative effects of dehydration (discussed next), so it is recommended that exercise be started in a euhydrated state.

DEHYDRATION

Dehydration refers to the loss of water from the body. For this discussion, it will also refer to hypohydration, the state of being in a body water deficit beyond the normal fluctuation in body water content (Sawka et al. 2007). The importance of dehydration is illustrated in the plethora of scientific literature devoted to the topic. This research has helped refine our understanding of the physiological considerations related to dehydration.

Under conditions of low volumes of body water loss, fluid is lost primarily from the extracellular space, while under conditions of high body water loss, fluid is lost more from the intracellular space (Sawka et al. 2001). Regardless, generally dehydration associated with exercise results in a hypertonic hypovolemia (Sawka 1992). Sweating results in hypotonic fluid loss, thereby rendering the vasculature hyperosmotic. In heat-acclimated persons, sweat is more hypotonic, and therefore the resultant plasma volume is more hypertonic relative to the intracellular and interstitial fluid spaces, so intravascular fluid volume is more efficiently defended in these individuals (Shibasaki et al. 2006). However, dehydration negates the benefits of heat acclimation because for a given metabolic intensity, sweat rate and skin blood flow are lower (likely because of elevated plasma osmolality and hypovolemia for sweating and skin blood flow, respectively) at a given core temperature (Montain et al. 1995; Sawka et al. 2001). These decrements in heat dissipating mechanisms result in less heat dissipation, greater heat storage, and higher core temperature for a given exercise intensity. This topic will be discussed in depth in a subsequent section of this chapter.

In addition to alterations in evaporative (sweating) and dry (skin blood flow) heat exchange, dehydration also results in elevated cardiovascular strain. This topic has been covered thoroughly in the scientific literature and is too extensive to be exhaustively covered here, but is highlighted in studies investigating the effect of dehydration on cardiovascular drift (progressive increase in heart rate and decrease in stroke volume during prolonged, constant-rate, submaximal intensity exercise). During prolonged (120 min) exercise in a warm environment (30°C), dehydration exacerbates the magnitude of cardiovascular drift and results in reduced peak oxygen uptake (Figure 11.1; Ganio et al. 2006).

Besides exacerbated cardiovascular drift, during exercise in hot conditions dehydration also reduces cardiac output, systemic vascular conductance, and active skeletal muscle blood flow relative to euhydration (Gonzalez-Alonso et al. 1999). This does not result in altered substrate delivery to muscle cells, but dehydration-associated elevated muscle temperature results in greater carbohydrate oxidation and muscle glycogenolysis (Gonzalez-Alonso et al. 1999; Logan-Sprenger et al. 2012). If carbohydrate and fluid availability are limited during exercise, this may result in premature fatigue.

To combat the intravascular fluid compartment deficits associated with dehydration, the kidneys release renin in response to increased renal sympathetic nerve

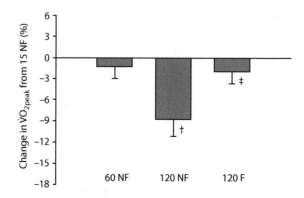

FIGURE 11.1 Mean ± SEM peak oxygen uptake ($\dot{V}O_{2peak}$), expressed as a percentage change from the value after cycling at 60% $\dot{V}O_{2peak}$ for 15 min with no fluid (15 NF), relative to values measured after cycling at 60% $\dot{V}O_{2peak}$ for 60 min with no fluid (60 NF), 120 min with no fluid, or 120 min with sufficient fluid to offset sweat losses (120 NF). † = significantly different from 15 NF; ‡ = significantly different from 120 NF. (From Ganio, M.S. et al. 2006. *Med Sci Sports Exerc* 38:901–909. With permission.)

activity, which starts a cascade of responses involving angiotensin and aldosterone that serve to conserve plasma sodium levels and thereby fluid volume. Additionally, in response to elevated plasma osmolality, the posterior pituitary gland releases antidiuretic hormone, which fosters fluid retention. In addition to fluid retention effects, these hormones also increase pre-capillary resistance and vasoconstriction in inactive tissues, which helps defend diminished blood volume by decreasing capillary hydrostatic pressure that then fosters greater net absorption.

REHYDRATION

Rehydration refers to the restoration of fluid to achieve a euhydrated state. In this context, this refers to fluid intake that occurs either during exercise or after exercise. The general rehydration goal is to avoid more than 2% dehydration or otherwise performance decrements will ensue (described in a subsequent section of this chapter).

Rehydration is driven largely by thirst, which is driven largely by plasma osmolality. Fluid regulating hormones, like antidiuretic hormone, will aid in minimizing water loss by the kidneys, but this system cannot restore fluid that has been lost (Mack 2012). Therefore, adequate thirst mechanisms must be in place to stimulate fluid replacement. Humans are generally slow rehydrators and as such often voluntarily dehydrate by consuming too little water after exercise-induced dehydration. This seems to be caused by electrolyte deficits in the intracellular and extracellular fluid spaces as well as retention of ingested fluid in the vascular space that curbs thirst (Mack 2012). As a result, elite athletes should consciously consume adequate sodium (which aids fluid retention) in post-exercise beverages and food, and they should consider ingesting beverages with flavor because this has been shown to maximize the rate of rehydration (Mack 2012). Approaches to developing individualized hydration plans are discussed in a later section of this chapter.

INFLUENCE OF HYDRATION STATUS ON BODY TEMPERATURE

In laboratory settings, when athletes perform intense aerobic exercise in the heat and become hypohydrated to a level ≥2% body mass loss (BML), there is a predictable increase in physiological strain and decrease in performance. For example, during exercise in the heat, body core temperature and heart rate (HR) increase by 0.12 to 0.2°C and 3 to 5 beats per minute, respectively, for every 1% of body mass lost (Buono and Wall 2000; Montain and Coyle 1992; Montain et al. 1998; Sawka et al. 1985). This graded core temperature increase with increasing water deficits suggests that physiological adjustments are both necessary and successful for preserving heat loss when skin blood flow is reduced. Evidence for the greater physiological strain and resultant compromised performance includes increased HR, decreased stroke volume, thermoregulatory strain, stress response, and perception of effort and anticipatory regulation of pace, hypovolemia, and hyperosmolality, among other factors (Casa et al. 2000a; Gonzalez-Alonso et al. 2000; Judelson et al. 2007; Maresh et al. 2001; Montain and Coyle 1992; Sawka et al. 2001; Turkevich et al. 1988).

Because exercise intensity is the single greatest influence on the rate of core temperature rise in the heat (Marino et al. 2004; Saltin and Hermansen 1966; Tucker et al. 2004), many of these laboratory studies controlled intensity. Also regulated in well-controlled studies were other variables that could compromise consistency among trials, including ambient temperature, humidity, length of exercise, time of day, nutritional intake, clothing, wind, and heat acclimatization status. Only when these variables are controlled can the influence of hydration status be isolated (Noakes et al. 1991).

Recent field studies also have examined the influence of hydration status on numerous physiological and performance outcomes, notably body core temperature and finishing time. Many of these studies have reported findings inconsistent with those of the laboratory studies noted previously: body temperatures did not increase with dehydration (Cheuvront et al. 2007; Davies 1979; Fowkes Godek et al. 2004, 2006; Laursen et al. 2006). Moreover, other performance outcomes were not related to hydration status and, in some cases, greater dehydration was associated with a performance advantage (Byrne et al. 2006; Laursen et al. 2006).

Variable intensity of exercise in field studies and not a lack of research quality in either setting is the cause of the different findings. Athletes who are allowed to perform an exercise task unsupervised may manipulate intensity based on physiological and psychological feedback. For instance, a severely dehydrated athlete may either decrease intensity in response to certain cues for self-protection or simply be limited by physiological constraints (Fudge et al. 2007; Gonzalez-Alonso et al. 2000; Judelson et al. 2007; Maughan et al. 1985; McNair et al. 1971; Sharwood et al. 2004). Thus, this person may actually have a lower body core temperature because intensity has decreased (Sampson and Kobrick 1980). Similarly, a euhydrated person can perform at a higher intensity for a longer period of time and, ironically, may have a higher body core temperature than a dehydrated counterpart (Marino et al. 2004). Both scenarios are possible in a field setting when intensity is not controlled. Thus, the premise that certain physiological responses (e.g., body core temperature) are not influenced by hydration status may, in fact, reflect uncontrolled intensity and not hydration status itself. Comparing field vs. laboratory findings has been made even more difficult by additional variables, such as the lack of crossover, within-subjects comparisons and uncontrolled weather conditions (temperature, humidity, solar, wind), and other factors in field studies. Therefore, it is important to assess field studies that control variables that may influence physiological strain (i.e., exercise intensity and hydration level).

Two such studies have been recently published (Casa et al. 2010; Lopez et al. 2011) that specifically controlled key variables in order to isolate the influence of hydration status on body temperature during a field study. The basic premise examined was, does the detrimental role of dehydration on exaggerated hyperthermic response during intense exercise in the heat that has been consistently shown in well-controlled laboratory studies exist in the field setting, or is some unique response in the field setting precluding the occurrence of this physiological outcome? The first study (Casa et al. 2010) controlled for finishing time in a submaximal effort while manipulating a small difference in hydration status (2% vs. 4% BML) in a crossover design in similar environmental conditions. They found that the relationship between level of dehydration and extent of hyperthermia was nearly identical to the previous laboratory findings. Specifically, they found an additional 0.22°C increase in body temperature and 6 beats per minute (BPM) increase in heart rate for every additional 1% BML. Additionally, they found that performance was enhanced when athletes were better-hydrated (~2% vs. 4% BML) when asked to run maximally in two other trials. Interestingly, whether in the sub-maximal or maximal effort, the runners exhibited less signs and symptoms of heat illness when better hydrated (even if they ran faster as in the maximal effort). A second recent study by Lopez et al. (2011) corroborated the findings of Casa et al. with a slight variation in the methodological design. They controlled two sub-maximal trials by matching heart rate (as compared to finishing time in the Casa et al. [2010] study) during the running event. They also utilized a crossover design comparing two levels of dehydration (2% vs. 4% BML). They also found results similar to the laboratory findings in that they reported a 0.17°C increase in core temperature for every additional 1% BML (see Table 11.1). In addition, they reported an increase in heat illness symptomatology and exaggerated Profile of Mood States (POMS) scores (Casa et al. [2010]

TABLE 11.1
Changes in Physiological Values for Each Additional 1% of BML: A Comparison of Field and Laboratory Studies

Physiological Value for Each Additional 1% BML	Field Studies		Laboratory Studies		
	Lopez et al. (2011)	Casa et al. (2010)	González-Alonso et al. (1997)	Sawka et al. (1985)	Montain and Coyle (1992)
Heart rate (b·min⁻¹)		6 ↑	1.5 ↑	4 ↑	4.5 ↑
Body temperature (°C)	0.17 ↑	0.22 ↑	0.25 ↑	0.15 ↑	0.23 ↑
Time (s)	44 ↓				

Source: Lopez, R.M. et al. 2011. *J Strength Cond Res* 25(11):2944–2954. With permission.

also found the same POMS responses) in the group that experienced just 2% additional BML. Therefore, the bottom line, whether it is field or laboratory settings, is that hydration plays a powerful, protective role in cooling the body during intense exercise in the heat. Additionally, it may play a role in preventing exertional heat illnesses.

In conclusion, it seems likely that the phenomenon related to exaggerated hyperthermia associated with dehydration that has been consistently shown in a laboratory setting exists when athletes perform intense athletic activities in the heat in a natural sport setting. The differences that have been noted between laboratory and field settings are linked to the methodological challenges in a field setting, which make it harder to isolate the effect, and not due to the absence of the physiological effect itself.

Two recent systematic reviews examined the influence of hydration on body temperature and heart rate. Huggins et al. (2012) and Adams et al. (2014) included 20 studies (both lab and field studies) that assessed the influence of hydration status on heart rate following variable or fixed intensity exercise in the heat and demonstrated an average increase of .22°C and 3 BPM for every additional 1% BML. The take-home for high-level athletes who care dearly about maximizing performance is that one of the best body cooling strategies they have at their disposal is to minimize the amount of dehydration during intense exercise in the heat. One such example of how dehydration may compromise performance during intense exercise in the heat is due to a decreased ability to accurately pace oneself during a maximal effort, as shown by Stearns et al. (2009) in a recent paper (Figure 11.2).

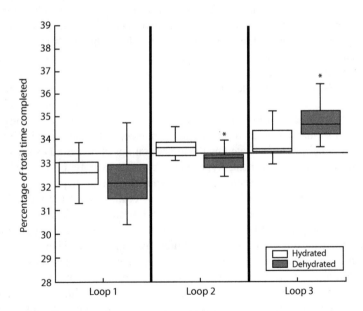

FIGURE 11.2 Percentage of total time completed per 2.5-mile loop. Represents the percentage of time each loop contributed to the total finishing time. *$p \leq .05$ when compared to hydrated trial at the same time point. The horizontal line at the 33.33% mark represents where an even pace for each loop would fall; therefore, a perfectly paced trial would have all three box plots along this line.

INFLUENCE OF HYDRATION STATUS ON EXERCISE PERFORMANCE

For over a century, athletes have noticed that exercise-induced dehydration has been linked to decreased exercise performance. Francisco Lázaro, a Portuguese marathon runner, was one of the first to notice that excessive sweating was making him slower. Therefore, he decided to stop dehydration by blocking sweating via application of wax over his skin during the 1912 Stockholm Olympics marathon. Unfortunately, he collapsed at the 30-km mark, and he died the next morning from complications of exertional heat stroke. Since the mid 1940s, scientists have also been interested in the effect of dehydration on exercise performance. For instance, in 1944, Pitts and his colleagues showed that dehydration, as a response to exercise in the heat, increased thermoregulatory strain and induced exhaustion (Pitts et al. 1944).

In 1980, Nadel and his colleagues found a significant decrease of stroke volume and cardiac output during exercise in the heat as a response to hypohydration (Nadel et al. 1980). A few years after, Armstrong et al. (1985) examined the effect of hypohydration on exercise performance. They studied the performance of eight trained, male runners on 1500 m, 5000 m, and 10,000 m while normally hydrated or hypohydrated on six separate occasions. Their running performance was reduced by 3.1%, 6.7%, and 6.3% in the 1500 m, 5000 m, and 10,000 m, respectively, as a response to hypohydration.

In the early 1990s, Montain and Coyle (1992) investigated the effect of graded hypohydration on temperature regulation and cardiovascular function. Eight trained individuals cycled in the heat for 2 h in four separate conditions while randomly receiving no, small, moderate, or large amounts of fluid in order to achieve a graded magnitude of hypohydration, ranging from −1% to −4% of their body mass. They concluded that the athletes' increase in heart rate and core temperature, as well as decline in stroke volume, was proportional to the degree of hypohydration during exercise. Similarly, Walsh and his colleagues, from the University of Cape Town in South Africa, investigated the effect of low levels of hypohydration on cycling performance in the heat (Walsh et al. 1994). They found that even a mild degree of hypohydration (−1.8% of body mass) decreased exercise performance, probably because of increased perception of fatigue, as indicated by the greater ratings of perceived exertion.

During exercise in the heat, hyperthermia and dehydration coincide, thereby making it difficult to examine whether hyperthermia or hypohydration limits exercise erformance. In 1997, González-Alonso et al. studied the individual and combined effects of hyperthermia and hypohydration on cardiovascular function (González-Alonso et al. 1997). They examined trained cyclists during 30 min of cycle ergometer exercise at 70% of maximal oxygen uptake. They demonstrated that both hyperthermia and hypohydration independently decreased cyclists' ability to maintain cardiac output during exercise. They also found that when these stress factors coincided, they had an additive effect on the decline of cardiac output similar to the sum of the decline for each factor alone. In a separate study, the same authors determined that during exercise in the heat, dehydration could markedly decrease blood flow to the exercising muscles by lowering perfusion pressure and systemic blood flow, rather than increasing vasoconstriction (González-Alonso et al. 1998).

Even though the effect of hypohydration has been mainly studied during exercise in the heat, it seems that even in a temperate environment hypohydration can limit exercise performance. In this regard, Cheuvront and his colleagues examined eight volunteers' cycling performance during a 30-min time trial, on four separate occasions, either while euhydrated or hypohydrated in a cold (2°C) or temperate (20°C) environment (Cheuvront et al. 2005). Their data indicated that hypohydration decreased performance only in the temperate, but not in the cold environment.

In some sports events (i.e., uphill cycling), athletes often believe that a decrease in body mass, even via dehydration, can enhance exercise performance by increasing the power to mass ratio. In this respect, Ebert et al. (2007) examined the effect of hypohydration during a hill cycling (8% grade) time exhaustion test in a warm environment at intensity equal to 88% of maximal aerobic power ($\dot{V}O_{2\,max}$) (Ebert et al. 2007). Prior to the performance, test subjects cycled for 2 h at 53% $\dot{V}O_{2\,max}$, while drinking different volumes of fluid in order to achieve the desired proportion of pre-exercise body mass (–2.5% vs. +0.3% of body mass). The results showed that even though cyclists were able to reduce their power requirements for any given cycling speed by lowering body mass, hypohydration had a significant detrimental effect on their performance.

Although hypohydration seems to negatively affect endurance exercise performance, at least in a laboratory setting, some scientists have argued that similar data are not found in real outdoors events. In 2010, Casa and his colleagues studied the effect of hypohydration on trail running in the heat (Casa et al. 2010). Seventeen male and female runners performed a 12-km trail run either euhydrated or hypohydrated at submaximal or maximal (race-like) intensities. The data indicated that during the maximal run, the performance was worse because of hypohydration. During the submaximal test, internal body temperature was greater during hypohydration. The authors concluded that even a small decrement in hydration state could impair physiological function and trail running performance in the heat. Likewise, Bardis et al. examined the effect of mild hypohydration during a short climbing cycling trial in the heat (Bardis et al. 2013a). Ten trained cyclists performed a 5-km outdoor hill cycling ride either euhydrated or hypohydrated by –1% of their body weight. The mild degree of hypohydration was linked to a 5.8% decrease in performance, as well as lower sweating and greater hyperthermia (see Figure 11.3).

Hypohydration has been also linked to declined skill performance in sports. Baker et al. (2007) examined the effect of hypohydration on 17 male basketball players in the heat during six separate conditions differing only by hydration status (two euhydrated and four hypohydrated by –1%, –2%, –3%, and –4% of body weight, respectively). Not only was the time to complete a basketball-specific movement drill slower, but also fewer shots were made when hypohydration reached –2% of body mass.

Recently, the effect of mild hypohydration on skeletal muscle metabolism was studied in nine females (Logan-Sprenger et al. 2012). Subjects cycled for 2 h at 65% of their $\dot{V}O_{2\,max}$ with or without fluid replacement. Progressive dehydration induced greater thermoregulatory and cardiovascular strain, as well as whole body carbohydrate oxidation and muscle glycogenolysis, evident from the –1% of body weight dehydration apparent during the first 1 h of cycling. Interestingly, Bardis et al. (2013b) examined the effect of mild hypohydration during a 30-km simulated-hill circuit course in a warm environment. The cycling course consisted of 3 bouts of

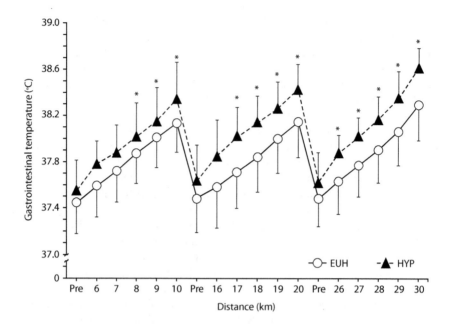

FIGURE 11.3   Gastrointestinal temperature (T_{GI}) of each kilometer during simulated-hill bouts (mean ± SD). *, Statistically significant differences, $p \le .05$ between trials at the same time point. (From Bardis, C. et al. 2013. *Med Sci Sports Exerc* 45:1782–1789. With permission.)

5 km at 50% of maximal power output and 5 km at an all-out-pace. Ten experienced cyclists rode either euhydrated or hypohydrated by –1% of their body mass, while drinking water to avoid significant change in their initial hydration status. Both mean cycling speed and power output were greater in the euhydrated trial due to lower body temperature and greater sweating sensitivity. There is some evidence that the act of drinking itself might have a beneficial effect on performance, probably due to activation of pharyngeal receptors (Arnaoutis et al. 2012).

INFLUENCE OF ERGOGENIC AIDS ON HYDRATION STATUS

Athletes take a large number of ergogenic aids in hopes of improving performance. This section will highlight three ergogenic aids that have consistently been shown to improve performance: caffeine, glycerol, and creatine. Although there are many other ergogenic aids, these deserve special attention because of their potential effect on hydration. Because dehydration can negatively affect performance, it is important for the athlete to understand if and how these ergogenic aids affect hydration status and ultimately their performance.

CAFFEINE

Caffeine is one of the most widely used substances taken by elite athletes. The high prevalence of use is likely due to caffeine's consistent beneficial effect on endurance performance and its legality at all levels of competition (Ganio et al. 2009). However, an underlying concern with caffeine is the possibility that it "promotes dehydration." Caffeine and its related compounds, theophylline and theobromine, have long been recognized as diuretic molecules that encourage excretion of urine via increased blood flow to the kidneys (Armstrong 2002). However, the effect of caffeine on whole-body water balance is dependent on a variety of factors such as caffeine dosing, timing of caffeine ingestion, and level of physical activity. The most salient question for the athlete should be: "Does using caffeine in a manner that improves performance result in dehydration?" If caffeine ingestion leads to dehydration, then any potential benefit of caffeine may be offset by the well-known deleterious effects of dehydration on performance.

A 70-kg individual needs ~210 to 420 mg of caffeine to improve performance (i.e., 3–6 mg/kg body mass) (Ganio et al. 2009). Ingesting that amount of caffeine may lead to increased urine output at rest. However, a recent review of 13 studies shows that fluid balance (i.e., volume of fluid consumed vs. urine volume) is similar when ingesting caffeine vs. a placebo fluid (Armstrong et al. 2007a; Figure 11.4). The reduction in renal blood flow and glomerular filtration rate during exercise may provide an explanation for why there is no diuretic effect of caffeine during exercise. A recent study confirmed that before, during, and after exercise, hydration status measured with a variety of hydration markers (e.g., plasma osmolality, urine specific gravity) is not different between caffeine and placebo fluid ingestion. Importantly,

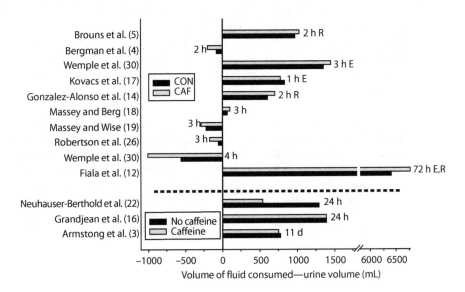

FIGURE 11.4 Mean fluid retention (above *dashed line*) when acutely consuming a control fluid (placebo or water) vs. a fluid containing caffeine or (below *dashed line*) when 24-h fluid intake (beverages + water content of food) contains caffeine vs. no caffeine. Negative values depict studies that report a net fluid loss. CAF = caffeine; CON = control fluid; E = exercise; R = rehydration after exercise. (From Armstrong, L.E. et al. 2007a. *Exerc Sport Sci Rev* 35(3):135–140. With permission.)

the caffeine dosing (6 mg/kg body mass) resulted in performance improvements (Ganio et al. 2010). Additionally, it is important to note that hydration status is not altered in physically active individuals who chronically ingest caffeine (Armstrong et al. 2005).

In conclusion, acute and chronic ingestion of caffeine at doses shown to improve performance (3–6 mg/kg body mass) do not promote dehydration at rest or during exercise. Thus, caffeine is a safe, legal drug to use for improving performance.

GLYCEROL

Because dehydration is detrimental to performance, starting hydrated and remaining hydrated throughout exercise is critical. However, *ad libitum* fluid intake is not sufficient to replace sweat losses during exercise. The mismatch between fluid losses and fluid intake results in dehydration and is termed "involuntary dehydration" because the physiological mechanisms inducing thirst are not sensitive enough to maintain euhydration. If adequate hydration cannot be maintained during exercise, starting hyperhydrated (i.e., greater than normal body water level) may provide an advantage. Hyperhydration prior to exercise may delay dehydration and its consequences (e.g., increased heart rate, increased core temperature, and decreased performance) (van Rosendal et al. 2010).

Hyperhydration can be achieved by ingesting large volumes of water, but the resulting plasma dilution leads to diuresis in a relatively short time. The addition of glycerol ($C_3H_8O_3$) to a water bolus prevents plasma dilution and leads to an expansion of blood volume without increased diuresis (Goulet et al. 2007; van Rosendal et al. 2010). Recent reviews conclude that individuals ingesting 1.1 g of glycerol per kilogram body mass in 24 mL/kg body mass of water will have a body fluid increase of 7.7 mL/kg body mass (Goulet et al. 2007; van Rosendal et al. 2010). This level of hyperhydration improves performance ~2.6% compared to hyperhydrating with water alone (Goulet et al. 2007).

Two important caveats to glycerol use are (1) some side effects from glycerol ingestion have been reported including nausea, gastrointestinal discomfort, and light-headedness (van Rosendal et al. 2010) and (2) glycerol is considered a "masking agent" by the World Anti-Doping Agency and therefore is banned from use. Despite these caveats, glycerol ingestion consistently hyperhydrates individuals and can improve performance, especially when exercise would otherwise result in dehydration (e.g., long-duration, high intensity exercise in the heat), but as noted in the Goulet review, not all of the glycerol studies noted performance benefit, even if it was intense exercise in the heat.

CREATINE

Creatine is one of the most popular nutritional supplements on the market. Athletes of all levels and sports use creatine for a variety of reasons (e.g., improved muscular power and recovery). However, there have been previous concerns that creatine supplementation may alter hydration status (Terjung et al. 2000). It is consistently observed that creatine supplementation increases total body water (TBW) (Lopez et al. 2009). Increased TBW with creatine use is primarily a result of increasedintracellular water stores; however, long-term use also increases extracellular fluid volumes (Lopez et al. 2009). The effects of creatine supplementation on other traditional markers of hydration status, such as urine specific gravity and plasma osmolality, are less known. This is important because changes in plasma osmolality, for example, elicit an abundance of cardiovascular, thermoregulatory, and endocrine responses. Watson and others (2006) observed that after 7 days of supplementation (21.6 g/day), resting urine specific gravity was not significantly different between those using creatine and those using a placebo. Plasma osmolality was slightly greater in the creatine vs. placebo group but remained at euhydrated levels (288 vs. 283 mOsm/kg H_2O, respectively). Likewise, fluid turnover at rest (fluid ingestion vs. urine production) is unaltered with 7 days of creatine supplementation. This provides evidence that creatine supplementation does not adversely affect hydration status, but future studies should carefully control fluid intake and measure fluid output while also measuring a variety of hydration status markers.

Also important to understand is if creatine supplementation affects cardiovascular and thermoregulatory responses during exercise. Alterations in these systems lead to direct impairments in performance, and these systems are largely influenced by hydration status. Short-term and long-term creatine supplementation does not impair the heart rate or core temperature responses to long duration (up to 80 min) exercise in the heat (30°C–37°C) (Watson et al. 2006). Further, creatine supplementation does not alter exercise heat tolerance, even when subjects begin exercise in a dehydrated state (Watson et al. 2006). A recent meta-analysis confirmed that when supplementing with creatine 5 to 28 days, there are no detriments in thermoregulation compared to placebo (Lopez et al. 2009).

In fact, it is possible that increased total body water with creatine supplementation (see previous section) leads to hyperhydration. This can delay dehydration, decrease cardiovascular strain, and improve thermoregulation during exercise as observed with glycerol ingestion (see previous section). Several studies have shown that creatine supplementation results in lower core temperature and heart rate during exercise in the heat (Easton et al. 2007). However, it should be noted that the magnitude of these improvements might not lead to performance improvements (Easton et al. 2007).

In summary, early concerns about creatine supplementation and exercise in the heat have been refuted by recent studies showing that creatine supplementation does not negatively alter hydration status. On the contrary, consistently observed increases in total body water with creatine supplementation may provide small cardiovascular and thermoregulatory benefits that may or may not improve performance.

CURRENT HYDRATION CONTROVERSIES

RUNNERS HAVE FASTER MARATHON TIMES WHEN THEY CONSUME LESS FLUID

This concept stems from two publications in particular (Knechtle et al. 2012; Zouhal et al. 2011) which reported, "The fastest runners lost the most weight." This concept has not been supported since appearing in print, and the findings of these publications can be debated for the following reasons. First, the published data involved a cross-sectional comparison of 643 marathon finishers (Zouhal et al. 2011) whose times ranged from about 150 to 310 min, and 210 finishers of a 100-km ultra-marathon (Knechtle et al. 2012) whose times ranged from about 7.5 to 20 h. The line of best fit (i.e., statistical linear regression) demonstrated that percentage of body weight loss accounted for only 4.7% and 2.6% of the variance in race time. Clearly, other factors were more important than body weight loss in determining exercise performance. Paradoxically, faster runners drank more fluid than slower runners did in one of these two studies (Knechtle et al. 2012). Second, due to differences in running speed, front runners consume fluids at a much different rate than back-of-the-pack runners. Fast marathon runners (i.e., finishing in less than 3 h) experience a high ventilation rate that precludes them from consuming water, out of concern for inhalation and coughing. Front runners also are conscious of time spent at aid stations. In contrast, slow runners typically spend more time at aid stations, drink more often, and walk during part of the race. Thus, an alternative concept (i.e., fast runners drink less than slow runners do) is superior to published statements such as, "the fastest runners lost the most weight" and "body weight loss in marathon runners may be ergogenic" (Zouhal et al. 2011). These final two statements should not be the basis of recommendations for endurance runners.

The question "Does dehydration affect exercise performance negatively?" is an important companion to the above concept. Numerous publications, dating back to the 1960s, have demonstrated decreased strength, maximal oxygen uptake, and endurance performance (Armstrong et al. 1985; Cheuvront et al. 2010; Sawka and Pandolf 1990), beginning when body weight loss reaches 1% to 2%. See the previous section, "Influence of Hydration Status on Exercise Performance."

Is "Drinking to Thirst" a Sound Approach to Rehydration?

Concerns about exertional hyponatremia (i.e., a medical emergency resulting from consuming too much water) have prompted some authorities to recommend that athletes rely on their sensory perceptions and "drink to thirst" (Noakes 2003), in the belief that relying on thirst is a natural way to avoid fluid overload. However, various professional organizations, such as the National Athletic Trainers' Association (NATA) (Casa et al. 2000a), have published guidelines regarding fluid replacement during exercise. These organizations agree that the goal of drinking during exercise is to prevent excessive dehydration, avoiding a body weight loss of more than 2%. For example, the current NATA Position Statement (Casa et al. 2000a) recommends that athletes develop an individualized plan. During exercise thirst can be a valuable tool for athletes who are dehydrated and should be heeded. Similarly, the current American College of Sports Medicine Position Stand (Sawka et al. 2007) mentions that athletes may benefit from drinking *ad libitum* (i.e., as much as they desire, whenever they choose to drink) assuming that they begin an event normally hydrated. The above recommendations illustrate the range of rehydration recommendations that are provided to athletes. Interestingly, virtually none of the studies that have supported drinking to thirst actually measured thirst during observations. Indeed, little direct evidence supports this practice.

Considering these facts, it is reasonable to ask, "How much fluid should be replaced?" The American College of Sports Medicine (Sawka et al. 2007) recommends that, *before* exercise, the goal is to begin physical activity in a euhydrated state and with normal plasma electrolyte levels. The athlete should slowly drink fluid at least 4 h before the exercise task. If he or she does not produce urine, or the urine is dark or highly concentrated, he or she should slowly drink more fluid about 2 h before the event. By hydrating several hours prior to exercise, urine output can return toward normal before starting the event. *During* high-intensity exercise events of 1 h or longer, as well as less intense exercise events sustained for longer periods, carbohydrate consumption can sustain performance. Carbohydrate intake at a rate of ~30–60 g/h maintains blood glucose. To achieve a carbohydrate intake sufficient to sustain performance, an individual could ingest 1/2 to 1 L of a conventional sports drink each hour (assuming 6%–8% carbohydrate), along with sufficient water to avoid dehydration greater than 2% body weight loss. *After* exercise, the goal is to fully replace any fluid and electrolyte deficit. The rate of fluid intake depends on the speed that rehydration must be accomplished and the magnitude of any fluid-electrolyte deficit. Consuming sodium during the recovery period will help retain ingested fluids and help stimulate thirst (Sawka et al. 2007). Ultimately thirst can be a valuable guide, but high level athletes should supplement thirst with individual needs and plans.

WHAT IS THE BEST METHOD TO ASSESS HYDRATION STATUS?

The turnover of body water is complex and dynamic. Thirst, drinking behavior, the kidneys, and sweat glands are involved to varying degrees, depending on the duration and intensity of exercise. Thus, all hydration assessment techniques (including bioelectrical impedance, body weight change, plasma concentration, plasma volume change, urine concentration, urine specific gravity, urine color, 24-h urine volume, saliva flow rate and concentration, and rating of thirst) are best viewed as singular measures of a complex and dynamic fluid matrix, containing interconnected compartments. This explains why a single method is not possible for all hydration assessment requirements (Armstrong 2007).

Yet, to ensure that they enter exercise well hydrated, and to ensure that they have effectively replaced the water in sweat, athletes require one or more techniques to assess their hydration state. The best techniques are easy-to-use, safe, portable, and inexpensive (Table 11.2). The three methods that meet these criteria are body weight change, urine specific gravity, and urine color. These are measured with a digital floor scale, a hand-held refractometer, and a urine color chart, respectively. In field settings, when an estimate of hydration status is needed or when a large body water loss is anticipated (i.e., prolonged endurance exercise), one should compare information from two or more hydration assessment methods.

Although thirst varies considerably from person to person, and is difficult to measure quantitatively, thirst provides clues to hydration status. That is, thirst is not sensed unless one is dehydrated by 1% to 2% of body weight. Thus, when thirst is recognized, a mild level of dehydration exists and the athlete should begin to rehydrate.

TABLE 11.2
Selected Characteristics of 13 Hydration Assessment Methods

Hydration Assessment Technique	Body Fluid Involved	Cost of Analysis	Time Required	Technical Expertise Required	Portability	Likelihood of Adverse Event
Stable isotope dilution	All (ECF and ICF)	3	3	3	3	2 or 3[b]
Neutron activation analysis	All	3	3	3	3	2 or 3[b]
Bioelectrical impedance spectroscopy (BIS)	Uncertain	2	2	2	2	2
Body mass change	All	1	1	1	1	1
Plasma osmolality	ECF	3	2	3	3	2
% Plasma volume change	Blood	2	2	3	3	2
Urine osmolality	Excreted urine	3	2	3	3	1
Urine specific gravity	Excreted urine	1	1	2	1	1
Urine conductivity	Excreted urine	2	2	2	3[c]	1
Urine color	Excreted urine	1	1	1	1	1
24-hour urine volume	Excreted urine	1	1	1	1	1

(Continued)

Hydration for High-Level Athletes

TABLE 11.2 (Continued)
Selected Characteristics of 13 Hydration Assessment Methods

Hydration Assessment Technique	Body Fluid Involved	Cost of Analysis	Time Required	Technical Expertise Required	Portability	Likelihood of Adverse Event
Salivary flow rate, osmolality, total protein	Whole, mixed saliva	2–3	2	3	2–3	1
Rating of thirst	Hypothalamus	1	1	1	1	1
Key ratings		1 = Small, little	1 = Small, little	1 = Small, little	1 = Portable	1 = Low
		2 = Moderate	2 = Moderate	2 = Moderate	2 = Moderate	2 = Moderate
		3 = Great, much	3 = Great, much	3 = Great, much	3 = Not portable	3 = High

Source: Armstrong, L.E. 2007. *J Am College Nutr* 26(5):575S–584S; Armstrong L.E. 2005. *Nutr Rev* 63:S40–S54. With permission.

Note: BIS = bioelectrical impedance spectroscopy; EFC = extracellular fluid; ICF = intracellular fluid.

a Modified and redrawn from Reference 7.
b Depending on the type of isotope involved (i.e., radioactive, stable, non-radioactive).
c Using a floor scare.
d Freezing point depression method.
e Portable, hand-held meters are available [4].

Developing Individualized Hydration Plans

Given all of the scientific evidence regarding the impact of hydration on physiological functioning, the value of a hydration plan during training and competition is
clear. Although the majority of water loss contributing to a state of hypohydration
occurs through sweat, many variables affect sweat rate and therefore water needs.
Factors that may alter water needs include but are not limited to age, acclimatization
status, intensity of exercise, sex, environmental conditions, hydration status, fitness
status, and barriers to sweat evaporation (such as protective equipment) (Armstrong
et al. 2007b). These factors emphasize the importance of creating an individualized
hydration plan, not only to account for individual variation, but also due to potential
variation within an individual over weeks and months. Therefore, to maximize training and performance, athletes should aim to replace their fluids based on their individual sweat rate for a given exercise intensity, environmental condition, and exercise
mode. Current recommendations state that an athlete should attempt to replace 80%
to 100% of the fluid that is lost through sweat, which should attenuate water losses
greater than 2% body mass loss as well as avoid body mass gains of more than 2%
for a majority of athletic events (Armstrong et al. 2007b). Longer events, such as a
marathon or longer triathlons, may challenge the ability of the athlete to keep up
with his or her sweat rate; nevertheless, every attempt should be made to minimize
these losses. Additionally, many sporting events may not allow free access to fluids
(i.e., soccer, tennis), which also challenges the athlete to appropriately time his or
her water intake.

Having an accurate understanding of an athlete's sweat rate is the first step to
establishing a successful hydration plan. This is a simple procedure and can be done
during any training session. This should be done in conditions as similar as possible to the event to which the athlete would like to apply these results. This means
performing the sweat rate testing in a similar weather environment, similar physical
fitness status, similar clothing, and similar exercise intensity to the event in which
he or she anticipates using this information. The athlete should ensure that he or she

TABLE 11.3
Steps to Determine Sweat Rate

Step	Actions to Take
1	Immediately before exercising, record a nude pre-workout weight to the 0.1 kg (or 0.1 lb is acceptable).
2	Exercise for 45–60 min at an intensity similar to the anticipated effort that will be performed, in the environment that is expected (air temperature and humidity), and in the clothing that you anticipate wearing.
3	Do not consume fluids or go to the bathroom during this exercise session. If you would like to consume fluids, you need to know the exact amount consumed.
4	Immediately after you complete the exercise session, record another nude weight. Be sure to wipe any extra sweat off with a towel before obtaining this weight.
5	See Table 11.4 for calculation of sweat rate.

TABLE 11.4
Calculation of Sweat Rate with Example Values

Calculation Steps		Example Values
1. Enter your pre-exercise weight in kilograms (if you have pounds, convert to kilograms by dividing pounds by 2.2)	_____kg	60 kg
2. Enter your post-exercise weight in kilograms	_____kg	58.5 kg
3. Subtract #2 from #1	_____kg	1.5 kg
4. Enter number of hours of exercise (60 min = 1 h, 45 min = 0.75 h)	_____h	0.75 h
5. If fluid was consumed during exercise, enter amount here in kilograms (1 kg = 33.8 oz or 4.2 cups)	_____kg	0.4 kg
6. Add the amount of fluid consumed (#5) to total weight lost (#3)	_____kg	1.9 kg
7. Divide #6 (or #3 if no fluid was consumed) by hours of exercise (#4)	_____kg/h	2.5 kg/h

Note: The result in #7 is your sweat rate as a function of kilograms per hour, which is also the same as liters per hour. To convert this to ounces or cups, multiply by 33.8 or 4.2, respectively.

is euhydrated when performing sweat rate testing. See Tables 11.3 and 11.4 for a step-by-step approach for determining sweat rate. Because items such as heat acclimatization, physical fitness, and environmental conditions will vary throughout a training season, it is also important to re-evaluate an athlete's sweat rate whenever there is a large change in any of these factors (e.g., once an athlete becomes acclimatized to exercising in the heat).

Once sweat rate is determined, an athlete will then need to determine how much fluid he or she will have access to during competition or training. If the athlete has unrestricted access, consuming the appropriate amount of fluid is relatively easy. However, if the athlete is participating in a marathon, for example, and there are a limited number of water stops, the athlete needs to predict how much he or she will consume at each station and how much he or she will lose throughout the race. For example, if the sweat rate for a female marathon runner who is expecting to finish the race in 3 h is 1.25 L/h, she would lose 3.75 L during the course of the marathon. If there were a water stop at every mile, where she consumes 4 oz (~0.12 L) of fluid, she would replace 3.12 L of water, leaving her 0.63 L in deficit. For a 55-kg athlete (121 lb), 0.63 L would equate to a dehydration level of 1.1%, which would be adequate to avoid the physiological consequences associated with dehydration levels greater than 2%. However, if there were only water breaks every 2 miles, she would have to consume twice as much fluid at each station or risk becoming more than 2% dehydrated. It is when scenarios begin to present this way that athletes must weigh the practicality of being able to consume these volumes of fluids with fewer opportunities. In scenarios where athletes only have a few, defined opportunities to drink (such as soccer), it is even more vital that the athlete begins the competition hydrated and maximizes opportunities to rehydrate throughout by projecting how much should be replaced at each opportunity to rehydrate.

An important consideration for developing a hydration plan is also gastric emptying rate. While the athlete theoretically may be able to consume adequate fluids, the athlete's stomach may not be able to process this volume of fluid during exercise. This explains why it is also important during training to practice consuming the volume and composition of fluids that an athlete plans to use in competition and fine-tune the amount the athlete can handle. It has been shown that, despite gastric upset on an initial exercise session where athletes replaced fluids based on their individual sweat losses, athletes who trained for just five exercise sessions repeating this fluid intake reported lower levels of gastric upset (despite a non-significant change in gastric emptying rate) (Lambert et al. 2008). In general, it has been found that athletes are able to tolerate consuming 80% of the fluids that are lost in sweat without gastric upset (Lambert et al. 2008); however, consideration should be given to longer endurance events where this mismatch could easily lead to dehydration levels greater than 2%. Practicing a hydration plan, and determining the athlete's tolerance to consume fluids (whether he or she is able to match 80%, 90%, or 100% of sweat losses) can help provide the athlete feedback as to what fluid intake his or her body can handle and also provide an opportunity to increase his or her tolerance to ingest fluids.

Other factors can also affect the stomach's ability to process fluid. Previous studies have demonstrated that dehydration between 4% and 5% in both cool (Neufer et al. 1989) and warm environments (Rehrer et al. 1990) impairs gastric emptying rate at rest. In addition, strictly exercising in a hot environment (49°C) impairs gastric emptying rate compared to a neutral environment (18°C) (Neufer et al. 1989). Other factors slowing gastric emptying include increased caloric content of fluids, temperature of the fluid, intense exercise (>70% $\dot{V}O_{2\,max}$), and increasing volume of fluid ingested (Maughan and Leiper 1999). All of these items highlight the need to practice a hydration plan and determine what an athlete is able to handle during exercise.

Lastly, in events lasting more than 4 h, the amount of electrolytes lost in sweat is significantly greater than shorter events and the risk for hyponatremia increases (Montain et al. 2006); therefore, it becomes important to understand an individual's sweat electrolyte composition and consequently the appropriate consumption of electrolyte supplements during endurance exercise greater than 4 h. Sweat electrolyte content will change based on an athlete's sweat rate and heat acclimatization status (Armstrong and Maresh 1991), thereby calling for periodic reassessment of sweat electrolyte content for accurate sweat electrolyte loss estimations when either of these factors might change. This should be performed in a qualified laboratory setting. It has been recommended that individuals who lose more than 3–4 g of sodium in their sweat should include sodium supplementation during competition or for athletes performing exercise bouts longer than 2 h (Coyle 2004). While sodium supplementation may be used as a preventative measure for hyponatremia, it is most important to avoid excessive fluid intake, which dilutes blood sodium levels, once again highlighting the need for an individual hydration plan (Montain et al. 2006).

Overall, it is very important to understand an individual's sweat rate and fluid ingestion tolerance in specific conditions, in addition to planning the appropriate timing of fluids given the anticipated opportunities. These strategies can lead to an optimal hydration plan that will help to attenuate overhydration and dehydration greater than 2%.

REFERENCES

Adams, W.M., E.M. Ferraro, R.A. Huggins, and D.J. Casa. 2014. Influence of body mass loss on changes in heart rate during exercise in the heat: A systematic review. *J Strength Cond Res.* 28(8):2380–2389.

Armstrong, L.E. 2002. Caffeine, body fluid-electrolyte balance, and exercise performance. *Int J Sport Nutr Exerc Metab* 12(2):189–206.

Armstrong, L.E. 2007. Assessing hydration status: The elusive gold standard. *J Am Coll Nutr* 26(5):575S–584S.

Armstrong, L.E., D.L. Costill, and W.J. Fink. 1985. Influence of diuretic-induced dehydration on competitive running performance. *Med Sci Sports Exerc* 17(4):456–461.

Armstrong, L.E., and C.M. Maresh. 1991. The induction and decay of heat acclimatization in trained athletes. *Sports Med* 12(5):302–312.

Armstrong, L.E., A.C. Pumerantz, M.W. Roti, D.A. Judelson, G. Watson, J.C. Dias, B. Sokmen, D.J. Casa, C.M. Maresh, H. Lieberman, and M. Kellogg 2005. Fluid, electrolyte, and renal indices of hydration during 11 days of controlled caffeine consumption. *Int J Sport Nutr Metab* 15(3):252–265.

Armstrong, L.E., D.J. Casa, C.M. Maresh, and M.S. Ganio. 2007a. Caffeine, fluid-electrolyte balance, temperature regulation, and exercise-heat tolerance. *Exerc Sport Sci Rev* 35(3):135–140.

Armstrong, L.E., D.J. Casa, M. Millard-Stafford, D.S. Moran, S.W. Pyne, and W.O. Roberts. 2007b. ACSM position stand: Exertional heat illnesses during training and competition. *Med Sci Sport Exerc* 39(3):556–572.

Arnaoutis, G., S.A. Kavouras, I. Christaki, and L.S. Sidossis. 2012. Water ingestion improves performance compared with mouth rinse in dehydrated subjects. *Med Sci Sports Exerc* 44:175–179.

Baker, L.B., K.A. Dougherty, M. Chow, and W.L. Kenney. 2007. Progressive dehydration causes a progressive decline in basketball skill performance. *Med Sci Sports Exerc* 39:1114–1123.

Bardis, C.N., S.A. Kavouras, G. Arnaoutis, D.B. Panagiotakos, and L.S. Sidossis. 2013a. Mild dehydration and cycling performance during 5-kilometer hill climbing. *J Athl Train* 48(6):741–747.

Bardis, C.N., S.A. Kavouras, L. Kosti, M. Markousi, and L. Sidossis. 2013b. Mild hypohydration decreases cycling performance in the heat. *Med Sci Sports Exerc* 45(9):1782–1789.

Bergman, E.A., L.K. Massey, K.J. Wise, and D.J. Sherrard. 1990. Effects of dietary caffeine on renal handling of minerals in adult women. *Life Sci* 47:557–564.

Brouns, F., E.M. Kovacs, and J.M. Senden. 1998. The effect of different rehydration drinks on post-exercise electrolyte excretion in trained athletes. *Int J Sports Med* 19:56–60.

Buono, M.J., and A.J. Wall. 2000. Effect of hypohydration on core temperature during exercise in temperate and hot environments. *Pflugers Arch* 440(3):476–480.

Byrne, C., J.K. Lee, S.A. Chew, C.L. Lim, and E.Y. Tan. 2006. Continuous thermoregulatory responses to mass-participation distance running in heat. *Med Sci Sports Exerc* 38(5):803–810.

Casa, D.J., L.E. Armstrong, S.K. Hillman et al. 2000a. National Athletic Trainers' Association Position Statement: Fluid replacement for athletes. *J Athl Train* 35(2):212–224.

Casa, D.J., C.M. Maresh, L.E. Armstrong et al. 2000b. Intravenous versus oral rehydration during a brief period: Responses to subsequent exercise in the heat. *Med Sci Sports Exerc* 32(1):124–133.

Casa, D.J., R.L. Stearns, R.M. Lopez et al. 2010. Influence of hydration on physiological function and performance during trail running in the heat. *J Athl Train* 45:147–156.

Cheuvront, S.N., R. Carter, J.W. Castellani, and M.N. Sawka. 2005. Hypohydration impairs endurance exercise performance in temperate but not cold air. *J Appl Physiol* 99:1972–1976.

Cheuvront, S.N., R.W. Kenefick, and S.J. Montain. 2007. Important insight from the 2003 Singapore half-marathon. *Med Sci Sports Exerc* 39(10):1883–1884.

Cheuvront, S.N., R.W. Kenefick, S.J. Montain, and M.N. Sawka. 2010. Mechanisms of aerobic performance impairment with heat stress and dehydration. *J Appl Physiol* 109:1989–1995.

Coyle, E.F. 2004. Fluid and fuel intake during exercise. *J Sport Sci* 22:39–55.

Davies, C.T. 1979. Influence of skin temperature on sweating and aerobic performance during severe work. *J Appl Physiol* 47(4):770–777.

Easton, C., S. Turner, and Y.P. Pitsiladis. 2007. Creatine and glycerol hyperhydration in trained subjects before exercise in the heat. *Int J Sport Nutr Exerc Metab* 17(1):70–91.

Ebert, T.R., D.T. Martin, N. Bullock et al. 2007. Influence of hydration status on thermoregulation and cycling hill climbing. *Med Sci Sports Exerc* 39:323–329.

Fiala, K.A., D.J. Casa, and M.W. Roti. 2004. Rehydration with a caffeinated beverage during the nonexercise periods of 3 consecutive days of 2-a-day practices. *Int J Sport Nutr Exerc Metab* 14:419–429.

Fowkes Godek, S., J.J. Godek, and A.R. Bartolozzi. 2004. Thermal responses in football and cross country athletes during their respective practices in a hot environment. *J Athl Train* 39(3):235–240.

Fowkes Godek, S., A.R. Bartolozzi, R. Burkholder, E. Sugarman, and G. Dorshimer. 2006. Core temperature and percentage of dehydration in professional football linemen and backs during preseason practices. *J Athl Train* 41(1):8–17.

Fudge, B.W., Y.P. Pitsiladis, D. Kingsmore, T.D. Noakes, and B. Kayser. 2007. Outstanding performance despite low fluid intake: The Kenyan running experience. In *East African Running: Toward a Cross-Disciplinary Perspective*, Y.P. Pitsiladis, J. Bale, C. Sharp, and T.D. Noakes, Eds. New York: Routledge, 63–84.

Ganio, M.S., J.E. Wingo, C.E. Carroll, M.K. Thomas, and K.J. Cureton. 2006. Fluid ingestion attenuates the decline in VO_{2peak} associated with cardiovascular drift. *Med Sci Sports Exerc* 38:901–909.

Ganio, M.S., J.F. Klau, D.J. Casa, L.E. Armstrong, and C.M. Maresh. 2009. Effect of caffeine on sport-specific endurance performance: A systematic review. *J Strength Cond Res* 23(1):315–324.

Ganio, M., E. Johnson, J. Klau et al. 2010. Effect of ambient temperature on caffeine ergogenicity during endurance exercise. *Eur J Appl Physiol* 1–12.

González-Alonso, J., R. Mora-Rodríguez, P.R. Below, and E.F. Coyle. 1997. Dehydration markedly impairs cardiovascular function in hyperthermic endurance athletes during exercise. *J Appl Physiol* 82:1229–1236.

González-Alonso, J., J.A. Calbet, and B. Nielsen. 1998. Muscle blood flow is reduced with dehydration during prolonged exercise in humans. *J Physiol* 513(Pt 3):895–905.

Gonzalez-Alonso, J., J.A.L. Calbet, and B. Nielsen. 1999. Metabolic and thermodynamic responses to dehydration-induced reductions in muscle blood flow in exercising humans. *J Physiol (Lond)* 520:577–589.

Gonzalez-Alonso, J., C.L. Heaps, and E.F. Coyle. 1992. Rehydration after exercise with common beverages and water. *Int J Sports Med* 13:399–406.

Gonzalez-Alonso, J., R. Mora-Rodriguez, and E.F. Coyle. 2000. Stroke volume during exercise: Interaction of environment and hydration. *Am J Physiol Heart Circ Physiol* 278(2):H321–H330.

Goulet, E.D., M. Aubertin-Leheudre, G.E. Plante, and I.J. Dionne. 2007. A meta-analysis of the effects of glycerol-induced hyperhydration on fluid retention and endurance performance. *Int J Sport Nutr Exerc Metab* 17(4):391–410.

Grandjean, A.C., K.J. Reimers, K.E. Bannick, and M.C. Haven. 2000. The effect of caffeinated, non-caffeinated, caloric and non-caloric beverages on hydration. *J Am Coll Nutr* 19:591–600.

Huggins, R.A., J. Martschinske, K. Applegate, L.E. Armstrong, and D.J. Casa. 2012. Influence of dehydration on internal body temperature changes during exercise in the heat: A meta-analysis. *Med Sci Sports Exerc* 44(5)S587:3019.

Judelson, D.A., C.M. Maresh, M.J. Farrell et al. 2007. Effect of hydration state on strength, power, and resistance exercise performance. *Med Sci Sports Exerc* 39(10):1817–1824.

Knechtle, B., P. Knechtle, A. Wirth, C.A. Rust, and T. Rosemann. 2012. A faster running speed is associated with a greater body weight loss in 100-km ultra-marathoners. *J Sports Sci* 30(11):1131–1140.

Kovacs, E.M., J.H.C.H. Stegen, and F. Brouns. 1998. Effect of caffeinated drinks on substrate metabolism, caffeine excretion, and performance. *J Appl Physiol* 85:709–715.

Lambert, G.P., J. Lang, A. Bull, J. Eckerson, S. Lanspa, and J. O'Brien. 2008. Fluid tolerance while running: Effect of repeated trials. *Int J Sports Med* 29:878–882.

Laursen, P.B., R. Suriano, M.J. Quod et al. 2006. Core temperature and hydration status during an Ironman triathlon. *Br J Sports Med* 40(4):320–325.

Logan-Sprenger, H.M., G.J. Heigenhauser, K.J. Killian, and L.L. Spriet. 2012. Effects of dehydration during cycling on skeletal muscle metabolism in females. *Med Sci Sports Exerc* 44:1949–1957.

Lopez, R.M., D.J. Casa, B.P. McDermott, M.S. Ganio, L.E. Armstrong, and C.M. Maresh. 2009. Does creatine supplementation hinder exercise heat tolerance or hydration status? A systematic review with meta-analyses. *J Athl Train* 44(2):215–223.

Lopez, R.M., D.J. Casa, K.A. Jensen et al. 2011. Examining the influence of hydration status on physiological responses and running speed during trail running in the heat with controlled exercise intensity. *J Strength Cond Res* 25(11):2944–2954.

Mack, G. 2012. The body fluid and hemopoietic systems. In *ACSM's Advanced Exercise Physiology*, P.A. Farrell, M.J. Joyner, and V.J. Caiozzo, Eds. Philadelphia, PA: Walters Kluwer Lippincott Williams & Wilkins, 529–550.

Maresh, C.M., J.A. Herrera-Sota, L.E. Armstrong et al. 2001. Perceptual responses in the heat after brief intravenous versus oral rehydration. *Med Sci Sports Exerc* 33(6):1039–1045.

Maresh, C.M., C.L. Gabaree-Boulant, L.E. Armstrong et al. 2004. Effect of hydration status on thirst, drinking, and related hormonal responses during low-intensity exercise in the heat. *J Appl Physiol* 97:39–44.

Marino, F.E., D. Kay, and N. Serwach. 2004. Exercise time to fatigue and the critical limiting temperature: Effect of hydration. *J Therm Biol* 29(1):21–29.

Massey, L.K., and T.A. Berg. 1985. The effect of dietary caffeine on urinary excretion of calcium, magnesium, phosphorus, sodium, potassium, chloride, and zinc in healthy males. *Nutr Res* 5:1281–1284.

Massey, L.K., and K.J. Wise. 1984. The effect of dietary caffeine on urinary excretion of calcium, magnesium, sodium and potassium in healthy young females. *Nutr Res* 4:43–50.

Maughan, R.J., and J.B. Leiper. 1999. Limitations to fluid replacement during exercise. *Can J Appl Physiol* 24(2):173–187.

Maughan, R.J., J.B. Leiper, and J. Thompson. 1985. Rectal temperature after marathon running. *Br J Sports Med* 19(4):192–195.

McNair, D., M. Lorr, and L. Droppleman. 1971. *Profile of Mood States Manual.* San Diego, CA: Educational and Industrial Testing Service, 1–23.

Montain, S.J., and E.F. Coyle. 1992. Influence of graded dehydration on hyperthermia and cardiovascular drift during exercise. *J Appl Physiol* 73:1340–1350.

Montain, S.J., W.A. Latzka, and M.N. Sawka. 1995. Control of thermoregulatory sweating is altered by hydration level and exercise intensity. *J Appl Physiol* 79:1434–1439.

Montain, S.J., M.N. Sawka, W.A. Latzka, and C.R. Valeri. 1998. Thermal and cardiovascular strain from hypohydration: Influence of exercise intensity. *Int J Sports Med* 19(2):87–91.

Montain, S.J., S.N. Cheuvront, and M.N. Sawka. 2006. Exercise associated hyponatremia: Quantitative analysis to understand the aetiology. *Brit J Sport Med* 40(2):98–105.

Nadel, E.R., S.M. Fortney, and C.B. Wenger. 1980. Effect of hydration state of circulatory and thermal regulations. *J Appl Physiol* 49:715–721.

Neufer, P.D., A.J. Young, and M.N. Sawka. 1989. Gastric emptying during exercise: Effects of heat stress and hypohydration. *Eur J Appl Physiol* 58:433–439.

Neuhauser-Berthold, M., S. Beine, S.C. Verwied, and P.M. Luhrmann. 1997. Coffee consumption and total body water homeostasis as measured by fluid balance and bioelectrical impedance analysis. *Ann Nutr Metab* 41:29–36.

Noakes, T.D. 2003. Overconsumption of fluids by athletes. *BMJ* 327(7407):113–114.

Noakes, T.D., K.H. Myburgh, J. du Plessis et al. 1991. Metabolic rate, not percent dehydration, predicts rectal temperature in marathon runners. *Med Sci Sports Exerc* 23(4):443–449.

Pitts, G., R. Jonson, and F. Consolazio. 1944. Work in the heat as affected by intake of water salt and glucose. *Am J Physiol* 142:253–259.

Rehrer, N.J., E.J. Beckers, F. Brouns, F. Ten Hoor, and W.H.M. Saris. 1990. Effects of dehydration on gastric emptying and gastrointestinal distress while running. *Med Sci Sport Exerc* 22(6):790–795.

Robertson, D., J.C. Frolich, R.K. Carr, J.T. Watson, J.W. Hollifield, D.G. Shand, and J.A. Oates. 1978. Effects of caffeine on plasma renin activity, catecholamines, and blood pressure. *N Engl J Med* 298:181–186.

Saltin, B., and L. Hermansen. 1966. Esophageal, rectal, and muscle temperature during exercise. *J Appl Physiol* 21(6):1757–1762.

Sampson, J.B., and J.L. Kobrick. 1980. The environmental symptoms questionnaire: Revisions and new field data. *Aviat Space Environ Med* 51(9 pt 1):872–877.

Sawka, M.N. 1992. Physiological consequences of hypohydration: Exercise performance and thermoregulation. *Med Sci Sports Exerc* 24:657–670.

Sawka, M.N., and K.B. Pandolf. 1990. Effects of body water loss on physiological function and exercise performance. In *Perspectives in Exercise Science and Sports Medicine, Volume 3. Fluid Homeostasis During Exercise*, Gisolfi C.V., and D.R. Lamb, Eds. Carmel: Benchmark Press, 1–38.

Sawka, M.N., A.J. Young, R.P. Francesconi, S.R. Muza, and K.B. Pandolf. 1985. Thermoregulatory and blood responses during exercise at graded hypohydration levels. *J Appl Physiol* 59(5):1394–1401.

Sawka, M.N., S.J. Montain, and W.A. Latzka. 2001. Hydration effects on thermoregulation and performance in the heat. *Comp Biochem Physiol A Mol Integr Physiol* 128(4):679–690.

Sawka, M.N., L.M. Burke, E.R. Eichner, R.J. Maughan, S.J. Montain, and N.S. Stachenfeld. 2007. American College of Sports Medicine position stand. Exercise and fluid replacement. *Med Sci Sports Exerc* 39(2):377–390.

Sharwood, K.A., M. Collins, J.H. Goedecke, G. Wilson, and T.D. Noakes. 2004. Weight changes, medical complications, and performance during an Ironman triathlon. *Br J Sports Med* 38(6):718–724.

Shibasaki, M., T.E. Wilson, and C.G. Crandall. 2006. Neural control and mechanisms of eccrine sweating during heat stress and exercise. *J Appl Physiol* 100:1692–1701.

Stearns, R.L., D.J. Casa, R.M. Lopez et al. 2009. Influence of hydration status on pacing during trail running in the heat. *J Strength Cond Res* 23(9):2533–2541.

Terjung, R.L., P. Clarkson, E.R. Eichner et al. 2000. American College of Sports Medicine roundtable. The physiological and health effects of oral creatine supplementation. *Med Sci Sports Exerc* 32(3):706–717.

Tucker, R., L. Rauch, Y.X. Harley, and T.D. Noakes. 2004. Impaired exercise performance in the heat is associated with an anticipatory reduction in skeletal muscle recruitment. *Pflugers Arch* 448(4):422–430.

Turkevich, D., A. Micco, and J.T. Reeves. 1988. Noninvasive measurement of the decrease in left ventricular filling time during maximal exercise in normal subjects. *Am J Cardiol* 62(9):650–652.

van Rosendal, S.P., M.A. Osborne, R.G. Fassett, and J.S. Coombes. 2010. Guidelines for glycerol use in hyperhydration and rehydration associated with exercise. *Sports Med* 40(2):113–129.

Walsh, R.M., T.D. Noakes, J.A. Hawley, and S.C. Dennis. 1994. Impaired high-intensity cycling performance time at low levels of dehydration. *Int J Sports Med* 15:392–398.

Watson, G., D. Casa, K.A. Fiala et al. 2006. Creatine use and exercise heat tolerance in dehydrated men. *J Athl Train* 41(1):18–29.

Wemple, R.D., D.R. Lamb, and K.H. McKeever. 1997. Caffeine vs. caffeine-free sports drink: Effects on urine production at rest and during prolonged exercise. *Int J Sports Med* 18:40–46.

Zouhal, H., C. Groussard, G. Minter et al. 2011. Inverse relationship between percentage body weight change and finishing time in 643 forty-two kilometer marathon runners. *Br J Sports Med* 45(14):1101–1105.

12 Minerals and Athletic Performance

Rachel C. Kelley, MS
Stella Lucia Volpe, PhD, RD, LDN, FACSM
Department of Nutrition Sciences, Drexel University,
Philadelphia, Pennsylvania

CONTENTS

INTRODUCTION

Minerals are required micronutrients involved in numerous metabolic reactions in the body, including glycolysis, lipolysis, proteolysis, enzymatic activity, structural components, and antioxidant defense systems. There are 7 major minerals and 11 trace minerals (Table 12.1). It would not be feasible to discuss all 18 minerals within this chapter; thus, the following minerals will be the focus of this chapter: calcium, magnesium, iron, and zinc.

CALCIUM

SIGNIFICANCE IN HUMAN PHYSIOLOGY AND HEALTH

Calcium is well known for its structural role of adding hardness and stiffness to bones and teeth. The majority of human bone, 90% to 98%, is a non-living mineral and protein complex with calcium comprising 37% to 40% of this mineral mixture (Heaney 2006). Not only does calcium in bone support the skeletal framework and allow for mechanical work, but it also acts as the reservoir for calcium ions for the rest of the human body. The amount of calcium in bone accounts for 99% of the body's supply of calcium, and acts as an important regulator of cell function (Weaver and Heaney 2006).

Although calcium is most often cited for its benefits to bone health, the maintenance of calcium levels in other cell types and in serum is crucial for a variety of physiological functions. For example, regulated changes in calcium levels in muscle fibers determine the initiation and cessation of muscle contraction. Calcium ions allow actin and myosin interactions to occur in skeletal muscle by binding troponin and exposing actin-binding sites (Widmaier et al. 2011). Calcium is also responsible for the actin-myosin binding in smooth muscle cells due to the ion's regulation of enzymes that phosphorylate myosin (Widmaier et al. 2011). Another example of

---

TABLE 12.1
Major and Trace Minerals

Major Minerals	Trace Minerals
Calcium	Iron
Phosphorus	Zinc
Potassium	Copper
Sulfur	Selenium
Sodium	Iodide
Chloride	Fluoride
Magnesium	Chromium
	Manganese
	Molybdenum
	Boron
	Vanadium

---

calcium's physiological importance is its role in nerve cell signaling. Calcium interacts with synaptotagmins, vesicle proteins in nerve synapses, and this binding leads to vesicle fusion and release of neurotransmitters (Widmaier et al. 2011). Because of the pervasiveness of calcium signaling in the human body, calcium influences countless cell processes like electrical conduction of neural impulses, hormone secretion, cell movement, and cell proliferation (Barrett et al. 2012). Furthermore, calcium ions interact with extracellular proteins, as well, and thus act as cofactors to proteases, blood-clotting enzymes, and other proteins (Weaver and Heaney 2006). Because of calcium's vital functions in cell signaling and protein activation, serum levels are maintained even at the expense of bone mineral density. Thus, proper dietary calcium intake will spare bone of mineral loss and prevent future risk of osteoporosis, fracture, and general frailty.

REGULATION IN THE HUMAN BODY

As stated previously, the metabolic functions of calcium demand that serum levels of this mineral remain within a particular homeostatic range (9–10 mg/dL). When cell-surface receptors detect calcium levels outside of this range, a series of events occur involving three calciotropic hormones: parathyroid hormone (PTH), vitamin D, and calcitonin. When calcium levels fall below 9 mg/dL, cell signaling causes the parathyroid gland to secrete PTH. The release of PTH results in increased calcium absorption in the kidneys, bone resorption of calcium via activation of osteoclasts, and the activation of vitamin D. Active vitamin D, calcitriol, increases calcium absorption in the intestine by increasing the expression of calbindin, a protein that binds calcium ions and transports them from the intestinal lumen to the bloodstream. Like PTH, calcitriol also increases renal absorption of calcium and osteoclastic activity in bone to raise serum calcium levels. On the other hand, when serum calcium levels are greater than 11 mg/dL, calcitonin counteracts the actions of PTH and active vitamin D, and the hormone triggers increased urinary excretion of calcium and osteoblastic activity in bone (Weaver and Heaney 2006).

CALCIUM REQUIREMENTS

The recommended calcium intake for athletes is the same as the amount listed in the Recommended Dietary Allowance (RDA) for the general population (Table 12.2) (Institute of Medicine, Food and Nutrition Board 2010). Calcium intakes for males and females, 9 to 18 years of age, are elevated (1300 mg/day) relative to other age ranges because peak bone mass attainment occurs during these peripubertal and pubertal years, especially in girls (Weaver and Heaney 2006). Men and women, 19 to 50 years of age, should consume 1000 mg/day of calcium, and females 51 to 70 years of age have a slightly elevated calcium requirement (1200 mg/day) than men of the same age range (1000 mg/day) to prevent further bone loss due to menopause. After age 70, both men and women should consume 1200 mg/day of calcium. Dairy products are the most common dietary sources of calcium, and calcium is highly bioavailable in these forms (Weaver and Heaney 2006). Other sources of calcium include broccoli, spinach, beans, and calcium-set tofu (Weaver and Heaney 2006). More sources of calcium are listed in Table 12.3.

TABLE 12.2
Recommended Dietary Allowances (RDA) for Calcium, Magnesium, Iron, and Zinc

Life Stage (Years of Age)	Calcium (mg/day)	Magnesium (mg/day)	Iron (mg/day)	Zinc (mg/day)
		Males		
9 to 13	1300	240	8	8
14 to 18	1300	410	11	11
19 to 30	1000	400	8	11
31 to 50	1000	420	8	11
51 to 70	1000	420	8	11
>70	1200	420	8	11
		Females		
9 to 13	1300	240	8	8
14 to 18	1300	360	15	9
19 to 30	1000	310	18	8
31 to 50	1000	320	18	8
51 to 70	1200	320	8	8
>70	1200	320	8	8

Source: Adapted from Institute of Medicine, Food and Nutrition Board. *Dietary Reference Intakes for Calcium and Vitamin D* (2010); *Dietary Reference Intakes for Calcium, Phosphorus, Magnesium, Vitamin D and Fluoride* (1997); *Dietary Reference Intakes for Vitamin A, Vitamin K, Arsenic, Boron, Chromium, Copper, Iodine, Iron, Manganese, Molybdenum, Nickel, Silicon, Vanadium, and Zinc* (2001). Washington, DC: National Academy Press.

TABLE 12.3
Food Sources of Calcium

Food	Calcium Content (mg)
1/2 cup of macaroni	8
1/2 cup of artichokes	51
1/2 cup of broccoli	88
1/2 cup of collards	152
1/2 cup of Swiss chard	184
1/2 cup of okra	92
1/2 cup of almonds	120
1/2 cup of baked beans	155

Source: Adapted from http://www.nal.usda.gov/fnic
/foodcomp/search/.

STATUS IN ATHLETES

Calcium intake in female athletes is a prolific field of study, and the majority of studies indicate that these athletes are not meeting calcium recommendations. Researchers collected 3-day diet records from female collegiate volleyball players at the beginning of the season, at peak training, and one week into postseason (Anderson 2010). Individual calcium intakes of the players varied considerably, but of the 15 participants, 50% were not meeting the RDA for calcium at the beginning of the season. Interestingly, this figure improved during training and in the postseason, when 25% of players were not meeting calcium requirements instead of 50%.

The incidence of calcium deficiency is more striking in female adolescent athletes (15.7 ± 0.7 years of age). A cross-sectional study analyzing food records of 33 junior elite female soccer players found that two-thirds of the girls did not consume 1100 mg/day of calcium (Gibson et al. 2011). Given that the most recent calcium Dietary Reference Intake (DRI) for adolescents has risen to 1300 mg/day, this statistic describing deficiency is probably greater than the reported 67%. Ferreira da Costa et al. (2013) also reported inadequate calcium consumption in adolescent female swimmers. Seventy-seven female swimmers, 11 to 19 years of age, completed questionnaires to evaluate the prevalence of disordered eating. After identifying disordered eating, scientists compared data from 3-day food records between athletes with or without the condition. They found that median intakes of calcium, zinc, and folate were inadequate across all swimmers, and calcium deficiency worsened with the presence of disordered eating in girls 15 to 19 years of age.

Most calcium status data on athletes is specific to females. This trend in the literature may stem from the fact that women experience osteoporosis more often than men (Iwamoto et al. 2010). However, recent work published by Iwamoto et al. (2010) suggests that male athletes also consume inadequate intakes of calcium and vitamin D. Food frequency data on Japanese professional baseball players demonstrated that these athletes, on average, consume inadequate amounts of calcium (459 mg/day) and vitamin D (9.9 mcg/day) (Iwamoto et al. 2010). Additionally, urine analysis indicated that low calcium and vitamin D in the diet of these baseball players were associated with increased levels of bone resorption biomarkers.

Juzwiak et al. (2008) analyzed 4-day food diaries in 44 competitive male tennis players, 10 to 19 years of age. Their data showed that 86.4% of these adolescent male athletes were consuming less than 1300 mg of calcium each day. Their results, however, did not demonstrate a relationship between insufficient calcium intake in males and declines in bone mineral density. They hypothesized that physical activity and lean muscle mass are better predictors of bone mineral density than calcium intake in male adolescents.

EXERCISE PERFORMANCE AND SUPPLEMENTATION

As with other micronutrients, the American College of Sports Medicine (ACSM), the Academy of Nutrition and Dietetics (AND), and Dietitians of Canada state that consuming calcium beyond the DRI has not been associated with ergogenic effects, but attainment of healthy calcium status may improve performance (Rodriguez et al.

2009). A review by Josse and Phillips (2013) supports the hypothesis that sufficient calcium and vitamin D intakes, in conjunction with resistance exercise, confer body composition changes that are beneficial to athletes. Milk as a supplement after resistance exercise appears to be the best choice to achieve these effects of lean mass gains and fat mass losses (Josse and Phillips 2013). The calcium and vitamin D in milk have been shown to increase lipolysis, decrease lipogenesis, and lead to the saponification and decreased absorption of fats in the gastrointestinal tract (Parikh and Yanovski 2003; Shi et al. 2001; Zemel 2003). The protein in milk provides the necessary amino acids for muscle growth. Josse et al. (2010) supplemented women with 500 mL of skim milk immediately following training and then another 500 mL of skim milk 1 h after training as part of a 12-week resistance exercise program. Women drinking milk after exercise experienced significantly greater gains in muscle mass and losses in fat mass compared to women who consumed a control beverage.

Calcium status may also improve muscle synthesis in males through a testosterone mechanism. Cinar et al. (2009) divided 30 healthy male athletes into three groups for four weeks: no exercise with a calcium gluconate supplement; 90 min/day of training with a calcium gluconate supplement; and 90 min/day of training without a supplement. The athletes performed a 20-min shuttle run pre-supplementation and post-supplementation and blood was drawn before and after this exercise. This study design allowed researchers to observe the independent effects of exercise and supplementation on testosterone levels, as well as to determine how exercise and supplementation interacted synergistically. After four weeks of treatment, males undergoing the exercise training had higher testosterone levels than the sedentary group and this increase was heightened in the exercise plus calcium supplementation group. However, Cinar et al. (2009) did not evaluate calcium intake of the athletes prior to supplementation; therefore, it is unclear if this effect on testosterone occurred due to correction of deficiencies or the presence of additional calcium. Furthermore, testosterone's effect on muscle growth remains controversial and requires more research, and the supplement used in this study was not calcium carbonate or calcium citrate, the more bioavailable forms of calcium supplementation (Volpe 2009).

In addition to possible ergogenic effects, achieving sufficient calcium intake in athletes, via either dietary changes or supplementation, may have a protective effect against stress fractures. Young female athletes, especially those participating in sports like running and gymnastics where pressures to limit weight exist, are at high risk for stress fractures (Tenforde et al. 2010). These athletes are prone to disordered eating, and this diet restriction is associated with nutrient deficiencies, menstrual irregularities, and hormonal changes that hinder their attainment of optimal bone mineral density (Tenforde et al. 2010). In their review on calcium status and stress fracture risk, Tenforde et al. (2010) cite two prospective studies documenting improved bone mineral density and decreased risk for stress fracture with increased calcium and vitamin D intake via diet (Nieves et al. 2010) or supplementation (Lappe et al. 2008). Nieves et al. (2010) used food frequency questionnaires, dual x-ray absorptiometry, and reports of stress fractures to assess dietary intake, bone mineral density, and stress fracture incidence, respectively, in 125 female competitive distance runners, 18 to 26 years of age. They reported that increased dairy consumption, especially skim milk, was the best predictor for protection from stress fractures and gains in bone mineral density of the total body and hip (Nieves et al. 2010).

Lappe et al. (2008) also highlighted the importance of increased calcium and vitamin D intake in active females by conducting a randomized clinical trial evaluating the effect of 2000 mg/day of calcium and 800 International Units (IU)/day of vitamin D on stress fracture risk. Their results indicated that female military recruits taking the supplement reduced their risk of stress fracture by 20% compared to recruits taking the placebo.

Recent data published by Moran et al. (2012) show that active men with calcium and vitamin D deficiencies are also at risk for developing stress fractures. Scientists evaluated dietary intake and serum calcium in 74 Israeli Defense Forces recruits before and during basic training. Orthopedic surgeons periodically examined the recruits for stress fractures. Of the 74 recruits who were tested before basic training, 12 developed stress fractures. The mean intakes of calcium (589 mg/day) and vitamin D (117.9 IU/day) of these 12 recruits before training were 38.9% and 25.1% lower, respectively, than those of the other 62 men who did not suffer from stress fractures. Additionally, after six months of training, there was a significant difference in mean serum calcium levels between recruits with stress fractures (9.5 mg/dL) and those without fractures (9.8 mg/dL). These findings suggest that calcium and vitamin D supplementation to correct deficiencies in male athletes should be investigated for possible protective effects.

Athletes should also be aware of increased calcium losses due to greater sweat volumes and higher protein intakes than other less active populations. Even though sodium is the electrolyte of primary concern with respect to loss via sweat, small amounts of calcium have also been detected in perspiration (Bergeron 2003; Kilding et al. 2009). After two training sessions, Kilding et al. (2009) collected absorbent sweat pads from 13 international level female soccer players and analyzed them with inductively coupled plasma atomic emission spectroscopy to determine mineral concentrations. They found that athletes lost 0.9 mmol/L of calcium in sweat. Scientists note that this amount is too small to contribute to muscle cramps (Bergeron 2003; Kilding et al. 2009), but increased sweating in athletes may contribute to a negative calcium balance. Athletes who choose to take protein supplements should also monitor their calcium intake. The recommended calcium to protein ratio is approximately 16 mg: 1 g, and protein intakes that skew this ratio can greatly increase urinary calcium loss (Weaver and Heaney 2006).

If nutrition assessment indicates that an athlete's calcium needs are not being met, supplementation could have beneficial effects on health and athletic performance. For best absorption, athletes who choose to take calcium supplements should take 500 mg in the morning and 500 mg at night every day with 400 IU of vitamin D with each dose (Volpe 2009). Importantly, calcium carbonate supplements are best absorbed when taken with food, but calcium citrate supplements can be consumed with or without food (Volpe 2009). Supplementation amounts for female athletes with disordered eating, amenorrhea, and risk for osteoporosis are increased to 1500 mg of elemental calcium and 400 to 800 IU of vitamin D daily (Rodriguez et al. 2009).

MAGNESIUM

SIGNIFICANCE IN HUMAN PHYSIOLOGY AND HEALTH

Magnesium (Mg) plays a crucial structural and regulatory role in over 300 metabolic reactions in the human body (Rude and Shils 2006; Volpe 2009). The mineral is especially important in energy utilization through the formation of a magnesium and adenosine triphosphate (Mg-ATP) complex. The Mg-ATP structure changes the orientation of the ATP molecule in a way that allows various kinases to bind the substrate and then use the phosphate groups to activate or inactivate downstream proteins (Rude and Shils 2006). Magnesium is also required for the action of key enzymes in energy-yielding pathways. The mineral activates creatine phosphoki-nase, pyruvate dehydrogenase, hexokinase, and cytochrome C; therefore, magne-sium aids in the utilization of phosphocreatine, function of the tricarboxylic acid cycle, efficiency of glycolysis, and productivity of oxidative phosphorylation, respec-tively (Carvil and Cronin 2010). Furthermore, magnesium acts as a regulator and signaling component in second messenger pathways such as those involving cyclic adenosine monophosphate (cAMP) and phospholipase C (Rude and Shils 2006). The fundamental process of gene expression also depends on proper magnesium status due to the mineral's influence on deoxyribonucleic acid (DNA) and ribonucleic acid (RNA) polymerases, exonucleases, and topoisomerase. Because magnesium ions have a positive charge, the mineral is also able to interact directly with negatively charged DNA and RNA molecules and stabilize these structures. Additionally, mag-nesium, like other cations, binds various structures on cellular membranes. These interactions affect membrane stability and permeability as well as transport systems for ions like calcium, sodium, and potassium (Rude and Shils 2006). Given all of these effects, magnesium impacts fuel catabolism, DNA, RNA, and protein syn-thesis, bone health, immune function, muscle relaxation and contraction, neuronal activity, and cardiac excitability (Brilla 2012; Rude and Shils 2006).

The percentage of the U.S. population not meeting the RDA for magnesium has decreased from 75% (Rude and Shils 2006) to 48% according to 2005 to 2006 National Health and Nutrition Examination Survey (NHANES) data (Rosanoff et al. 2012). Despite this improvement, inadequate magnesium intakes remain a genuine health concern given the detrimental effects of magnesium deficiency. Symptoms of severe magnesium deficiency include hypocalcemia, seizures and other neuromus-cular dysfunctions, hypokalemia, muscular weakness and wasting, cardiac arrhyth-mia, and myocardial infarction (Rude and Shils 2006). Since the manifestation of these conditions is not widespread, the current hypothesis is that many individu-als, and thus many athletes, may be suffering from marginal magnesium deficiency. Long-term suboptimal magnesium intake has been linked to chronic health concerns such as type 2 diabetes mellitus, metabolic syndrome, hypertension, atherosclerotic vascular disease, and osteoporosis (Rosanoff et al. 2012; Volpe 2013).

MAGNESIUM HOMEOSTASIS DURING EXERCISE

Serum levels of magnesium are poor indicators of magnesium status; only 1% of the magnesium in the human body is found in serum/plasma, 50% to 60% resides in bone and supports skeletal structure, and the remaining magnesium is intracellular and participates in signaling and enzymatic reactions (Rude et al. 2009). For this reason, serum magnesium concentration is not the ideal indicator of magnesium status, but it remains the most practical and widely used method. The changes that occur in serum magnesium levels during various training regimens, however, may illustrate the adequacy of magnesium stores and how well the body can mobilize the mineral to tissues of need. Magnesium is required for neuromuscular function and energy utilization, so distribution of this mineral will vary depending on the intensity, duration, and type of exercise, and how these characteristics influence cellular demands (Nielsen and Lukaski 2006).

MAGNESIUM REQUIREMENTS

It is recommended that athletes consume foods rich in magnesium to meet the RDA for this mineral (Table 12.4) (Institute of Medicine, Food and Nutrition Board 1997). Magnesium requirements increase with age and are higher for men than for women. The recommended magnesium intake for pre-pubescent males and females is 240 mg/day, and this increases to 410 mg/day and 360 mg/day in males and females, respectively, 14 to 18 years of age. The increase would aid in the high metabolic demands during this period of significant growth. Men and women, 31 years of age or older, should consume 420 mg/day and 320 mg/day, respectively, of magnesium. Whole grains, legumes, and dark-green, leafy vegetables are high sources of magnesium (Office of Dietary Supplements, National Institutes of Health 2009). Fruits like bananas and raisins as well as dairy products are other sources of magnesium.

TABLE 12.4
Food Sources of Magnesium

Food	Magnesium Content (mg)
Halibut, cooked, 3 oz	90
Almonds, dry roasted, 1 oz	80
Cashews, dry roasted, 1 oz	75
Soybeans, mature, cooked, 1/2 cup	75
Spinach, frozen, cooked, 1/2 cup	75
Cereal, shredded wheat, 2 rectangular biscuits	55
Potato, baked w/skin, 1 medium	50
Peanut butter, smooth, 2 tablespoons	50
Wheat Bran, crude, 2 tablespoons	45
Black-eyed peas, cooked, 1/2 cup	45
Yogurt, plain, skim milk, 8 fluid oz	45
Bran flakes, 1/2 cup	40

Source: Adapted from http://www.nal.usda.gov/fnic/foodcomp/search/.

STATUS IN ATHLETES

Previous research and current studies conclude that poor magnesium status in athletes has been and continues to be an issue in sports nutrition (Bohl and Volpe 2002; Imamura et al. 2013; Matias et al. 2010; Santos et al. 2011). Due to the severity of magnesium deficiency symptoms, it is unlikely that athletes capable of participating in training and competition suffer from this condition. Nonetheless, marginal magnesium deficiency, defined as consuming 260 mg/day or less in men and 220 mg/day or less in women, is a practical concern for active individuals (Nielsen and Lukaski 2006). Because strenuous exercise has been shown to increase magnesium loss in urine and sweat (Bohl and Volpe 2002), as well as increase magnesium utilization in energy production and muscle contraction (Carvil and Cronin 2010), an insufficient magnesium intake may be more of a concern for athletes than for sedentary individuals.

In a review of older magnesium studies, Bohl and Volpe (2002) assert that magnesium intakes of athletes range from exceeding dietary guidelines in populations like highly trained runners, to falling short of adequate consumption such as in wrestlers and gymnasts. Analyses of more recent studies, however, indicate that the current trend in athletes is insufficient dietary magnesium (Anderson 2010; Gibson et al. 2011; Imamura et al. 2013; Matias et al. 2010; Santos et al. 2011). Food frequency data on Japanese collegiate male rugby players indicated that the mean intakes of rugby forwards (311 mg/day) and rugby backs (283 mg/day) were below both the Japanese, United States, and Canadian recommendations (Imamura et al. 2013).

Santos et al. (2011) evaluated 7 days of 24-hour diet recalls from elite male basketball, handball, and volleyball players, and concluded that the average daily magnesium intake of 244.7 mg was significantly below the RDA. Female athletes have also been found to consume diets poor in magnesium (Anderson 2010; Gibson et al. 2011). Three-day food records from collegiate volleyball players indicated that 75% of the women did not meet the RDA for magnesium at the beginning of the season, and this figure rose to 87.5% at the peak of their training (Anderson 2010). In direct contrast to these findings, Heaney et al. (2010) reported that food frequency data on elite Australian female athletes participating in a variety of sports demonstrated a mean intake of magnesium above the RDA. Nevertheless, 20% of these female athletes did not meet the RDA, suggesting that suboptimal magnesium consumption should remain a nutritional concern even if only a subset of athletes are at risk.

EXERCISE PERFORMANCE AND SUPPLEMENTATION

Magnesium status may play a pivotal role in an individual's response to aerobic exercise due to the mineral's effects on muscle contraction, ATP utilization, and carbohydrate metabolism. In an exquisitely controlled study by Lukaski and Nielsen (2002), the performance of postmenopausal women on submaximal exercise tests corresponded with their magnesium intake (Lukaski and Nielsen 2002). The researchers included three dietary phases: an equilibrium or control phase, a magnesium depletion phase, and a magnesium repletion phase. Registered dietitians prepared a low-magnesium diet for the women, and the participants consumed this diet with 200 mg/day of supplemental magnesium during the 35-day control phase, followed this diet without supplementation during the 93-day depletion phase, and then returned to eating the low-magnesium diet along with supplemental magnesium in the 49-day repletion phase. In each of the three periods, researchers analyzed blood samples and muscle biopsies, and found that the women had significantly lower red blood cell and muscle magnesium concentrations, as well as a downward trend in serum magnesium concentrations during the depletion phase vs. the control and repletion periods. During each phase, the women also performed a submaximal exercise test until reaching a previously determined intensity. The women exhibited significantly higher peak and total oxygen consumption, cumulative net oxygen utilization, and heart rate during magnesium restriction. Therefore, the same exercise became more taxing when magnesium was not consumed in adequate amounts, and energy production was less efficient. Although this study included non-athlete participants, the elegant design allowed each participant to be her own control, linked magnesium intake to cellular magnesium status, and then connected low magnesium intake to impaired cardiorespiratory and cardiovascular responses during exercise. Older studies in adolescent, competitive swimmers (Conn et al. 1988) and trained male athletes (Lukaski et al. 1983) documented positive correlations between maximal oxygen consumption and serum magnesium, and these findings support a role for magnesium in aerobic performance. Additionally, male triathletes receiving magnesium supplements showed better running, cycling, and swimming times vs. triathletes receiving a placebo (Golf et al. 1998). Magnesium supplementation in other active populations has also elicited improvements in aerobic performance (Brilla and Gunter 1995; Ripari et al. 1989).

Animal studies have sought to elucidate mechanisms through which magnesium could exert these advantageous effects on athletic performance. Chen et al. (2009) separated gerbils into two groups; one group received an injection of magnesium sulfate 30 min before a forced swimming test, and the control group received a saline injection. The gerbils who received the magnesium supplement had greater swim duration times than the controls. Blood collection data illustrated that the magnesium-supplemented gerbils exhibited higher levels of plasma magnesium during exercise, which corresponded with better mobilization of glucose and an attenuated blood lactate increase. These physiological changes could explain how the supplemented gerbils achieved longer swim times before exhaustion (Chen et al. 2009). These findings parallel human data showing reduced lactate levels at rest and at exhaustion in individuals who were supplemented with magnesium before exercise (Cinar et al. 2006).

The efficacy of magnesium supplementation in inducing improvements to aerobic capacity, however, is contended in the literature. Finstad et al. (2001) conducted a randomized, double-blind, placebo-controlled, crossover study and reported that magnesium supplementation did not elicit physiological improvements in active women during aerobic or anaerobic treadmill tests (Finstad et al. 2001). The researchers acknowledged that the supplement used in the study, 212 mg/day of magnesium oxide, is small compared to other supplementation studies, and that some of the women who were determined to have low serum magnesium levels before treatment actually improved their magnesium status throughout the course of the experiment independent of supplementation. These characteristics of the study could have reduced the supplement's potential to improve magnesium status, and thus, performance. Other data from magnesium supplementation in swimmers (Ruddel et al. 1990) and athletes with low to normal serum magnesium concentrations (Weller et al. 1998) have also found no effect of magnesium supplementation on aerobic capacity. Because research on magnesium supplementation as an ergogenic aid has been equivocal, the current hypothesis is that supplementation will not benefit athletes who meet magnesium recommendations through diet. Improvements may be seen if the athlete supplements during a magnesium-poor state.

Recent athlete studies suggest that magnesium supplementation may also support strength performance in active individuals who were previously deficient. A common practice among elite judo athletes is severe diet and hydration restriction prior to a competition to qualify for their weight category (Matias et al. 2010). A dehydrated state coupled with strenuous exercise can produce a magnesium deficit due to high sweat losses (Matias et al. 2010). Matias et al. (2010) measured intracellular water (a measure of hydration status), dietary intake, body composition, serum and urinary magnesium levels, and power output in 20 elite judo athletes in a baseline hydrated state and then again prior to competition. None of the judo athletes met magnesium intake recommendations at either measurement, but the athletes experienced greater dehydration (intracellular water losses at or above 2%) before competition and demonstrated significantly greater reductions in serum magnesium concentration. Along with lower serum magnesium levels, the dehydrated athletes scored lower on hand grip and upper-body power tests when compared to judo athletes who did not experience significant hydration changes before their event. In a similar study, Santos et al. (2011) concluded that there was a significant positive correlation between magnesium intake and scores on a variety of strength tests (e.g., maximal isometric flexion, handgrip, and jumping tests) in elite male basketball, handball, and volleyball players. These elite male athletes were not meeting the RDA for magnesium, but the less deficient they were, the better their strength performance.

Both of these aforementioned studies highlight an association between the magnitude of magnesium deficiency and anaerobic performance, but clinical trials are needed to support a causative relationship. The two studies also only report magnesium intakes and failed to include data on other possible deficiencies that may contribute to this reduction in anaerobic performance. Nevertheless, this association between magnesium status and strength, along with previous data linking magnesium supplementation to greater gains in lean mass and higher power output of quadriceps (Brilla and Haley 1992), suggest that the mineral could enhance muscle growth in athletes.

The literature has yet to reach a consensus on whether to prescribe magnesium supplements to athletic populations. However, individuals participating in high intensity exercise on a regular basis should be aware that their magnesium needs are 10 to 20% greater than sedentary persons' needs due to greater losses in sweat and urine (Nielsen and Lukaski 2006). If dietary intake analysis finds that an athlete is not meeting magnesium recommendations, magnesium supplementation may improve performance. In a comparison of various oral magnesium supplements, magnesium chloride and magnesium lactate supplements exhibited greater bioavailability than magnesium oxide (Firoz and Graber 2001). In addition to the supplement's bioavailability, the amount of elemental magnesium in each dose should also be considered. Magnesium oxide supplements currently contain the highest percentage (60%) of elemental magnesium when compared to other magnesium salts (Office of Dietary Supplements, NIH 2009); however, magnesium oxide typically results in diarrhea and less absorption of magnesium. Current evidence supports a conservative prescription of 100 mg of magnesium/day (Carvil and Cronin 2010) and no greater than 350 mg of magnesium/day (Calbert et al. 2011). For athletes, specific benefits of maintaining adequate magnesium status include efficient oxygen utilization, reduced damage from oxidative stress during and following exercise, improved energy production, enhanced protein synthesis, and better regulation of muscle contraction (Carvil and Cronin 2010).

IRON

SIGNIFICANCE IN HUMAN PHYSIOLOGY AND HEALTH

Iron is found in every living cell. Total body iron is about 5 g; however, this varies due to body weight, hemoglobin concentration, sex, and size of iron storage compartments. The general functions of iron include oxygen transport in red blood cells and tissues, ATP generation, prevention of lipid peroxidation (although it can act as a pro-oxidant if too much iron is consumed), storage and transport, and thyroid hormone function (iron is required for the functioning of 1,5'-deiodinase, which converts triiodothyronine to thyroxine). Normal serum iron ranges from 20 to 52 mcg/dL.

Iron deficiency is the most common nutritional deficiency in the world. It is a major concern for approximately 15% of the world's population. Iron deficiency manifests itself as alterations in immune function, cognitive performance, energy metabolism, and exercise or work performance.

REGULATION IN THE HUMAN BODY

Although iron is abundant in the human body and in nature, it is tightly regulated in the body. The total amount of iron in the human body is 40 to 50 mg/kg of body weight; nonetheless, research using stable isotopes of iron has shown that the labile iron pool has about 70 mg of iron (Himmelfarb 2007). Only 1 to 2 mg of iron is lost from the body on a daily basis because iron is recycled and used again (Himmelfarb 2007). Iron is tightly regulated because, although iron can act as an antioxidant, it can also act as a pro-oxidant, causing DNA and lipid and protein oxidation. Thus, the body sequesters iron via binding it to transferrin, the transferrin receptor and ferritin, preventing iron from increasing free radical damage to the body (Himmelfarb 2007).

One of the key regulators of iron into the circulation is by the protein hepcidin. Hepcidin is a peptide hormone produced mainly in the liver, and is encoded by the HAMP gene. It decreases dietary iron absorption by decreasing iron transport across the intestinal mucosa, as well as decreasing iron exit from macrophages and the liver. Hepcidin achieves this by decreasing the transmembrane iron transporter ferroportin (Ganz 2003). Ferroportin is a transmembrane protein. Its main role is to transport iron from inside the cell to outside the cell.

Because exercise is a stressor and causes inflammation, and hepcidin levels increase as part of the inflammatory response, serum iron levels will decrease because iron is trapped within the macrophages and liver cells (Ganz 2003). This cascade of events could lead to iron deficiency anemia due to an insufficient quantity of serum iron being present to develop red blood cells. Conversely, when hepcidin concentrations are below normal levels, such as in hemochromatosis (a genetic disorder with excess iron absorbed and stored in the body), iron overload ensues because of excessive iron influx, facilitated by ferroportin (Ganz 2003).

Iron Requirements

The RDA for iron is 8 mg/day for males 19 to >70 years of age and females 51 to >70 years of age, and 18 mg/day for females 19 to 50 years of age (Table 12.2) (Institute of Medicine, Food and Nutrition Board 2001). The tolerable upper intake levels (UL) for iron have been established as 45 mg/day for these same age groups. See Table 12.5 for food sources of iron.

Status in Athletes

It has been reported that increased serum and urine concentrations of hepcidin have been found in athletes after working out, with concomitant decreases in iron status found after long periods of training. McClung et al. (2013) conducted an observational study to examine the effects of military training on iron status, inflammation, and serum hepcidin concentrations. They studied 21 Norwegian soldiers who were participating in 7 days of winter training. They reported that military training increased serum hepcidin concentrations, as well as interleukin (IL)-6, an inflammatory marker; however, iron status was not affected by training.

In another study where iron status was evaluated, Govus et al. (2014) assessed if acute hypoxic exercise influenced IL-6 and hepcidin concentrations and iron status in 13 moderately trained endurance athletes. These athletes were required to perform five 4-min intervals at 90% of their peak oxygen consumption (VO_{2peak}) in

---

TABLE 12.5
Food Sources of Iron

Food	Iron Content (mg)
Beef liver, braised, 3 oz	5.8
Lean sirloin, broiled, 3 oz	2.9
Lean ground beef, broiled, 3 oz	1.8
Skinless chicken breast, roasted, 3 oz	0.9
Fortified breakfast cereal, 1 cup	4.5 to 18
Boiled spinach, 1/2 cup	3.2
Firm tofu, 1/2 cup	2.0

Source: Adapted from http://www.nal.usda.gov/fnic/foodcomp/search/.

---

normoxic and hypoxic conditions. They reported that acute exercise hypoxia did not affect IL-6 and hepcidin concentrations, as well as iron status. Therefore, acute exercise performed at the same relative intensity in hypoxia did not result in an increased risk to iron status compared with exercise in normal oxygen conditions.

Peeling et al. (2014) sought to examine the iron status and acute post-exercise hepcidin concentrations in athletes. They grouped their 54 athletes into four groups, based on serum ferritin concentrations: <30 mcg/L, 30 to 50 mcg/L, 50 to 100 mcg/L, or >100 mcg/L. Each athlete completed one of the following five running sessions: (1) 8 × 3 min at 85% VO_{2peak}; (2) 5 × 4 min at 90% VO_{2peak}; (3) 90 min of continuous exercise at 75% VO_{2peak}; (4) 40 min of continuous exercise at 75% VO_{2peak}; and (5) 40 min of continuous exercise at 65% VO_{2peak} (Peeling et al. 2014). They found no within or between group differences for baseline or post-exercise serum iron or IL-6 concentrations; however, post-exercise IL-6 concentrations were significantly increased from baseline within each group ($p < 0.05$). As serum ferritin levels increased, baseline and 3-h post-exercise hepcidin concentrations were consecutively greater ($p < 0.05$). Nonetheless, post-exercise hepcidin concentrations were only significantly increased in three of the four groups (serum ferritin levels of 30 to 50, 50 to 100, and >100 mcg/dL; $p < 0.05$). Iron stores may regulate baseline hepcidin concentrations and the level of post-exercise hepcidin response. Low iron stores blocked post-exercise hepcidin concentration increases, likely superseding any inflammatory-driven elevations that resulted from exercise (Peeling et al. 2014).

Exercise Performance and Supplementation

Because iron is required for thyroid hormone metabolism, and therefore, metabolic rate, Harris Rosenzweig and Volpe (2000), in a case study, evaluated the effect of iron supplementation on thyroid hormone concentrations and resting metabolic rate (RMR) in two college female athletes. Two iron deficient anemic female athletes, 18 (A1) and 21 (A2) years of age, were supplemented for 4 months with 23 mg/day of elemental iron, as ferrous fumarate. Thyroid hormone status and RMR were evaluated at 0, 8, and 16 weeks. The iron deficiency anemia was clinically corrected in both participants (via measures of hemoglobin and hematocrit) from baseline to 16 weeks. However, 4 months of iron supplementation did not fully replete iron stores because serum ferritin concentrations were not fully restored. Although statistical analyses could not be conducted because this was a case study, participant A1 had an increase in throxine concentrations and RMR, while participant A2 showed a decline in these measures. Although others have reported improvements in thyroid hormone function and RMR (Beard et al. 1990, 1998), more research needs to be conducted in larger samples to definitively establish this response.

In a more recent study, Burden et al. (2014) conducted a meta-analysis to evaluate whether iron supplementation improves both the iron status and aerobic capacity of endurance athletes who had iron deficiency without anemia. The authors used 17 studies they deemed eligible for their criteria. They included studies where the researchers measured iron supplementation on serum ferritin, serum iron, transferrin saturation, and hemoglobin concentrations. Burden et al. (2014) reported that iron supplementation improved the iron status and aerobic capacity of endurance athletes who were iron deficient, but not anemic; however, supplementation greater than 80 days did not affect serum ferritin concentrations further.

In an effort to establish if iron-fortified bread would improve the iron status of female runners, Alaunyte et al. (2014) asked 11 recreational female runners to replace their usual bread with iron-rich bread as part of their regular diet for 6 weeks. The women were about 32 years of age, exercised 239 ± 153 min per week, with 161 ± 150 min of those total minutes composed of running. The researchers collected 24-h dietary recalls, as well as blood levels of serum transferrin, serum transferrin receptor, serum ferritin, totally iron binding capacity, and transferrin receptor/ferritin log index.

At baseline, the women did not consume sufficient dietary iron (10.7 ± 2.7 mg/ day); more than one-third of the participants had iron depletion, with a serum ferritin level of <12 mcg/L. The intervention resulted in a significantly higher iron consumption of 18.5 mg/day ($p < 0.05$), and improvements in iron status, but not iron stores. A longer intervention may have resulted in increased serum ferritin stores. Nonetheless, the use of high iron bread is a viable way to improve iron status in female athletes.

Della Valle and Haas (2014) conducted a randomized, placebo-controlled 6-week trial with iron supplementation on iron status and exercise performance in 31 female rowers who had iron deficiency without anemia (15 were given an iron supplement [100 mg/day of ferrous sulfate], 16 were given a placebo). Della Valle and Haas (2014) measured the following variables at baseline and the end of 6 weeks: hemoglobin, serum ferritin, soluble transferrin receptor, and blood lactate concentrations, as well as a 4-km rowing time trial and VO_{2peak}. All rowers significantly improved their lean body mass and VO_{2peak} from baseline to end of study ($p < 0.001$). Rowers in the iron-supplemented group had an increase in their serum ferritin concentrations ($p = 0.07$), and significant improvements in their lactate response ($p = 0.05$). Iron supplementation improved iron status and lactate response in female rowers with iron deficiency without anemia.

ZINC

SIGNIFICANCE IN HUMAN PHYSIOLOGY AND HEALTH

Zinc is required for more than 300 metabolic reactions in the body. There are five stable isotopes of zinc: ^{64}Zn, ^{66}Zn, ^{67}Zn, ^{68}Zn, and ^{70}Zn. Zinc is usually in its divalent state (Zn^{2+}) in biological systems and it readily complexes with amino acids, peptides, proteins, and nucleotides. About 60% of total body zinc is found in the muscle, 30% in bone, and less than 1% is found in the plasma. The liver and plasma represent the readily exchangeable zinc pools, while bone represents the slowly exchangeable zinc pool.

Zinc acts as a metalloenzyme with alcohol dehydrogenase, carboxypeptidase, carboxyanhydrase, pyruvate carboxylase, alkaline phosphatase and copper, and zinc-superoxide dismustase, to name a few. These enzymes indicate zinc's diverse roles within the body: metabolism of alcohol, protein metabolism, acid-base balance, carbohydrate metabolism, bone metabolism, and antioxidant functions. Zinc is also involved in growth, wound healing, reproduction, and taste acuity.

Zinc fingers are "small protein structural motifs" that denote any number of structures related by their management of a zinc ion. Zinc fingers are usually repeated cysteine- and histidine-containing domains that bind zinc in a tetrahedral configuration. Zinc finger proteins include transcription factors for DNA.

ZINC REGULATION DURING EXERCISE

Plasma zinc concentrations have been shown to decline with acute stress, which is thought to be related to an increased uptake of zinc by the liver and bone marrow for synthesis of acute phase proteins. Strenuous exercise is a stressor and induces an acute phase response. Others have reported both declines and increases in plasma zinc levels following strenuous exercise (Anderson et al. 1984; Mundie and Hare 2001). In the first study of its kind, Volpe et al. (2006) examined the effect of acute exhaustive exercise vs. rest on short-term zinc kinetics in males, using stable isotopes of zinc. It was a crossover design study, where they evaluated 12 healthy, sedentary males, 25 to 35 years of age. Volpe et al. (2006) measured fasting blood concentrations of plasma zinc, serum creatine kinase, and serum cortisol. After baseline blood samples were obtained, an intravenous stable isotope of 0.1 mg ^{70}Zn was infused via a butterfly catheter into the opposite arm of the blood draws. Blood was sampled at the following intervals post-isotope infusion: 2, 5, 10, 15, 30, 45, 60, 75, 90, and 120 min. They also measured plasma volume changes to account for hemoconcentration post-exercise (during the exercise protocol). The researchers provided participants with the same meal the night before prior to each trial, to ensure food intake did not have an effect on zinc kinetics. The participants were 74.6 ± 12.9 kg with a body mass index (BMI) of 22.4 ± 3.4 kg/m^2 and a percentage body fat of 16.9 ± 7.0% (via hydrostatic weighing).

Volpe et al. (2006) found that plasma zinc concentrations significantly decreased 40 min post-exercise until the end of blood draws. With respect to the zinc kinetics, the plasma pool of zinc significantly increased with exercise, compared to rest conditions ($p = 0.05$), while there was a trend for the liver zinc pool to increase ($p = 0.12$). The increase in the plasma zinc pool may be explained by a shift of plasma zinc into the interstitial fluid and uptake of zinc by the liver. The researchers stated that some possible mechanisms include increased cytokine activity and sequestering of zinc into the liver or changes in oncotic pressure with exercise. These results may reflect the acute stress response of strenuous exercise.

REGULATION IN THE HUMAN BODY

Zinc homeostasis is tightly regulated by metallothionein, a cysteine-rich, low molecular weight protein (Peroza et al. 2009). Metallothionein is located within the intestinal mucosa, and its synthesis increases with increased zinc intake. Within the intestinal mucosa, metallothionein will bind with zinc, forming a zinc-metallothionein complex. When zinc is required by the body, metallothionein releases it in the blood, where it typically is carried by albumin.

ZINC REQUIREMENTS

The RDA for zinc is 8 and 11 mg/day for women and men, 19 to greater than 70 years of age, respectively (Table 12.2) (Institute of Medicine, Food and Nutrition Board

TABLE 12.6
Food Sources of Zinc

Food	Zinc Content (mg)
Oysters, cooked, breaded, and fried, 3 oz	74.0
Beef chuck roast, braised, 3 oz	7.0
Crab, Alaska king, cooked, 3 oz	6.5
Beef patty, broiled, 3 oz	5.3
Breakfast cereal, fortified with 25% of the Daily Value for zinc, 3/4 cup serving	3.8
Lobster, cooked, 3 oz	3.4
Pork chop, loin, cooked, 3 oz	2.9
Baked beans, canned, plain or vegetarian, 1/2 cup	2.9
Chicken, dark meat, cooked, 3 oz	2.4
Yogurt, fruit, low fat, 8 oz	1.7
Cashews, dry roasted, 1 oz	1.6

Source: Adapted from http://www.nal.usda.gov/fnic/foodcomp/search/.

2001). The tolerable (UL) for zinc is 40 mg/day for women and men of the aforementioned age ranges. Food sources of zinc are listed in Table 12.6.

Status in Athletes

The zinc status of athletes has been evaluated by a number of researchers, with mixed results. Wierniuk and Wlodarek (2013) examined the energy and nutritional intake in 25 male athletes, 19 to 25 years of age, who were practicing aerobic sports, who were students at two different universities in Poland. They weighed 80.6 ± 9.6 kg, with a BMI of 23.01 ± 1.70 kg/m^2. The researchers evaluated dietary intake based on 3-day dietary records. These athletes did not take dietary supplements. Their overall energy intake was below requirements, as denoted by low carbohydrate and protein intake, despite a higher than required fat intake. Although dietary intakes of vitamins A, C, and D, as well as folate and magnesium were below normal levels, the athletes consumed adequate amounts of zinc. These data indicate a need for sports nutrition counseling in collegiate male athletes (Wierniuk and Wlodarek 2013).

Zalcman et al. (2007) examined the nutritional status of 24 adventure race athletes (18 men, 6 women), 24 to 42 years of age, via their dietary intake (3-day food record), body composition (plethysmography), and biochemical markers. Both men and women consumed higher than required protein and fat, while male athletes consumed carbohydrate at the lower recommended limit. Although Zalcman et al. (2007) reported adequate intake of most vitamins and minerals, these athletes did not consume adequate dietary zinc, once again demonstrating that these athletes need to be counseled and educated on proper sports nutrition habits for their overall health and performance.

Giolo De Carvalho et al. (2012) measured plasma zinc status in eight state and national level male swimmers, 18 to 25 years of age, who had been at these elite levels for at least 5 years. They evaluated zinc status in swimmers three times over a 14-week period by assessing plasma, erythrocyte, urine, and saliva zinc concentrations, as well as anthropometric measures and 3-day food records. The researchers reported that, aside from salivary zinc, which did not correlate with any other zinc measures, all other measures of zinc were significantly below normal values. Giolo De Carvalho et al. (2012) concluded that these elite swimmers were zinc deficient, and that salivary zinc is not a good measure of zinc status.

EXERCISE PERFORMANCE AND SUPPLEMENTATION

Zinc supplementation studies in athletes have been varied in participants, study design, and outcome measures. Not all have focused on exercise performance. Kara et al. (2011) evaluated the effects of exercise and zinc supplementation on cytokine release in young wrestlers and non-athletes. Forty male participants were separated into four groups: zinc-supplemented athletes, non-supplemented athletes, zinc-supplemented sedentary participants, and non-supplemented sedentary participants. Blood samples were collected at baseline and the end of the 8-week study for serum tumor necrosis factor-α (TNF-α), interleukin-2 (IL-2), and interferon-γ levels (IFN-γ). Kara et al. (2011) reported significantly higher concentrations of TNF-α, IL-2, and IFN-γ in the two zinc-supplemented groups compared to the two non-supplemented groups ($p < 0.01$). This is likely a result of zinc's role in the inflammatory response.

Because puberty associated with intense exercise will result in greater oxidative stress, de Oliveira Kde et al. (2009) assessed the effect of zinc supplementation on antioxidant, zinc, and copper status in adolescent male football players, 13 ± 0.4 years of age. In this 12-week study, 21 players were supplemented 22 mg of zinc gluconate, while 26 players were given a placebo.

After 12 weeks, plasma zinc and erythrocyte iron concentrations significantly increased ($p < 0.05$) in both groups. Urinary zinc concentrations significantly increased ($p < 0.001$) in the zinc supplemented group, while erythrocyte zinc significantly decreased ($p = 0.002$) in the placebo group. Plasma iron and copper concentrations significantly decreased ($p = 0.01$ and $p = 0.015$, respectively) in the zinc supplemented group. As far as measures of antioxidant status, the researchers reported that plasma ferric-reducing ability and plasma conjugated dienes increased, but erythrocyte osmotic fragility decreased in both groups, although the changes in plasma conjugated dienes and erythrocyte osmotic fragility were significantly lower in the zinc supplemented group compared to the placebo group ($p < 0.01$). Supplementation of zinc in healthy adolescent football players improved antioxidant status, but impaired copper and iron status.

SUMMARY

Calcium, magnesium, iron, and zinc are 4 of the 18 required minerals. They all play significant roles in the body. Research conducted in the area of calcium, magnesium, iron, and zinc has shown mixed results with respect to nutritional status and improving exercise performance. Although results have been mixed, it is important that athletes consume the proper amount of minerals to prevent deficiencies and improve physical performance. Longer-term supplementation studies are required to definitively ascertain the effects minerals can have on exercise performance.

REFERENCES

Alaunyte, I., V. Stojceska, A. Plunkett, and E. Derbyshire. 2014. Dietary iron intervention using a staple food product for improvement of iron status in female runners. *J Int Soc Sports Nutr* 11(1):50.

Anderson, D.E. 2010. The impact of feedback on dietary intake and body composition of college women volleyball players over a competitive season. *J Strength Cond Res* 24:2220–2226.

Anderson, R.A., M.M. Polansky, and N.A. Bryden. 1984. Acute effects of chromium, copper, zinc, and selected clinical variables in urine and serum of male runners. *Biol Trace Elem Res* 6:327–336.

Barrett, K.E., S. Boitano, S.M. Barman, and H.L. Brooks. 2012. *Ganong's Review of Medical Physiology*, 24th ed. New York: McGraw-Hill Medical.

Beard, J.L., M.J. Borel, and J. Derr. 1990. Impaired thermoregulation and thyroid function in iron-deficiency anemia. *Am J Clin Nutr* 52(5):813–819.

Beard, J.L., D.E. Brigham, S.K. Kelley, and M.H. Green. 1998. Plasma thyroid hormone kinetics are altered in iron-deficient rats. *J Nutr* 128(8):1401–1408.

Bergeron, M.F. 2003. Heat cramps: Fluid and electrolyte challenges during tennis in the heat. *J Sci Med Sport* 6:19–27.

Bohl, C.H., and S.L. Volpe. 2002. Magnesium and exercise. *Crit Rev Food Sci Nutr* 42:533–563.

Brilla, L.R. 2012. Magnesium influence on stress and immune function in exercise. *J Sports Med Doping Stud* 2:1–3.

Brilla, L.R., and T.F. Haley. 1992. Effect of magnesium supplementation on strength training in humans. *J Am Coll Nutr* 11:326–329.

Brilla, L.R., and K.B. Gunter. 1995. Effect of magnesium supplementation on exercise time to exhaustion. *Med Exerc Nutr Health* 4:230–233.

Burden, R.J., K. Morton, T. Richards, G.P. Whyte, and C.R. Pedlar. 2014. Is iron treatment beneficial in, iron-deficient but non-anaemic (IDNA) endurance athletes? A meta-analysis. *Br J Sports Med* doi: 10.1136/bjsports-2014-093624. Epub ahead of print.

Calbert, J.A., F.C. Mooren, L.M. Burke, S.J. Stear, and L.M. Castell. 2011 A-Z of nutritional supplements: Dietary supplements, sports nutrition foods and ergogenic aids for health and performance: Part 24. *Br J Sports Med* 45:1005–1007.

Carvil, P., and J. Cronin. 2010. Magnesium and implications on muscle function. *Strength Cond J* 32:48–54.

Chen, Y., H. Chen, W. Wang et al. 2009. Effects of magnesium on exercise performance and plasma glucose and lactate concentrations in rats using a novel blood-sampling technique. *Appl Physiol Nutr Metab* 34:1040–1047.

Cinar, V., M. Nizamhoglu, and R. Mogulkoc. 2006. The effect of magnesium supplementation on lactate levels of sportsmen and sedenter. *Acta Physiol Hung* 93:137–144.

Cinar, V., A.K. Baltaci, R. Mogulkoc, and M. Kilic. 2009. Testosterone levels in athletes at rest and exhaustion: Effects of calcium supplementation. *Biol Trace Elem Res* 129:65–69.

Conn, C.A., R.A. Schemme, B.W. Smith, E. Ryder, W.W. Henser, and P.K. Ku. 1988. Plasma and erythrocyte magnesium concentrations and correlations with maximal oxygen capacity. *Magnesium* 7:27–36.

Della Valle, D.M., and J.D. Haas. 2014. Iron supplementation improves energetic efficiency in iron-depleted female rowers. *Med Sci Sports Exerc* 46(6):1204–1215.

de Oliveira Kde, J., C.M. Donangelo, A.V. de Oliveira, Jr., C.L. da Silveira, and J.C. Koury. 2009. Effect of zinc supplementation on the antioxidant, copper, and iron status of physically active adolescents. *Cell Biochem Funct* 27(3):162–166.

Ferreira da Costa, N., A. Schtscherbyna, E.A. Soares, and B.G. Ribeiro. 2013. Disordered eating among adolescent female swimmers: Dietary, biochemical, and body composition factors. *Nutrition* 29:172–177.

Finstad, E.W., I.J. Newhouse, H.C. Lukaski, J.E. McAuliffe, and C.R. Stewart. 2001. The effects of magnesium supplementation on exercise performance. *Med Sci Sports Exerc* 33:493–498.

Firoz, M., and M. Graber. 2001. Bioavailability of US commercial magnesium preparation. *Magnes Res* 14:257–262.

Ganz, T. 2003. Hepcidin, a key regulator of iron metabolism and mediator of anemia of inflammation. *Blood* 102(3):783–788.

Gibson, J.C., L. Stuart-Hill, S. Martin, and C. Gaul. 2011. Nutrition status of junior elite Canadian female soccer athletes. *Int J Sport Nutr Exerc Metab* 21:507–514.

Giolo De Carvalho, F., F.T. Rosa, V. Marques Miguel Suen, E.C. Freitas, G.J. Padovan, and J.S. Marchini. 2012. Evidence of zinc deficiency in competitive swimmers. *Nutrition* 28(11–12):1127–1131.

Golf, S.W., S. Bender, and J. Grüttner. 1998. On the significance of magnesium in extreme physical stress. *Cardiovas Drugs Ther* 12:197–202.

Govus, A.D., C.R. Abbiss, L.A. Garvican-Lewis et al. 2014. Acute hypoxic exercise does not alter post-exercise iron metabolism in moderately trained endurance athletes. *Eur J Appl Physiol* 114(10):2183–2191.

Harris Rosenzweig, P., and S.L. Volpe. 2000. Effect of iron supplementation on thyroid hormone levels and resting metabolic rate in two college female athletes: A case study. *Int J Sport Nutr Exerc Metab* 10(4):434–443.

Heaney, R.P. 2006. Bone biology in health and disease. In *Modern Nutrition in Health and Disease*, 10th ed., M.E. Shils, M. Shike, A.C. Ross, B. Caballero, and R.J. Cousins, Eds. Baltimore, MD: Lippincott William & Wilkins, 1314–1325.

Heaney, S., H. O'Connor, J. Gifford, and G. Naughton. 2010. Comparison of strategies for assessing nutritional adequacy in elite female athletes' dietary intake. *Int J Sport Nutr Exerc Metab* 20:245–256.

Himmelfarb, J. 2007. Iron regulation. *J Am Soc Nephrol* 18(2):379–381.

Imamura, H., K. Iide, Y. Yoshimura et al. 2013. Nutrient intake, serum lipids and iron status of collegiate rugby players. *J Int Soc Sports Nutr* 10:1–9.

Institute of Medicine, Food and Nutrition Board. 1997. *Dietary Reference Intakes for Calcium, Phosphorus, Magnesium, Vitamin D and Fluoride.* Washington, DC: National Academy Press.

Institute of Medicine, Food and Nutrition Board. 2001. *Dietary Reference Intakes for Vitamin A, Vitamin K, Arsenic, Boron, Chromium, Copper, Iodine, Iron, Manganese, Molybdenum, Nickel, Silicon, Vanadium, and Zinc.* Washington, DC: National Academy Press.

Institute of Medicine, Food and Nutrition Board. 2010. *Dietary Reference Intakes for Calcium and Vitamin D.* Washington, DC: National Academy Press.

Iwamoto, J., T. Takeda, K. Uenishi, H. Ishida, Y. Sato, and H. Matsumoto. 2010. Urinary levels of cross-linked N-terminal telopeptide of type I collagen and nutritional status in Japanese professional baseball players. *J Bone Miner Metab* 28:540–546.

Josse, A.R., J.E. Tang, M.A. Tarnopolsky, and S.M. Phillips. 2010. Body composition and strength changes in women with milk and resistance exercise. *Med Sci Sports Exerc* 42:1122–1130.

Josse, S.M., and A.R. Phillips. 2013. Impact of milk consumption and resistance training on body composition of female athletes. *Med Sport Sci* 59:94–103.

Juzwiak, C.R., O.M. Amancio, M.S. Vitalle, M.M. Pinheiro, and V.L. Szejnfeld. 2008. Body composition and nutritional profile of male adolescent tennis players. *J Sports Sci* 26:1209–1217.

Kara, E., M. Ozal, M. Gunay, M. Kilic, A.K. Baltaci, and R. Mogulkoc. 2011. Effects of exercise and zinc supplementation on cytokine release in young wrestlers. *Biol Trace Elem Res* 143(3):1435–1440.

Kilding, A.E., H. Tunstall, E. Wraith, M. Good, C. Gammon, and C. Smith. 2009. Sweat rate and sweat electrolyte composition in international female soccer players during game specific training. *Int J Sports Med* 30:443–447.

Lappe, J., D. Cullen, G. Haynatzki, R. Recker, R. Ahlf, and K. Thompson. 2008. Calcium and vitamin D supplementation decreases incidence of stress fractures in female navy recruits. *J Bone Miner Res* 23:741–749.

Lukaski, H.C., and F.H. Nielsen. 2002. Dietary magnesium depletion affects metabolic responses during submaximal exercise in postmenopausal women. *J Nutr* 132:930–935.

Lukaski, H.C., W.W. Bolonchuk, L.M. Klevay, D.B. Milne, and H.H. Sandstead. 1983. Maximal oxygen consumption as related to magnesium, copper, and zinc nutriture. *Am J Clin Nutr* 37:407–415.

Matias, C.N., D.A. Santos, C.P. Monteiro et al. 2010. Magnesium and strength in elite judo athletes according to intracellular water changes. *Magnes Res* 23:138–141.

McClung, J.P., S. Martini, N.E. Murphy et al. 2013. Effects of a 7-day military training exercise on inflammatory biomarkers, serum hepcidin, and iron status. *Nutr J* 4;12(1):141.

Moran, D.S., Y. Heled, Y. Arbel et al. 2012. Dietary intake and stress fractures among elite male combat recruits. *J Int Soc Sports Nutr* 9:1–7.

Mundie, T.G., and B. Hare. 2001. Effects of resistance exercise on plasma, erythrocyte, and urine Zn. *Biol Trace Elem Res* 7:923–928.

Nielsen, F.H., and H.C. Lukaski. 2006. Update on the relationship between magnesium and exercise. *Magnes Res* 19:180–189.

Nieves, J.W., K. Melsop, M. Curtis et al. 2010. Nutritional factors that influence change in bone density and stress fracture risk among young female cross-county runners. *PM&R* 2:740–750.

Office of Dietary Supplements, National Institutes of Health. 2009. Dietary supplement fact sheet: Magnesium. http://ods.od.nih.gov/factsheets/Magnesium-HealthProfessional/.

Parikh, S.J., and J.A. Yanovski. 2003. Calcium intake and adiposity. *Am J Clin Nutr* 77:281–287.

Peeling, P., M. Sim, C.E. Badenhorst et al. 2014. Iron status and the acute post-exercise hepcidin response in athletes. *PLoS One* 9(3):e93002.

Peroza, E.A., R. Schmucki, P. Guntert, E. Freisinger, and O. Zerbe. 2009. The beta(E)-domain of wheat E(c)-1 metllothionein: A metal-binding domain with a distinctive structure. *J Mol Biol* 1:207–218.

Ripari, P., G. Pieralisi, M.A. Giamberardino, and L. Vecchiet. 1989. Effects of magnesium pico-linate on some cardiorespiratory submaximal effort parameters. *Magnes Res* 2:70–74.

Rodriguez, N.R., N.M. DiMarco, and S. Langley. 2009. Position of the American Dietetic Association, Dietitians of Canada, and the American College of Sports Medicine: Nutrition and athletic performance. *J Am Diet Assoc* 109:509–527.

Rosanoff, A., C.M. Weaver, and R.K. Rude. 2012. Suboptimal magnesium status in the United States: Are the health consequences underestimated? *Nutr Rev* 70:153–164.

Ruddel, H., C. Werner, and H. Ising. 1990. Impact of magnesium supplementation on perfor-mance data in young swimmers. *Magnes Res* 3:103–107.

Rude, R.K., and M.E. Shils. 2006. Magnesium. In *Modern Nutrition in Health and Disease*, 10th ed., M.E. Shils, M. Shike, A.C. Ross, B. Caballero, and R.J. Cousins, Eds. Baltimore, MD: Lippincott William & Wilkins, 223–247.

Rude, R.K., F.R. Singer, and H.E. Gruber. 2009. Skeletal and hormonal effects of magnesium deficiency. *J Am Coll Nutr* 28:131–141.

Santos, D.A., C.N. Matias, C.P. Monteiro et al. 2011. Magnesium intake is associated with strength performance in elite basketball, handball and volleyball players. *Magnes Res* 24:215–219.

Shi, H., A.W. Norman, W.H. Okamura, A. Sen, and M.B. Zemel. 2001. 1α, 25-Dihydroxyvitamin D3 modulates human adipocyte metabolism via nongenomic action. *FASEB J* 15:2751–2753.

Tenforde, A.S., L.C. Sayres, K.L. Sainani, and M. Fredericson. 2010. Evaluating the relationship of calcium and vitamin D in the prevention of stress fracture injuries in the young athlete: A review of the literature. *PM&R* 2:945–949.

Volpe, S.L. 2009. Minerals—Calcium, magnesium, chromium, and boron. In *Nutritional Concerns in Recreation, Exercise, and Sport*, J.A. Driskell, and I. Wolinsky, Eds. Boca Raton, FL: Taylor & Francis Group, 123–143.

Volpe, S.L. 2013. Magnesium in disease prevention and overall health. *Adv Nutr* 4(3):378S–383S.

Volpe, S.L., N.M. Lowe, L.R. Woodhouse, and J.C. King. 2006. Effect of maximal exercise on the short-term kinetics of zinc metabolism in sedentary men. *Br J Sports Med* 41(3):156–161.

Weaver, C.M., and R.P. Heaney. 2006. Calcium. In *Modern nutrition in health and disease*, 10th ed., M.E. Shils, M. Shike, A.C. Ross, B. Caballero, and R.J. Cousins, Eds. Baltimore, MD: Lippincott William & Wilkins, 194–210.

Weller, E., P. Bachert, H. Meinck, B. Friedmann, P. Bartsch, and H. Mairbaurl. 1998. Lack of effect of oral Mg-supplementation on Mg in serum, blood cells, and calf muscle. *Med Sci Sports Exerc* 30:1584–1591.

Widmaier, E.P., H. Raff, and K.T. Strang. 2011. *Vander's Human Physiology: The Mechanisms of Body Function*, 12th ed. New York: McGraw-Hill.

Wierniuk, A., and D. Włodarek. 2013. Estimation of energy and nutritional intake of young men practicing aerobic sports. *Rocz Panstw Zakl Hig* 64(2):143–148.

Zalcman, I., H.V. Guarita, C.R. Juzwiak et al. 2007. Nutritional status of adventure racers. *Nutrition* 23(5):404–411.

Zemel, M.B. 2003. Mechanisms of dairy modulation of adiposity. *J Nutr* 133:252S–256S.

Index

Page numbers followed by f and t indicate figures and tables, respectively.

A

Absorption, drug
  exercise-drug interaction, 213–214
  exercise training adaptation, 216
  paracellular pathway, 208
  transcellular pathway, 208
Academy of Nutrition and Dietetics (AND), 279
Acceptable Macronutrient Distribution Range of Dietary Reference Intakes, 135
Acceptable macronutrient distribution ranges (AMDR), 82
Acetaminophen, 219, 221–222
Acetyl CoA, 18, 19
Acetyl-CoA oxidation, 40
Acquired immune system, 229f, 230–231, 230t; see also Immune system
ACSM, see American College of Sports Medicine (ACSM)
Actin-myosin binding, calcium and, 276
Activation energy, 13, 20
Active tubular secretion, 213
Activities of daily living (ADL), 8, 9t; see also Total energy expenditure (TEE)
Acute infection and illness, see Infection and illness, acute
Acute supplementation protocols, 124t
"Adaptive microtrauma," 237
Adenosine diphosphate (ADP), 14, 17f, 90
Adenosine triphosphate (ATP), 14–16, 14f, 15f, 16f, 49; see also Energy release/consumption in chemical reactions
  high energy need, 90
  in muscle contraction, 15f
  production from energy sources, 15f
Adenosine triphosphate (ATP)-phosphocreatine (PCr) system overview, 17, 17f
Ad libitum, 121
  fluid, 250, 260, 262
Adulteration of dietary supplement, deliberate, 201
Aerobic capacity, iron status and, 289–290
Aerobic endurance exercise tests, 57
Aerobic exercise, 38
Aerobic processes, 14, 15

Aesthetic athletes
  about risks/benefits of ergogenic aids, 183
  sports drinks/bars for, 183
  vitamin/mineral supplements for, 183
  weight-loss dietary supplements, use of, 182
Aesthetic sports, 112; see also Nutrition for aesthetic/weight-class sport athletes
  about, 132
  athletes, dietary supplements of, 181–183
  dancers, 136–141, 137t–140t
  energy requirements for, 133
  figure skating, 141–149, 143t–148t
  gymnastics, 149–157, 150t–155t
  pre-exercise carbohydrate recommendations for, 134
  synchronized swimming, 157–159, 158t
Age and basal metabolic rate, 7f
Albumin, drug binding with, 210, 212, 218
Alcohol intake
  in sports clubs, 114
Alpha-acid glycoprotein, 218
Amenorrhea (AM), 141
American College of Sports Medicine (ACSM), 25, 279
American College of Sports Medicine Position Stand, 262
Aminoacidemia, 76
Amino acids
  β-alanine, 94
  catabolism, 70
  and deamination, 19
  for energy production, 22f
  proteins and, 39–40; see also Nutrition for endurance athletes
Amphetamines, 219, 220
Anabolic agents, 197
Anabolic compounds, 48
Anaerobic exercise, 24
Anaerobic performance, magnesium and, 286
Anaerobic processes, 14, 15
AND, see Academy of Nutrition and Dietetics (AND)
Androstenedione, 198
Anorectic agents, 197
Antibodies, 230